This book is dedicated to the tens of millions of world citizens who have died of AIDS or are HIV-positive, and their loved ones. Also to the pioneering spirit of the Nkosi Johnsons, Jonathan Manns, Mechai Viravaidyas, Larry Kramers, Betinhos, Ashok Pillais, Yusuf Hamieds, Suniti Solomons, and Pimjai Intamoons, who have battled incessantly to break the world's silence on AIDS.

Combating AIDS
Communication Strategies in Action

Arvind Singhal
Everett M. Rogers

Sage Publications
New Delhi ■ Thousand Oaks ■ London

First published in 2003 by

Sage Publications India Pvt Ltd
M-32 Market, Greater Kailash-I
New Delhi 110 048

Sage Publications Inc
2455 Teller Road
Thousand Oaks, California 91320

Sage Publications Ltd
6 Bonhill Street
London EC2A 4PU

Published by Tejeshwar Singh for Sage Publications India Pvt Ltd, typeset at InoSoft Systems in 10 pt Book Antiqua and printed at Chaman Enterprises, Delhi.

Library of Congress Cataloging-in-Publication Data

Singhal, Arvind, 1962-
    Combating AIDS: communication strategies in action / Arvind Singhal, Everett M. Rogers.
        p. cm.
    Includes bibliographical references and index.
        1. AIDS (Disease)—Prevention. 2. Communication in medicine.
3. Health behavior. I. Rogers, Everett M. II. Title.
    RA643.8 R646   616.97'9205–dc21   2003   2002151739

ISBN: 0-7619-9727-X (US-Hb)   81-7829-212-2 (India-Hb)
       0-7619-9728-8 (US-Pb)   81-7829-213-0 (India-Pb)

Sage Production Team: Aruna Ramachandran, Proteeti Banerjee, Rajib Chatterjee, N.K. Negi, and Santosh Rawat

Contents

List of Tables

List of Tables

List of Figures

List of Plates

Preface

■

One must meet a person living with AIDS, especially one of the many individuals in developing countries who cannot afford anti-retroviral drugs, in order to understand the debilitating effects of the disease. Anthony is a 30-something Kenyan who lives in a gloomy 10-by-10-foot room in a concrete block apartment building in the Kayole slum on the outskirts of Nairobi. His living space has no windows and opens onto an unlit corridor. Anthony took care of his wife, who died from AIDS three months before our visit. Now Anthony lies on a narrow bed, dying himself. His two children, the youngest also HIV-positive, were sent back to his village to live with relatives. Anthony's father takes care of him now, a strange situation in which grandparents are responsible for their children and grandchildren (one grandparent in Africa is caring for 31 grandchildren, all AIDS orphans).

We met Anthony in June 2001, after walking a mile through the crowded slum to his room, accompanied by two outreach workers from a health clinic operated by Women Fighting AIDS in Kenya (WOFAK). One outreach worker, a pleasant young woman, told us that she was HIV-positive. The other woman had lost both parents to AIDS, and her sister was living with HIV. Everyone in Kayole has family members dead or dying from AIDS, and many, perhaps 30 percent of all adults, are HIV-positive. The outreach workers visit people living with HIV/AIDS in their homes because they are too weak to come to the clinic. Also, individuals who present themselves at the clinic are stigmatized by community members who suspect them of being HIV-positive.

The two outreach workers visit Anthony every two weeks. During our visit, Anthony choked down some pills for his opportunistic infections of the lungs and throat. He coughed incessantly, a deep hack, and complained of chest pain. The outreach workers helped Anthony swallow sips of oral rehydration therapy (ORT, composed of sugar, salt, and water). It would help prevent dehydration of his body due to diarrhea. The workers gave Anthony herbal therapies, all that the WOFAK clinic can afford to provide. The women cooked tomatoes and onions over a kerosene burner, foods soft enough for Anthony to swallow.

Anthony could barely whisper, and even these attempts seemed painful. Anthony and his father spend the day sitting in his darkened room, listening to the radio. Essentially, they wait for him to die. As we walked slowly back to the clinic, the outreach workers commented on how much Anthony had weakened since their previous visit. They hoped that he might live for another two or three of their visits.

The purpose of this book is to synthesize critical lessons learned about effective HIV/AIDS prevention programs, with a major emphasis on communication strategies. Here we map future directions for more effective AIDS control programs, so that these programs can be improved and so that the worldwide epidemic can be controlled.

The world is now more than 20 years into the HIV/AIDS crisis with no vaccine in sight, and with relatively few effective and sustainable prevention programs. While numerous programs have been mounted throughout the world since the first AIDS cases were reported in the early 1980s, the AIDS epidemic is out of control in many nations of Africa and Asia. Over 65 million people have been infected with HIV, of which over 25 million have died of AIDS. Worldwide, some 14,000 people are infected every day, 95 percent of them in developing countries (Lamptey, 2002). Although the rates of HIV infection and AIDS deaths have declined in the richer nations of the developed world, infection rates are soaring in developing countries. AIDS is now the leading cause of death in Africa, and the fourth leading cause of death globally. In seven Sub-Saharan African nations, more than 22 percent of the population aged 15 to 49 is infected with HIV. Africa accounts for 83 percent of all AIDS deaths worldwide. In South Africa, AIDS deaths are so widespread that small children now play a new game called "Funerals." In Zimbabwe, the AIDS epidemic has shortened life expectancy by 22 years, rolling back the gains achieved in previous decades. Two out of every three Zimbabweans aged between 15 and 39 are HIV-positive!

AIDS was relatively slow in coming to Asia, and until the late 1980s, no Asian nation had experienced a major epidemic. However, Thailand and India then became important centers for the AIDS epidemic. Thailand is one of the world's first success stories in controlling the epidemic, as we detail in Chapter 2. In contrast, India is a nation where not nearly enough was done about AIDS during the first years of the epidemic. Today, India has an estimated four million commercial sex workers. HIV prevalence among commercial sex workers in Mumbai is 70 percent, and each sex worker provides services to an average of seven clients per night. The AIDS epidemic has become a conflagration on the Indian subcontinent. While the Indian government is mainly concerned with other matters, over four million people in India are estimated to be HIV-positive, a number that is second perhaps only to South Africa's.

AIDS affects many more people than it infects. The epidemic impoverishes families as they try to meet the costs of patient care and of funerals. AIDS leaves behind orphans with a dim future. And the epidemic reverses many of the hard-won development gains of past decades.

Despite this growing crisis, the world is making poor use of behavior change communication strategies for HIV/AIDS prevention. The authors' experience, gained over the past 15 years, of advising the Centers for Disease Control and Prevention (CDC, the leading U.S. agency responsible for fighting the epidemic), UNAIDS, and other international health organizations, suggests a major underestimation by such agencies of the role that communication can play in HIV prevention, care, and support. Many HIV/AIDS intervention programs are led by medical doctors, who certainly know all about the virus and its effects on the human body, but are often ill-prepared for developing and evaluating communication strategies to combat the spread of the virus. Many egregious mistakes have been made in AIDS communication. Prevention is shortchanged, despite the facts that no cure for AIDS has been found, and the cost of anti-retroviral therapy is out of the reach of most of those who need it. Few communication activities are guided by an effective strategy, so resources are used inefficiently (Ratzan, 1993). Formative research is not conducted or its results are disregarded, so that communication messages frequently miss their mark. Many communication activities are not culturally appropriate, so they may offend, which is easy to do when dealing with a sensitive topic like HIV/AIDS that involves sex, stigma, and death. In short, most HIV/AIDS communication interventions are flying blind.

Here, we build upon our past work on HIV/AIDS prevention. Our experience includes Singhal's involvement in UNAIDS deliberations on the role of communication in HIV/AIDS, his work on the advisory committee for Soul City in South Africa, and on Family Health International's AIDSCAP Project in the mid-1990s, and his investigation, with Dr. Peer Svenkerud, of the relative effectiveness of 80 HIV prevention programs in Bangkok. Rogers conducted a parallel investigation, with Professor Jim Dearing, of 100 HIV prevention programs in San Francisco in 1993–95. Previously, again with Professor Dearing, Rogers had studied how the issue of AIDS climbed the national media agenda in the United States. The agenda-setting process for the epidemic proceeded very slowly, and was delayed by four years after the first AIDS cases were identified. The basic strategy for fighting an epidemic should be to move immediately to throw every possible weapon at the disease. The four lost years in the United States (1981–85) were later to become a lingering catastrophe, not just in North America but throughout the world.

The authors of the present volume also studied the effects of entertainment-education radio and television programs on HIV prevention in Tanzania, India, Thailand, and China. We feel that the entertainment-education strategy of communication, detailed in Chapter 7, offers great promise for disease prevention, as documented by our field experiment in Tanzania from 1993 to 1997, and as illustrated by South Africa's *Soul City*.

Our history of collaboration in communication research and writing has led to three books, *India's Information Revolution* (Sage, 1989), *Entertainment-Education: A Communication Strategy for Social Change* (Lawrence Erlbaum Associates, 1999), and *India's Communication Revolution: From Bullock Carts to Cyber Marts* (Sage, 2001), and many journal articles and chapters in edited books. While each of us brings somewhat different perspectives to the present task, we collaborate here to produce an integrated volume that we hope benefits from the strengths of each.

During 2001 we visited five fairly representative nations heavily involved in the struggle to slow the epidemic: Brazil, South Africa, Kenya, Thailand, and India. We had worked previously in each of these countries, and our study benefited from our personal contacts in each nation. We gathered relevant literature and personally interviewed key officials and observers. For instance, in Brazil we conducted 30 in-depth interviews with key officials, representatives of non-governmental organizations (NGOs), and community leaders, and visited a dozen HIV prevention, care, and support programs. We reviewed available research results, and sought to identify promising communication strategies.

How did we identify the key individuals and organizations to interview in each country? We typically began with UNAIDS officials that we already knew (largely through Singhal's work with UNAIDS): Michael Fox, Bunmi Makinwa, Dan Odallo, and Werasit Sittitrai. We e-mailed individuals and organizations suggested by UNAIDS, and then followed a snowballing process of tracing other relevant contacts. Warren Feek, Director of The Communication Initiative; Neill McKee, Johns Hopkins University's Center for Communication Programs (JHU/CCP); Uttara Bharath, Deputy Chief of Party, JHU/CCP's Zambia Field Office; Dr. Bella Mody, Professor of Telecommunication, Michigan State University; Dr. William J. Brown, Dean, College of Communications and the Arts, Regent University; and Aarthi Pai, M.A. student in the Communication and Development Studies Program at Ohio University, provided additional contacts. We attended conferences of HIV/AIDS organizations in Brazil and in Thailand, where we made further contacts and arranged additional interviews. Fortunately for us, the world of HIV/AIDS professionals is highly networked within nations, and internationally. We were fortunate to meet personally with some of the well-known heroes of the worldwide battle to control the epidemic, ranging from Senator Mechai Viravaidya in Thailand, to Dr. Yusuf Hamied, President of Cipla in Mumbai (Bombay), to Dr. Suniti Solomon, the Indian medical doctor who identified the first HIV-infected individuals in India in 1986. Here we seek to give a voice to these world figures, as well as to local champions like Mrs. Pimjai Intamoon in a village near Chiang Mai, Thailand, and to the handful of enthusiastic young Indians in Chennai who have presented street theater on HIV/AIDS to over a million villagers in recent years.

Corinne L. Shefner-Rogers accompanied us on each of the five country visits. Dr. Rafael Obregon, at that time, Professor of Social Communication, Universidad del Norte, Baranquilla, Colombia, participated in our Brazil visit, and Dr. Pat Chatiketu and Dr. Piyanart Chatiketu joined us in our work in Thailand. We thank each of these key collaborators. Four eminent scholars critiqued the present book manuscript: Dr. Rafael Obregon; Dr. Scott Ratzan, Editor, *Journal of Health Communication*, and Vice-President (Government Affairs) of Johnson and Johnson's European operations; Dr. Shereen Usdin, co-founder of the Soul City Institute for Health and Development Communication, South Africa; and Dr. Collins Airhihenbuwa, Professor of Bio-behavioral Health, Penn State University, and a consultant to UNAIDS. Dr. Shaheed Mohammed at Marist College contributed a Caribbean flavor to this book.

We acknowledge the following leaders and officials who gave generously of their time when we visited their organizations:

1. In Brazil: Dr. Veriano Terto, Executive Director, Associação Brasileira Interdisciplinar de AIDS (ABIA), Rio de Janeiro; Geraldinho Veira, Executive Director, and Veet Vivarta, Coordinator of Youth Programs, News Agency for Children's Rights (ANDI), Brasília; Miguel Sanchez, Assistant to the Director, Centro Franciscano de Lucha contra SIDA (CEFRAM), São Paulo; Regina Figueiredo, Centro Vergueiro de Atenção a Saúde da Mulher e Produção de Materiais Educativos (CEVAM), São Paulo; Ellen Zita Ayer, Coordinator, Disque Saúde, Ministry of Health, Brasília; Dr. Paulo Roberto Proto de Souza, Executive Director, Family Health International, Brasília; Silvana Mosias, Carla Formiga, and Vinicius Rodarte, Grupos de Apoyo a PLWAs (GAPA), State of Minas Gerais, Belo Horizonte; Dr. Jorge Beloqui, Co-director, Grupo Pella Vida (GIV), São Paulo; Rubens Duda, Executive Director, HIV/AIDS NGO Forum, São Paulo; Denisse Pires, HIV/AIDS/STDs Program, Secretariat of Health, Rio de Janeiro; Dr. Fábio Mezquita

and Gabriela Calasanz, HIV/AIDS Program, City of São Paulo; Father Valeriano Paitoni, Bishop, Paróquia Nossa Senhora de Fátima, Imirim, São Paulo; Mauro Nunes, Coordinator, Médicines Sans Frontières, Rio de Janeiro; Eliane Izolan, Rosemary Muñoz, Mauro Figueiredo, Katia Galvinski, Anna Lucia Ribeiro de Vasconcelos, Paulo Guilherme Meireles, Ranulfo Cardoso, Jr., José Roberto Gribosi, José Luis Leão Dos Santos, Wellington Vilela, and Jhoney Barcarolo, National AIDS Program, Ministry of Health, Brasília; Valeria Saraceni, Manager, HIV/AIDS Program, City of Rio de Janeiro; Maria Etelvina Reis de Toleco Barros, Country Program Advisor, UNAIDS, Brasília.

2. In South Africa: Sharon Ekambarum, Advocacy Officer, AIDS Consortium, Braamfontein; Glen Mabuza, Project Director, AIDS Counseling Care and Training, Chris Hani Baragwanath Hospital, Soweto; Warren Parker, Director, Center for AIDS Development, Research and Evaluation (CADRE), Johannesburg; Theo Steele, Campaigns Coordinator, Congress of South African Trade Unions (COSATU), Braamfontein; Sister Sue Roberts, Helen Joseph Polyclinic, Johannesburg; Lungi Morrison, Advocacy Initiatives, loveLife, Melrose; Jenny Marcus and Lauren Jankelowitz, CARE, Houghton; Dr. Garth Japhet, Executive Director, Dr. Shereen Usdin, Dr. Sue Goldstein, Savera Kalideen, Sally Ward, Harriet Perlman, Agnes Shabalala, Thuli Shongwe, and Joel Sebolao, Soul City, Parkstown.

3. In Kenya: Mary Ann Burris, Program Officer, Ford Foundation, Nairobi; Anne A. Owiti, Director, Kibera Community Self-help Program (KICOSHEP), Nairobi; Michelle Folsom, Karen Schmidt, and Maina Kiranga, Program for Appropriate Technology in Health (PATH), Nairobi; Catherine Canungo and Doreen Odida, Women Fighting AIDS in Kenya (WOFAK), Nairobi.

4. In Thailand: Senator Jon Ungpakorn, Chairman, AIDS Access Foundation, Bangkok; Dr. Parichart Sthapitanonda-Sarabol, Chulalongkorn University,

Bangkok; Niwat Suwanphatthana, Project Officer, AIDS Network Development Foundation, Chiang Mai; Ricky Tan, Director, Care Corner Orphanage Foundation, Chiang Mai; Dr. Surasing Visrutaratna, Chiang Mai Public Health Office; Mrs. Pimjai Intamoon, Director, Community Health Project, Chiang Mai; Chantawipa (Noi) Apisuk, EMPOWER Foundation, Nonthaburi; Phra Phongthep Dhammagaruko, Director, Friends for Life Center, Chiang Mai; Dr. Katherine Bond, Usasinee Rewthong, and Pawana Wienrawee, PATH, Bangkok; Senator Mechai Viravaidya, Chairman, Population and Community Development Association, Bangkok; Mrs. Nittaya Promporchuenboon, Director, Duang Prateep Foundation, Klong Toey, Bangkok; Amporn Boontan, Executive Director, Thai Youth AIDS Prevention Project, Chiang Mai; Dr. Wiwat Rojanapithayakorn, UNAIDS, Bangkok (formerly Director of the 100 Percent Condom Program, Ministry of Public Health).

5.   In India: Dr. Anand Malaviya, formerly Professor of Medicine at the All India Institute of Medical Sciences; Mrs. Usha Bhasin, Prasar Bharati (Broadcasting) Corporation; Dr. Bimal Charles, Director, Dr. V. Sampath Kumar, Intervention Officer, Dr. Arvind Kumar, Industrial Intervention, and Dr. Lakshamibai, Research, AIDS Prevention and Control Project, Voluntary Health Services, Chennai; K. Vaidyanathan, AIDS Prevention and Control Project for Maharashtra (AVERT), Wadala, Mumbai; Peter Gill, Executive Producer, Lori McDougall, Sangeeta Sharma Mehta, and Dr. Jyoti Mehra (former Technical Consultant, Healthy Highways Project), BBC World Service Trust, New Delhi; Dr. Bhupendra Sheoran, Project Manager, Center for AIDS Prevention Studies (CAPS), Sion Hospital, Mumbai; Akhila Shivdas, Director, and Sumita Thapar, Program Coordinator, Center for Advocacy and Research (CFAR), New Delhi; Dr. N. Bhaskara Rao, Chairman, and P.N. Vasanti, Director, Center for Media Studies, Saket, New Delhi; Dr. P. Manorama, President, Community Health Education Society (CHES), Kodambakkam, Chennai;

Dr. Yusuf K. Hamied, Chairman, and Dr. Jaideep A.
Gogtay, Medical Services, Cipla, Mumbai Central; Ashok
Pillai, President, Indian Network for People Living with
HIV/AIDS (INP+), Chennai; Sangeeta Parmeswaran,
Project CHILD (Children of HIV+ People Living in
Dignity), Mumbai; Sanjay R. Chaganti, Program
Manager, HIV/AIDS Prevention, and Arupa Shukla,
Project Manager, HIV/AIDS Project, PSI, Mumbai;
Neelam Kapur, Joint Director IEC, National AIDS Control
Organization (NACO), New Delhi; Harini, R.
Jeevanandham, P. Oyya, M. Raviraj, M. Sampath, and
Nithya Balaji, Nalamdana, Chennai; S. Ramasundaram,
Joint Secretary, Ministry of Commerce and Industry,
New Delhi (formerly Director, Tamil Nadu AIDS Control
Society, Chennai); R.C. Gandhi, Director, Tamil Nadu
AIDS Control Organi-zation, Chennai; Dr. Suniti
Solomon, Director, Dr. N. Kumarasamy, Chief Medical
Officer and Clinical Researcher, and A.K. Srikrishnan,
NIMH Project, Y.R.G. Center for AIDS Research and
Education (Y.R.G. CARE), Chennai.

At the time that we visited the five countries, important events had
just occurred in the worldwide AIDS epidemic. Brazil was leading
the world in overcoming the drug companies' patent laws that
protected their intellectual property rights to anti-retroviral drugs
(the "triple cocktail"). The government of Brazil provides these
drugs at no cost to all HIV+ persons. The improvement in these
patients' quality of life and the corresponding drop in death rates
and in new HIV infection rates were spectacular (although new
communication problems came with the free triple cocktails, such
as providing information about the correct dosage of up to 35 pills
taken daily by some individuals). Shortly before our arrival in
Brazil in March 2001, the legal controversy about the drug patents
had erupted into a major issue involving the World Trade
Organization (WTO), the U.S. government, pharmaceutical
companies, and various advocacy groups (this controversy is
detailed in Chapters 1 and 3). Eventually, in November 2001, the
WTO voted to cease its resistance to the manufacture of low-priced
generic drugs by developing nations. Dr. Yusuf Hamied and the
Cipla Company of Mumbai, India, caused a revolution in 2001

when they announced a many-fold drop in the price of anti-retrovirals, to only $350 per person per year. Even this price, however, has not helped most HIV-positive people in developing nations, where the cost of the anti-retrovirals is still prohibitive.

While President Fernando Henrique Cardoso and the national government of Brazil were wrestling with the AIDS epidemic in an effort to slow it down, President Thabo Mbeki and the South African government were mismanaging this vast problem (an unbelievable 22 percent of adults in South Africa were HIV-positive in 2002). During a memorable presentation by the late Nkosi Johnson, the lovable little 11-year-old boy then living with AIDS, at the 2000 International AIDS Conference in Durban, President Mbeki rose from his seat and left the auditorium. This symbolic act was poor public relations in front of the world community of AIDS researchers, officials, and activists. Mbeki questions whether HIV causes AIDS, insisting that poverty is the real cause (it is indeed a strong contributory factor).

When we were in Nairobi in June 2001, Kenyan president Daniel Arap Moi was calling attention to the epidemic in every speech he gave, whatever the topic and whoever the audience. The president, when inaugurating a new kindergarten, urged his audience of small children to avoid becoming seropositive. Moi even urged Kenyans to abstain from sex for two years in order to curb the spread of AIDS. Earlier, in the 1980s, Moi had spent several years denying the problem, insisting that there was no AIDS in Kenya. Foreign journalists who wrote about AIDS in Kenya in the late 1980s were escorted to Nairobi's Jomo Kenyatta Airport and sent home. Today, the Ministry of Health estimates that 700 Kenyans die every day from AIDS. Such death rates are all the more tragic because they can be avoided, as the case of Thailand suggests.

After five years of neglect, while the epidemic ran wild through Thailand's numerous brothels, in 1991–92 a dynamic, no-nonsense leader, Mechai Viravaidya, took charge of the AIDS control program. Mechai was the architect of Thailand's highly effective family planning program in the 1970s and 1980s. After just 20 months of concerted effort in 1991–92, Thailand was on its way to becoming the first nation in the world to control HIV/AIDS effectively. Our study of five nations shows clearly that the political will of top policy-makers is a key factor in controlling the epidemic. Minister Mechai and Presidents Cardoso and Itamar Franco have displayed such commitment, President Mbeki has not, and President Moi didn't, but now appears to be doing so. Commitment to controlling the epidemic is not just an individual matter of presidents and prime ministers, however. National AIDS policies result from a communication-based agenda-setting process in which advocacy groups and others play a crucial role.

During our five-nation exploration in 2001, the week-long United Nations session on AIDS drew world attention to the epidemic. A lighted red ribbon, 50 meters high, was prominently displayed on the UN building in Manhattan, a somber sign of the world's pandemic. We recognize the important role of national policies regarding the epidemic, and explain the crucial role of communication in the national agenda-setting process through which such policies are formed. The AIDS epidemic is very much a political process, one in which communication can play a strong role. Such policies, of course, must be implemented effectively, or they do not matter.

The epidemic is also an issue of economics. AIDS is increasingly concentrated in poor countries, and the poorest of the poor in these countries are the most vulnerable. Today, thanks to the virus, low socioeconomic status is a death sentence for many HIV+ individuals. The triple cocktail can prolong life and return the bedridden to active work, but the anti-retroviral drugs cost $15,000 per year in the United States. If the person living with AIDS resides in the United States or in Brazil, the government, or a health insurance company, generally bears this expense. But for someone living in a huge urban slum like Kibera in Nairobi, Klong Toey in Bangkok, or in a township like Soweto in South Africa, the drugs are simply unaffordable. So, eventually, after a lingering, painful illness, the individual dies. Alleviating poverty and advancing economic development are important steps toward improving health, because higher income is strongly associated with access to health services. Profiteering on the part of international drug companies, while poor people living with HIV/AIDS cannot afford to buy anti-retroviral drugs, is problematic.

Fighting the AIDS epidemic involves more than political will and socioeconomic factors. HIV/AIDS prevention programs are everywhere in the world today. There are hundreds of such programs in most large cities, and thousands in most developing countries. Their outreach workers and counselors, many of whom live with the virus themselves, are at the frontline of the war on AIDS. If these programs could make better use of communication strategies, lives could be saved. A *communication strategy* is a formula for changing the behavior of individuals and systems that is based on communication theories that provide a framework for designing and implementing communication interventions.

Our partner in preparing this book is Population Communications International (PCI), an NGO headquartered in New York. Population Communications International is known for its pioneering role in mounting entertainment-education radio and television broadcasts to encourage family planning and HIV/AIDS prevention in developing nations. Over recent decades, we collaborated with PCI in India, Tanzania, and China in studying the effects of PCI-assisted entertainment-education interventions. We thank David J. Andrews, President; Kate Randolph, Vice-President, International Programs; and the PCI representatives in the nations that we visited, like Dr. Kimani Njogu in Nairobi, for their helpfulness. Our travel costs were supported by PCI, who also made valuable inputs to this book at every step of its development. Susan Rhodes, PCI's Senior Program Officer, provided detailed editorial comments on each chapter.

Several people at Ohio University aided us in the preparation of this book: Peggy Sattler, Lars Lutton, and Lara Neel helped with our photographs and artwork; graduate students Li Wang and Pei-Wen Lee provided research assistance; Dr. Greg Shepherd, Director of the School of Interpersonal Communication, and Dr. Kathy Krendl, Dean of the College of Communication, encouraged our research; and Dr. Steve Howard, Director of African Studies, helped with our visits to Kenya and South Africa.

Family members — Anuja, Aaryaman, and Anshuman Singhal in Ohio, and Mahendra and Shashi Singhal in New Delhi — believed in this project, providing support throughout the research and writing process.

This book is written for global, national, and local policy-makers; project officials and practitioners in international development agencies, NGOs, and local governments; scholars and teachers of public health, communication, and development studies; activists and socially conscious entrepreneurs; and for the general reader who desires a critical synthesis of the efforts to control the world's gravest health threat. For purposes of clarity, we utilize such terminology as "high-risk" groups, "AIDS orphans," and "promiscuity," while acknowledging that some experts on the epidemic object to these terms. The individuals in high-risk groups are more accurately described as "vulnerable populations engaged in high-risk behaviors," a much more cumbersome term. Even though AIDS orphans have lost both of their parents, their extended families of aunts and uncles may take care of them, at least in some cultures. "Multiple sexual partners" may be a less judgmental terminology than "promiscuity." But in each of these cases, we side with simplicity and clarity.

Our objective here is not small. Through more effective communication strategies, the world can reduce the incidence of HIV/AIDS in the countries of Latin America, Africa, and Asia. Clear understanding of a social problem is the first essential step toward its solution. We hope that you will profit from reading our account of the epidemic today. It is not a happy story. But it contains seeds of hope.

ARVIND SINGHAL
Athens, Ohio

EVERETT M. ROGERS
Albuquerque, New Mexico

1

History of the AIDS Epidemic

■

AIDS is the most serious threat the world faces today. If it isn't checked now, it will do unbelievable damage.

> Richard Holbrooke, former U.S. ambassador to the United Nations, and president of the Global Business Council on AIDS (quoted in Neary, 2001, p. 4).

At the moment, education and communication are the only weapons we have against HIV/AIDS.

> The late Dr. Jonathan Mann, former director of WHO's Global Program on AIDS, at the Asia-Pacific AIDS Conference, New Delhi, November 1992.

In 1996, Govind Singh, a 25-year-old migrant worker, left the village of Churcher in the Indian state of Uttar Pradesh to find employment in Mumbai. Like many of his fellow migrant workers, he slept with commercial sex workers. In 1999, when he began to feel tired and to lose weight, he went to Mumbai's Laksh Deep Hospital for a check-up. He was HIV-positive. Govind Singh's fellow migrant workers, many of whom belonged to Churcher, wrote home to their kin that Singh had AIDS and that "nobody should touch, talk with, or see him" (Mishra, 2000, p. 40). Too weak to work, when Singh returned to his village in April 2000, seeking shelter and care, he was shunned by his neighbors and family members, including his wife. Villagers dragged Singh into a *gote*, an enclosure for cattle and goats (Plate 1.1). His captivity became a center of attraction for Churcher's villagers, who peeped into the *gote*, teasing him about his promiscuity. Twice a day, the villagers threw food into his cold, wet, foul-smelling enclosure. As his condition worsened, Singh lay on the floor, and was often stepped on by the animals.

On 5 July 2000, Singh was found dead, and given a hurried cremation at a site outside the village. Since his death, Singh's wife, Devaki, and their two young children have become social outcastes in Churcher. Govind Singh was not the only victim of the AIDS epidemic and of anti-AIDS stigma in Churcher. In 1999, two other returned migrant workers, both HIV-positive, met with the same fate (Mishra, 2000). AIDS patients, and their families, represent India's new class of "untouchables."

Govind Singh's life, cut short by HIV and by his own community, symbolizes the multiple challenges faced by the world in addressing the HIV/AIDS pandemic: Could Singh's HIV infection have been prevented? Could the social stigma associated with HIV have been reduced, so that Singh could have lived, and died, with dignity? Can affordable AIDS drug therapy be provided to poor, illiterate migrant workers like Singh?

∎

Just like the cunningly lethal Human Immunodeficiency Virus (HIV), which changes its profile with deceptive flexibility to cause disability and death through pneumonia, skin cancer, tuberculosis, and other opportunistic infections, the characteristics of infected people and the main means of transmission typically change over time in a nation. In the United States and in most other countries, the epidemic first spread among gay men, injecting drug users, and commercial sex workers (CSWs) in large cities. Later, the epidemic broke out of these initial high-risk groups and was feminized by spreading to women through their infected husbands, pauperized by devastating the poorest and the most vulnerable individuals, and interiorized by spreading from cities to remote and rural areas through truck drivers, migrant workers, and the return of people

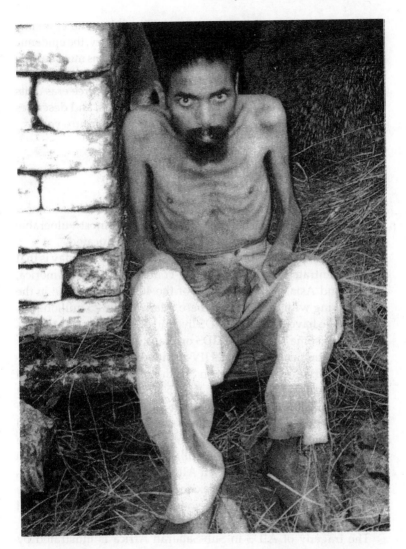

Plate 1.1   The Death of Govind Singh in an Indian Village *Gote*

Singh, a migrant worker in Mumbai, returned to his home village of Churcher, in Uttar Pradesh, where he faced extreme stigma due to AIDS. The villagers forced him to live in an animal pen, a *gote*, until his death.

Source: *India Today.*

living with AIDS to their birth homes. Thereafter, the epidemic posed a risk to the general population. In every country, the epidemic has been ever-changing, so that AIDS control programs must flexibly adapt their strategies.

This chapter profiles the AIDS epidemic by the three eras of its development that have occurred in most countries, and describes some rays of hope for controlling the epidemic in future years.

Vulnerability to the Epidemic

This book highlights the dire global, national, and local consequences of AIDS, especially among the world's most vulnerable people: women, children, the poor, and the uneducated.

The first key fact to know about the AIDS epidemic today is that it is concentrated in the developing countries of Latin America, Africa, and Asia, with 95 percent of the 40 million people in the world living with HIV located there. Many of the 25 million plus people who have died from AIDS lived in developing countries, as do most of some 14 million AIDS orphans in the world today. Of the 40 million people who are HIV-positive, 28 million are in Sub-Saharan Africa, 6 million are in South and Southeast Asia, and 1 million are in North America. Of the 5 million new infections that occurred in 2001, 3.4 million were in Sub-Saharan Africa. Some 3 million people died of AIDS-related causes during 2001. The total number of HIV-positive people in the world rose from 10 million in 1990 to 28 million in 1996, 34 million in 2000, and to 40 million in 2002. As Dr. Bette Korber, an AIDS researcher at Los Alamos National Laboratory (in New Mexico), stated: "The AIDS epidemic is not just about people dying; so are entire nations" (personal interview, 21 February 2002).

The tragedy of AIDS in Sub-Saharan Africa is illustrated by Arthur Chinaka's life (Schoofs, 1999). In 1990, when Arthur was 17-years-old and taking his high school examinations in Uganda, the school principal told him that his father had died of pneumonia, an opportunistic infection brought on by AIDS. In 1992, Arthur's uncle Edward died of AIDS. In 1994, his uncle Richard died of the disease. In 1996, his uncle Alex died of AIDS. Then, in 1999, his fourth uncle and his aunt Eunice died of AIDS. All were buried on the family farm near Mutare, Uganda. AIDS has wiped out entire families and communities in several Sub-Saharan African countries.

The Human Immunodeficiency Virus surfaced in Africa, and moved somehow to the United States, where it was first detected decades later. The rate of HIV infection and deaths due to AIDS first increased rapidly during the 1980s in the United States and in western Europe. Then, with more effective prevention programs based on widespread knowledge about how HIV transmission occurred and with the growing practice of safer sex, death rates in the United States dropped, starting in 1994. While the epidemic is far from unimportant in these rich nations today (by 2001, 438,795 Americans had died from AIDS, more than the number of those who died during World War I and World War II combined), AIDS is not the galloping killer that it is in poor countries (Garrett, 1992). For example, while more than 22 percent of adults in South Africa are HIV-positive, the comparable figure for the United States is less than 1 percent. Why have some nations been capable of controlling the AIDS epidemic but not others? Our book seeks to answer this question. It is a matter of cultural beliefs, available resources, how and when they are utilized, and the political will of national governments. If a developing nation does not have a high degree of political commitment to controlling the epidemic, little else matters.

Acquired Immune Deficiency Syndrome (AIDS) occurs when an HIV-positive individual has such lowered immune levels that he/she falls prey to a variety of opportunistic infections (Elwood, 1999). One basic reason why AIDS is mostly a disease of poor countries is due to the unbalanced distribution of health resources. Public spending on health in the developing countries of Latin America, Africa, and Asia averages less than 1 percent of gross domestic product, compared to 6 percent in wealthy nations (Olson, 2000). In the United States, more than 10 percent of gross domestic product is spent on health costs, and this proportion keeps rising. Money spent on disease *prevention* saves more lives than money spent on hospitals, high-technology medical equipment, and other expensive *treatment* facilities (Garrett, 2000). But in developing countries, an overall lack of funding means that relatively little is spent on prevention. The United Nations estimates that $7–10 billion a year is needed for mounting HIV/AIDS prevention efforts in developing nations. Unfortunately, 95 percent of all AIDS prevention money is spent in *developed* nations, while 95 percent of HIV-infected people live in *developing* countries. So funding for prevention of the AIDS epidemic does not match the location of the problem.

The Poor

Not only is the epidemic devastating the populations of poor countries in Latin America, Africa, and Asia, it especially affects the poorest people in these poor countries. For example, 74 percent of the infected individuals in Brazil are illiterate or have only an elementary school education. In South Africa, where race and socioeconomic status are closely linked, the epidemic is mainly (98 percent) concentrated among the black population, which makes up 90 percent of the total population of 43 million. In part, this connection between race and AIDS is due to the decades of Apartheid ("separateness") rule, when the white government of South Africa paid scant heed to the epidemic that was killing predominantly black people. Apartheid broke down family relationships, as many men migrated for work in the gold and the diamond mines, living in "dormitories" in segregated, all-black rural townships. This vast movement of the workforce led to a booming commercial sex industry in these townships. Sadly, the governments of Nelson Mandela and Thabo Mbeki, elected with much optimism in the immediate post-Apartheid period, have not been able to combat the silent killer of the very people who put them in office (Figure 1.1).

Poverty and HIV infection march side by side throughout the world. Why? One explanation is that the epidemic cuts down the economically weak who do not have access to basic health services and who cannot afford the expensive anti-retroviral drugs that can prolong life for an HIV-positive individual. A rich country with a relatively small percentage of its population infected (like the United States) can afford to provide these drugs to everyone. But HIV-positive individuals living in the rural townships of Soweto or Alexandra in South Africa (Soweto has an estimated three million inhabitants), in poverty-stricken villages in northern Thailand, or in the *busties* (slums) of Mumbai (Bombay), are doomed to an early death by economic factors. Neither they, nor their nations, can afford the anti-retrovirals. Nor do most developing nations provide effective large-scale HIV prevention programs. They lack adequate resources to do so.

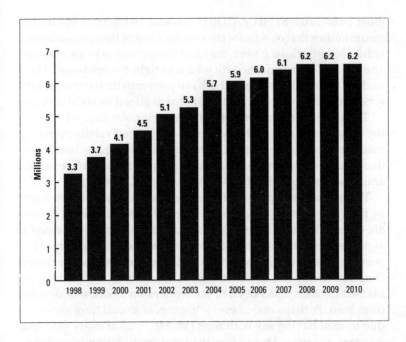

Figure 1.1   The Number of HIV-positive People in South Africa

The number of people living with HIV in South Africa rose rapidly in the years before 2002 to reach 22 percent of the adult population. The numbers begin to level off in future years (this on the assumption that more effective prevention interventions will be launched).

Source: Whiteside & Sunter (2000, p. 53).

Poverty creates vulnerability. When their crops fail, Cambodian farmers borrow money from moneylenders, who charge an exorbitant interest rate—up to 100 percent a month. When farmers fall behind on loan payments, sex traffickers offer a way out: "Sell your daughter and we'll help you repay the loan." Reluctantly, the poor farmers agree, perpetuating both vulnerability and the risk of HIV infection.

The Weak and Vulnerable

Poor people, women, and children (especially AIDS orphans, child laborers, street children, and those at risk for prostitution) are the most vulnerable to HIV/AIDS (Fumento, 1990). Individuals and communities that constitute the bottom rung of the socioeconomic ladder have the least power, the most limited access to information, and the fewest resources with which to fight the epidemic. These underprivileged of society also have poor nutritional status, little access to health care, and are least able to afford medical services.

The developing nations of Latin America, Africa, and Asia are the most vulnerable to the epidemic, given their relative poverty, malnutrition, unemployment, illiteracy, and inadequate health care, due to rural–urban migration, income inequality, gender inequality, and other exacerbating factors (Melkote et al., 2000).

Women in developing countries are expected to prove their worth by marrying, having children, and caring for their families. Women are especially vulnerable to HIV, and are the least empowered to avoid being at risk. Women are more stigmatized if they become HIV-positive. The vast majority of cases of HIV transmission in developing countries today are heterosexual. While female sex workers are blamed for the spread of HIV, sex work exists because of demand from men. Perhaps one in every 10 cases of sexual transmission is due to men having sex with men (MSM). Four of every five drug injectors are men. More often than not, men determine whether sexual intercourse takes place and whether a condom is used (Foreman, 1999). Worldwide, women are today contracting HIV at a faster rate than men. Women with the virus can pass it along to their future children at birth or through breast-feeding. At home and in the hospital, women assume greater responsibility in caring for those sick with the opportunistic infections due to AIDS.

In countries such as India, women's powerlessness is glorified in a *pativrata* (dedication to the husband) image, which projects women as loyal and subordinate to their husbands, even when neglected, ill-treated, or deserted (Mane & Maitra, 1992). The *pativrata* woman, unfortunately, dutifully engages in unprotected sex with her husband, despite knowing her partner's HIV-positive status.

Women are more likely to be blamed for becoming HIV+, even if they have led monogamous lives and were infected by their promiscuous partners. Mothers are often blamed when their infants become infected with HIV. As a result of this blame-the-victim stigma, many women who are offered HIV tests refuse such testing because of the difficulties they would face were they to test positive for HIV. Women's economic dependence on men, violence against women, and the greater acceptability of male promiscuity combine to leave women at particularly high risk for HIV infection. So gender relationships should be at the heart of communication strategies for HIV/AIDS prevention. How can communication experts attend more closely to issues of gender relations in formulating strategies for preventing the epidemic?

Stigma

The stigma of HIV/AIDS is especially pronounced because many of the sufferers, at least in the early stages of the epidemic, were homosexuals, injecting drug users, or the poor. *Stigma* is prejudice and discrimination against people who are regarded and treated in a negative way. Throughout the world, anti-AIDS stigma is a barrier to the humane treatment of infected individuals. In India, and in many other nations, HIV-positive people are stereotyped as having behaved immorally, and they are punished accordingly.

In Chapter 6, we tell of people in India, Thailand, South Africa, and other countries who have been fired by their employers and evicted by their landlords, who have been lynched, or committed suicide. The civil rights of HIV-positive people are routinely violated in every nation. People living with HIV/AIDS (PWAs) are beginning to organize for social change. Thus, PWAs become empowered to fight stigma, to lobby for making anti-retrovirals more widely available, and to seek other policies that benefit people living with HIV/AIDS.

Era 1: Urban Beginnings

Twenty years ago, HIV/AIDS did not exist, at least in the sense that almost no one knew of its existence. Today it is to be found everywhere in the world. As the epidemic invaded each nation, it usually passed through three time periods: (*a*) beginning among high-risk populations in urban centers; (*b*) breaking out from these high-risk groups of commercial sex workers and injection drug users; and (*c*) an interiorization era as the epidemic spread throughout the nation.

The Nature of HIV

No one knows exactly where the Human Immunodeficiency Virus originated, or the conditions that led to its spread among humans in the early 1980s. It may have existed in a latent form for very many years. Probably it lived in an animal host.

HIV-1 was identified in 1983 by Dr. Robert Gallo and other medical scientists at the National Cancer Institute in Bethesda, Maryland. At about the same time, Dr. Luc Montagnier of the Pasteur Institute in Paris isolated HIV-2 from AIDS patients. These two human HIV viruses are distinguishable by their genome make-up today, but are believed to have had a common ancestor in Africa. Scientists think that HIV-2 was transmitted to humans from a simian source, probably the sooty mangabeys that are hunted for food in Senegal, Guinea, the Ivory Coast, and Gambia. Perhaps a mangabey bit the hunter while it was being killed for food.

HIV-1, which is much more lethal, is most closely related to SIVcpz, Simian Immunodeficiency Virus, and was transmitted from the Central African chimpanzee, *Pan troglodytes troglodytes.* HIV-1 mutates very rapidly, and Simian Immunodeficiency Virus crossed over to humans (on at least three separate occasions) as Human Immunodeficiency Virus. As the result of mutation, 11 different subtypes of HIV-1 have been identified, and are designated as A through K. Subtype B is found in the Americas, Japan, and Europe, while subtype C predominates in South Africa and India (and is responsible for 55 percent of all HIV-1 infections globally). Subtype E is found in Thailand. A new genetic subtype will probably be identified in the future, as the virus continues to mutate. Thus, a much more virulent and rapidly spreading form of the HIV may someday emerge, a very somber thought indeed. What if airborne transmission like in the case of the common cold were possible?

The word "virus" is Latin for "poison," an appropriate name since no cure exists for any virus (although preventive vaccines have been developed for such viruses as the measles, polio, and hepatitis B). The HIV virus, which is so small that 16,000 can sit on the head of a pin, invades a living white blood cell, and reprograms it to reproduce the virus. The infected cell now becomes a miniature virus factory. One HIV virus can make an astounding 10 billion copies of itself in a day, with a mutation rate of 1 in 10,000

(Gaitonde, 2001, p. 179). This notorious rate of random mutation can make HIV resistant to drugs. The rapid mutation also makes the development of a vaccine very difficult. The HIV infects a type of white blood cells known as T lymphocytes, also called T helper cells. They protect the human body against infections. The CD4 count measures the strength of an individual's immune system. A healthy adult has between 700 and 1,500 CD4 cells per cubic milliliter of blood. Over a period of years, the T cell count of an HIV-positive individual drops to a critical level, below 500, a sign of a depressed immune system. Below 200, the individual usually develops opportunistic infections. At this point, perhaps 10 years after infection (or sooner), the individual is said to have AIDS. An individual's viral load is measured as the number of viruses, expressed in log (tenfold changes) per milliliter of blood. During the lengthy incubation period, the individual appears to be healthy but can infect other people.

The current strains of the virus are very fragile organisms, unable to survive for more than a few seconds under room temperature when not inside the human body. This fragility means that the virus cannot spread by means of a handshake, kiss, or a sneeze, nor by means of a mosquito bite. Sharing of food, drinking glasses, or clothes will not transmit the virus. The main means of transmission worldwide is human sexual intercourse in which bodily fluids like semen or blood are exchanged. This is the reason why the sexually active age group from 15 to 45 is most at risk. HIV/AIDS, even more than some other diseases, is a network kind of malady. Individuals infect other individuals through the most intimate of interpersonal relationships, mainly sexual intercourse. The sex drive, one of the most basic of human needs, provides the main channel for the spread of the epidemic.

Also important in HIV transmission is the sharing of unclean needles, such as between injection drug users, and, in rare instances, the virus is transmitted by means of accidental needle-sticks. Occasionally a medical doctor, nurse, or dentist has been infected in this way. Infected blood can transmit the virus through transfusions, although many countries have made great progress in keeping their blood supply free of HIV.

Mother-to-child transmission (also called MTCT, or "vertical transmission") is common today, resulting in millions of pediatric AIDS cases. The chances of a baby born to an HIV+ mother being infected are about 40 percent. Because mother-to-child HIV trans-mission can be so easily prevented (or at least minimized) by an anti-retroviral drug costing a few cents, infected infants are an especially painful problem for the world. Mother-to-child transmission could be minimized with very little effort, cutting down these transmission rates at least by half. However, in many countries, hundreds of babies are born HIV+ every day.

A single exposure to the virus may or may not infect an individual. For example, certain commercial sex workers in some nations (like Kenya and Gambia), who are repeatedly exposed to the virus, somehow do not become infected (Kaul et al., 2000). Perhaps they have built up a kind of immunity to HIV infection (an interpretation with hopeful leads for attempts to someday find an HIV/AIDS vaccine). On the other hand, many infections are caused by a single sexual contact. Evidently there are wide individual differences in susceptibility to HIV infection.

The chances of a woman being infected by one act of sexual intercourse with an HIV+ man are about one in 100. The chances of a man being infected by one act of sexual intercourse with an HIV+ woman are about one in 1,000, but this probability may increase considerably if one of them has an STD (Moses et al., 1991). Sexually transmitted diseases (STDs) act as a co-factor in HIV transmission by increasing susceptibility to HIV (Jha et al., 2001). Lesions on the genitals caused by STDs increase the likelihood of HIV infection for both men and women. A project in the Mwanza region of Tanzania, along Lake Victoria, found that preventing and curing STDs reduced the incidence of HIV infection by 40 percent (Gilson et al., 1997; Grosskurth et al., 1995). Further, there is evidence that male circumcision protects against HIV infection in Africa (Moses et al., 1990). Uncircumcised men in Africa are twice as likely to be infected as circumcised men (Weiss et al., 2000).

Beginnings

In the late 1970s, the first clues of a strange new disease began to turn up in certain European hospitals. A Danish doctor, Dr. Grethe Rask, had practiced medicine in a remote hospital in Zaire. Rask became ill in 1975, returned to Denmark, and died in 1977, gasping for breath. A biopsy showed that the cause of death was the rare

Pneumocystis carinii pneumonia (PCP), a type of pneumonia carried by birds! Other mysterious cases of PCP presented themselves to doctors, especially in hospitals in Paris. A handsome young Air Canada flight steward frequently visited Paris during this period. His name was Gaetan Dugas (Shilts, 1987). He was later to become famous for his role in transmitting the virus in the United States.

Years later, when much more was known about HIV/AIDS, scientists tried to trace the origins of the epidemic. A dozen AIDS cases were retrospectively identified in 1978–79. Scattered cases of HIV infection or AIDS were identified in the United States and Haiti between 1972 and 1976 (Korber et al., 2000). The earliest known case of HIV-1 has been identified in one of 1,213 stored blood samples that were gathered in 1959 in Africa. The individual, designated "L70," was an adult male with a sickle-cell trait and a glucose deficiency, living in Kinshasa, Democratic Republic of Congo, then called Leopoldville, Belgian Congo (Zhu et al., 1998). Using sophisticated mathematical models and computer tools, and knowing that L70's infection probably had ancestors in the B, D, and F subtypes of HIV-1, biologists estimate that the first HIV case occurred in Africa in the 1930s (ibid.).

So HIV/AIDS lay relatively dormant for many decades. Then, for unknown reasons, it burst out of its African origins, and to date has become the scourge of 40 million people worldwide, plus 25 million more who have died.

The CDC Cluster Study

The first documented case of AIDS in the United States was identified in 1980 by a young immunologist, Dr. Michael S. Gottlieb, at the University of California, Los Angeles. His first patient sought medical care because of weight loss. He had candidiosis, a thick, white coating in his mouth (Gottlieb, 1998). One week later, this patient was readmitted to the UCLA Medical Hospital with fever and with *Pneumocystis carinii* pneumonia. Soon, local physicians in Los Angeles referred several more patients with weight loss, fever, and candidiosis to Gottlieb. All were young gay men. Their opportunistic infections led Gottlieb to suspect problems with their immune systems, and he found that the men indeed had a deficiency of T lymphocytes (Gottlieb, 2001). In Gottlieb's prior experience, immunodeficiency was found in infants and in patients on cancer chemotherapy. "In this age and type of otherwise healthy patient, oral thrush is as rare as hen's teeth . . . . " (Fettner & Check, 1984, p. 12).

Gottlieb's first patient presented him with a particularly puzzling constellation of symptoms. The UCLA Medical Hospital had a state-of-the-art laboratory for studying T cells, and Gottlieb had colleagues specializing in immunology with whom he discussed his puzzling cases. They performed a lung biopsy on the first patient. In this process of medical exploration, Gottlieb began to suspect that he was encountering an entirely new disease. He telephoned the Centers for Disease Control and Prevention (CDC, the U.S. government agency responsible for combating epidemics), but his news was greeted with disbelief and ironic laughter. Gottlieb persisted and eventually his report about the first five AIDS (this name for the epidemic was not used at the time) cases was published on 5 June 1981 in the CDC's weekly medical surveillance report, *Morbidity and Mortality Weekly Report (MMWR)*. Epidemiologists immediately began to search for the causes and means of transmission of this strange new disease of immune suppression.

One month later, the *MMWR* of 3 July 1981 reported a cluster of cases of Karposi's Sarcoma (KS), a rare type of skin cancer usually found among elderly men of Mediterranean ancestry. These cases were identified in New York and San Francisco (Maclure, 1998; Ng, 1991). The KS patients had blue, purple, or brownish patches on their skin. All of the individuals in the cluster were young gay men. The fact that the epidemic's first victims appeared at the same time in three locations (Los Angeles, New York, and San Francisco) was disquieting, and ominous. We know now that many thousands of individuals at scattered locations around the world were already HIV-positive at this time, although they had not yet shown the symptoms of AIDS. Many of the young men had Karposi's Sarcoma while others had pneumonia (also an unusual illness among otherwise healthy young men in the United States). Within weeks, yet more cases were reported to the CDC. Four Haitians in Miami died of opportunistic infections. They had low levels of T lymphocytes. Surprisingly, the Haitians were not gay.

The new disease was very puzzling, and it was starting to spread rapidly. Epidemiologists of the CDC galvanized into action, seeking to understand the new epidemic. It was spreading like a biological chain letter.

Patient Zero

The CDC investigators identified the first 40 patients in the United States to be diagnosed with AIDS symptoms. At this stage the disease did not have an official name, although some people called it GRIDS, for Gay-Related Immune Deficiency Syndrome. The CDC epidemiologists found that, of the 40 men, the 19 who lived in Los Angeles were linked through sexual contacts with the 21 other patients who resided in San Francisco, New York, and elsewhere in the United States. Clearly, something that caused the human immune function to fail to protect the body from opportunistic infections was being transmitted from man to man via sexual contact. Was it caused by some type of lubricant used in gay sex? Was it a drug (like poppers, an inhalant) frequently taken at that time in the U.S. gay community?

The first 40 patients with the mysterious disease had one quality in common, a high degree of sexual activity. They reported sexual contacts with an average of 227 different individuals per year. One patient consulted his little black book, and said that he had had 1,560 sexual contacts! The CDC epidemiologists identified one of the 40 AIDS cases, whom they dubbed "Patient Zero," as playing a particularly key role in the network of AIDS patients. Patient Zero had had sexual contacts with eight of the 39 other men, and he was one of the first of the 40 men to be infected. Further, he linked the Los Angeles cluster with the New York cluster.

Patient Zero was Gaetan Dugas, an Air Canada flight attendant. Dugas traveled widely, was strikingly attractive, and had a hyperactive sex drive. These characteristics represented a deadly combination of factors for the early transmission of AIDS. Patient Zero's eight direct sexual contacts led to eight other men with AIDS, who in turn led to 10 more of the 40 men. So in three steps, Patient Zero had infected 26 (63 percent) of the 39 other individuals with AIDS

(Klovdahl, 1985). Dugas's lymph nodes had been swollen since 1979. A year later, he noticed a small purple splotch on his face. His doctor diagnosed it as Karposi's Sarcoma. Dugas was 28 years old and he had the rare skin cancer associated with AIDS.

Even after he was diagnosed with AIDS, Patient Zero continued having unprotected sex, infecting individuals in an expanding network. If Gaetan Dugas had not been homosexual, perhaps the AIDS epidemic might not have afflicted mostly gays in its initial era. But that is only speculation, as many different individuals might have played the "Typhoid Mary" role in launching the AIDS epidemic (Mary Malone was an Irish immigrant cook in New York in 1909, who continued to work as a cook in a maternity hospital, infecting more people, even after she was diagnosed with typhoid; eventually she was banished for life to an institution).

Costly Delays

The CDC epidemiologists assumed that a virus was being transmitted through sexual contact among the 40 men, and that it caused an immune deficiency in the human body, which allowed various infections to then run unchecked. A year or two later, after this conclusion was supported by other evidence, AIDS was given its name, Acquired Immune Deficiency Syndrome. At this stage, the virus causing AIDS, HIV, was mainly being transmitted by the exchange of bodily fluids among gay men when they engaged in unprotected anal intercourse. Being HIV-positive usually led, after a latency period of several years, to diagnosis with AIDS symptoms. Death then followed a few years later. Indeed, Gaetan Dugas died from AIDS in 1984, four years after he was identified by the CDC. He was just a month past his thirty-second birthday.

From the beginning, it was recognized that the epidemic spread through sexual networks in an alarming exponential process. The implication for public health prevention was obvious: Stamp out the epidemic before it spread more widely. But the scientific evidence gathered by the CDC epidemiologists was ignored by high-ranking U.S. government officials, for reasons of anti-gay stigma, conflicting budget priorities, and bureaucratic inertia. One high-level government health official, the U.S. Secretary of Health and Human Services, who said publicly that AIDS was the number one health problem facing America, was "promoted" the next day to an obscure diplomatic post in a very small nation. The U.S. president Ronald Reagan went out of his way to avoid mentioning the epidemic, even when his personal friend, Hollywood actor Rock Hudson, died from AIDS four years after the epidemic was first identified in the United States.

The mass media did not frame the AIDS issue as an important human problem. *The New York Times* failed to play its usual influential role in setting the news agenda for AIDS, in part because its managing editor was homophobic (Dearing & Rogers, 1996). Individuals became infected. They developed AIDS. People died. Their deaths were duly reported by the CDC each month as dull statistics. The U.S. mass media largely ignored the epidemic that was spreading through the gay population of American cities, and the issue of AIDS did not climb the national agenda. A popular book about this early era of the AIDS epidemic in the United States was titled *And the band played on* (Shilts, 1987), referring to the sinking of the *Titanic* on its maiden voyage when it hit an iceberg in the North Sea. The ship's captain ordered the orchestra to play on, a kind of denial that also characterized the AIDS epidemic in its early years.

The San Francisco Experience

The first metropolitan center for the AIDS epidemic in the United States was San Francisco, which had become a haven for gay men in the decade prior to the epidemic. After suffering from stigma and discrimination in small towns and in other U.S. cities, thousands of gay men migrated to this tolerant northern California city, where they could live openly as gay. They organized gay men's associations, gained political power, and elected a gay politician to the City Council. The San Francisco Police Department was ordered to stop hassling patrons in the city's gay bars. Many gay men lived along Castro Street or were concentrated in nearby urban neighborhoods in San Francisco. By 1981, an estimated 40 percent of the city's male population was gay, the largest such population of any city in the world. Public bathhouses provided convenient locations for anonymous gay sex, which was celebrated by many in the gay community as part of their new-found freedom.

These conditions in San Francisco meant that HIV spread rapidly among the dense population of sexually promiscuous men. All but seven of the 122 individuals in a photograph of the Gay Men's Chorus of San Francisco, taken in 1993, had died since 1981. This dramatic photograph, widely published in U.S. newspapers, helped convey the lethal impact of the epidemic (Plate 1.2).

The San Francisco Model: An approach to HIV/AIDS prevention called the "San Francisco model" emerged in the city, based on a successful intervention, STOP AIDS (see Chapter 4). A key component of this model was the belief that prevention programs needed to be non-judgmental, to avoid stigmatizing the particular lifestyles or other behaviors of individuals targeted for prevention activities, even if they were drug abusers or commercial sex workers. For example, the term "drug user" was used by prevention program staff, rather than "drug abuser," a slight change in terminology that conveyed a world of meaning.

The STOP AIDS campaign was mounted by gay men for other individuals like themselves. The speakers at the small group meetings organized by STOP AIDS were perceived as highly credible, in part because they were HIV+, and their messages were culturally and linguistically appropriate for audience members. The speakers were selected because they were opinion leaders in the gay community, respected by their peers. At the end of each group meeting, the members were asked to make a commitment to practicing safer sex and to volunteer to organize and lead other small group meetings (Wohlfeiler, 1998). Thus, a multiplication factor was built into the small group meetings. Further, the HIV prevention programs were targeted at high-risk individuals, an effective communication strategy for an epidemic that was spreading through sexual networks among a certain population.

A massive change in sexual behavior occurred in San Francisco during the mid-1980s. For example, 50 percent of monogamous men and 71 percent of non-monogamous men reported that they practiced unprotected anal intercourse in 1983–84. Four years later, these figures had dropped to 12 percent and 27 percent respectively (McKusick et al., 1990). This rapid change resulted (*a*) from intensive

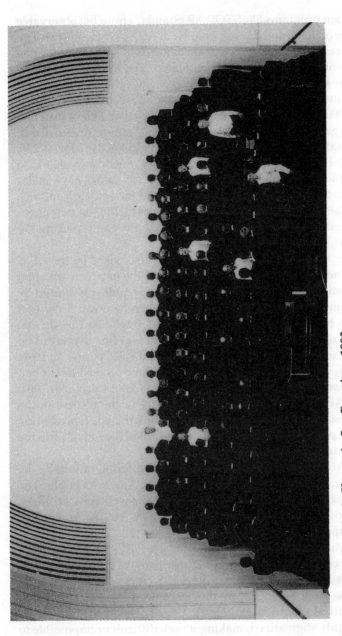

Plate 1.2   The Gay Men's Chorus in San Francisco, 1993

All but seven of the 122 members of the San Francisco Gay Men's Chorus are dressed in black and face away from the camera. They represent the members of the Chorus who had died from AIDS-related causes since 1981.

Source: *San Francisco Chronicle*. Photograph by Eric Luse.

prevention programs like STOP AIDS, and (*b*) from the observable presence of death and disease from HIV/AIDS. When several of an individual's friends have died or are dying from AIDS, the adoption of preventive behavior is self-motivated. The human cost of the epidemic in San Francisco was indeed terrible. By 1993, 48 percent of all homosexual and bisexual men in the city were HIV+ (Dearing et al., 1996). After the mid-1990s, when more than half of the HIV-positive gay men in San Francisco were taking anti-retroviral drugs, the annual death rate from AIDS dropped from 1,600 to a low of 250.

While the U.S. mass media did not carry much news about the AIDS epidemic until 1985, the San Francisco media gave major attention to this issue from the beginning of the epidemic in 1981, led by the city's five gay newspapers. Eventually, the two major newspapers and other San Francisco media began reporting the epidemic.

Public awareness of the epidemic was also raised by the AIDS quilt panels that were created for many of the gay men who had died from AIDS in San Francisco. The AIDS quilt was started by Cleve Jones in San Francisco in 1986, when he created the first panel to honor his friend Marvin Feldman, who had died from AIDS at age 33. The AIDS Memorial Quilt was first displayed on the Mall in Washington, D.C., in 1987; it had 1,920 panels. In 1996, when the quilt was displayed for the last time on the Mall, it had 40,000 panels and covered 26 football fields. By 1 December 2001, World AIDS Day, on the 20th anniversary of the disease in the United States, 45,000 panels had been constructed, representing about 10 percent of the 448,060 people who had died of AIDS in the United States.

The AIDS quilt symbolized the human suffering caused by the epidemic, and helped convey this pain to the American public. The individuals dying from AIDS in San Francisco were sons, brothers, and friends. Increasingly, they were women, African Americans, and Hispanics.

Unfortunately, the San Francisco model for HIV/AIDS prevention could not be adopted elsewhere because many of the preconditions were missing. Many gay men in other U.S. cities were not yet living openly as gays. Seldom were they organized in associations that had political clout (Adam, 1997). Usually, infected individuals were highly stigmatized, making it very difficult or impossible to communicate with them about AIDS prevention (Perloff, 2001). But the San Francisco experience showed the world that slowing down the epidemic was possible, at least under very special conditions. In the early 1990s, the San Francisco model offered some hope that prevention strategies could be effective.

Eventually, in the United States, as in other wealthy nations, the epidemic was brought under a greater degree of control. However, even during 1995, some 50,610 Americans died from AIDS. Thereafter, the number of deaths per year dropped sharply, and by 2001 it was less than one-third of the 1995 rate, with 15,000 deaths. Any human death is a tragedy, but this downward trend, a product of the anti-retroviral drugs and of effective prevention activities, is remarkable (although 40,000 Americans were infected with HIV in 2001). Unfortunately, the high-cost American interventions are not affordable in Latin America, Africa, and Asia, where the epidemic is spreading exponentially. The cost to the United States of combating the AIDS epidemic is considerable, even though it is a rich nation. Had effective HIV/AIDS interventions begun several years earlier, the total cost would have been a fraction of its eventual amount. The research funding alone, which is a small portion of the total cost of prevention, testing, treatment, and care for AIDS, is staggering. AIDS research funding provided just to the National Institutes of Health (NIH), after a slow start in the early 1980s, has increased at a 45 degree rate of growth, reaching $2.5 billion in 2002 (Folkers & Fauci, 2001). So waiting on an epidemic is costly.

Era 2: Breaking Out of High-Risk Populations

One of the authors involved the students in a class at the University of New Mexico in playing the AIDS Game. Each of the 20 students was given a glass half filled with water, and a spoon. One of the glasses was heavily dosed with salt. The students were instructed to pair off randomly at each of the six generations of the game. Each pair of students exchanged three spoonfuls of water in each generation of the AIDS Game. After six rounds of the exercise, to the amazement of the students, they *all* had a glass of salty water! The rate of infection proceeded in exponential order: 1, 2, 4, 8, 16, 32.

An epidemic spreads through interpersonal networks from a relatively small number of central nodes. The best opportunity for controlling an epidemic exists for only a brief window, before the epidemic breaks out of these nodes. If one plots the cumulative number of infected individuals over time, the distribution forms an S-shaped curve (Rogers, 1995). After a certain number of years, the rate of infection takes off and rises rapidly as the epidemic spreads into the general population (Figure 1.2). In the case of AIDS, this take-off period, when the epidemic breaks out of high-risk groups,

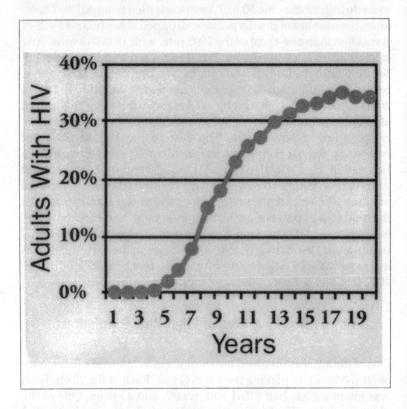

Figure 1.2   The S-shaped Curve of an Epidemic's Growth

Initial efforts to combat the HIV/AIDS epidemic in a nation center on prevention programs targeted to such high-risk groups as commercial sex workers, truckers, migrant workers, and injecting drug users. If this specialized effort is not successful in halting the further spread of the epidemic, it breaks out into the general population as the rate of infection "takes-off."

Source: UNAIDS.

generally occurs when around 1 percent of pregnant women visiting antenatal clinics test HIV-positive (this indicator is often used as a measure of the spread of HIV in a city or a nation). The history of the worldwide AIDS epidemic is mainly an unfortunate story of failure to grasp an early opportunity for halting the further spread of the virus.

The epidemic began at about the same time (the early 1980s) in many countries (Table 1.1). Often, the first people with HIV/AIDS were injecting drug users, commercial sex workers, or gay men in urban areas, but soon the epidemic spread to other populations by heterosexual or other means of transmission. For instance, some gay men were bisexual, and infected their wives or commercial sex workers. In Bangkok, the rate of HIV infection among injecting drug users rose from 1 percent in 1987 to 24 percent in 1998, and to 39 percent in 1999. While HIV spreads among the members of a high-risk group, like injecting drug users or commercial sex workers, the epidemic often crosses over to other high-risk groups and into the general population. In the early 1980s, HIV-positive men in San Francisco and other cities donated blood to the Red Cross, and hemophiliacs like Indiana schoolboy Ryan White were infected through the blood supply. The African American tennis star Arthur Ashe received two blood transfusions during heart surgery, and was infected with HIV. Some 5,000 hemophiliacs in Japan were infected by blood imported from the United States. Transmission through the blood supply, it was soon learned, could be eliminated by (a) testing blood donors for HIV, and (b) heating the blood to a high temperature for a brief time.

Also, once women were infected, it was discovered that mothers could transmit the virus to their children at birth. In certain countries today, such mother-to-child transmission (MTCT) is widespread. Some 40 percent of all seropositive people in South Africa are pregnant women, most of whom were infected by their husbands and male partners. Frequently, in these patriarchal cultures, once the husband becomes aware that his wife is seropositive, he accuses her of infidelity, and throws her out of their home. This unfair process of blaming-the-victim leads to mothers with children becoming homeless, as her parents often will not provide help. Infected wives lead to an increasing number of AIDS orphans, many of whom are HIV-positive. Their infection can be prevented in many cases by a one-time oral dose of Nevirapine for the mother

Table 1.1

A Comparison of the AIDS Epidemic in Six Selected Nations as of the End of 2001

Nation	Total Population	Per Capita GNP	Date Epidemic Began	First High-Risk Group	Number of HIV+ People	Number of AIDS Orphans	Number of AIDS Deaths
South Africa	43M	$3,210	1983	Gays	4.7M	500K	300K
Kenya	30M	$340	1983	CSWs	2.3M	730K	200K
Brazil	167M	$5,029	1981	Gays	0.58M	45K	200K
Thailand	63M	$1,700	1984	CSWs, Gays	700K	85K	300K
India	1,015M	$370	1986	CSWs	4M	75K	300K
Cambodia	12M	$280	1991	CSWs	0.23M	15K	18K
World	6B	–	1981	Gays	40M	14M	25M

Source: Based on UNAIDS and other data sources.

during delivery, and for the newborn child after delivery (and by bottle-feeding the baby instead of breast-feeding it after it is born). Nevirapine costs about $4 per birth, and is now provided free of cost in many developing countries by certain drug companies, as Cipla does in India (Chapter 3).

Commercial sex workers became infected with the virus early in the unfolding of the epidemic, and the red-light districts of metropolitan centers like Mumbai (Bombay), Chennai (Madras), Kolkata (Calcutta), Bangkok, Nairobi, and other mega-cities in developing nations became key nodes in the expanding networks of infection. These HIV infection centers catered especially to men who were seasonal urban migrant workers, who in turn infected their wives when they returned home. Thus began the interiorization process of the epidemic in many countries.

Sex tours to places like Bangkok and Nairobi carried the virus across international boundaries. Kenya denied the seriousness of its AIDS epidemic, out of fear that such news would damage the tourist industry, an important source of national income. For several years in the late 1980s, President Daniel Arap Moi insisted that there was no AIDS in his country. A foreign newsperson in Nairobi who reported on the epidemic was immediately sent home. Kenyan newspeople who wrote about AIDS were jailed. During these years of repression in Kenya, the epidemic continued to spread rapidly, as it broke out of the original nodes of vulnerable groups.

Such a national policy of denial is to be found in many countries in the early years of the epidemic. This situation, however, changed suddenly in Thailand in the late 1980s. Until then, Thais had defined the AIDS epidemic as mainly a foreign disease that had infected a few commercial sex workers in Bangkok and Chiang Mai. Then, in June 1989, a government surveillance survey in Chiang Mai found that a startling 44 percent of all CSWs in the city's brothels were HIV-positive. Thais began to realize that AIDS was not just a disease of foreign sex tourists, but rather an epidemic that was spreading among the Thai population. In 1991–92 the outspoken Mechai Viravaidya, who was at the time both the director of Thailand's AIDS program and chairman of its Tourist Authority, stated in a television interview: "Sperm Tours. I suggest they [sex tourists] don't buy a ticket to Thailand. They should buy rat poison and stay home and take it instead" (D'Agnes, 2001, p. 345). At the time, a high percentage of commercial sex workers in Bangkok were

HIV-positive, and the epidemic was radiating out from Thailand to other nations, and, through sex customers, to the general population of Thailand. Something had to be done, and quickly. Mechai led the way in 1991–92, in the first successful AIDS control program in a developing nation.

Truck stops along main travelways in developing countries became nodes in the expanding networks of the virus. A 1992 study by the African Medical Research and Education Federation (AMREF) in Tanzania found that half of the commercial sex workers at the truck stops on the Trans-African Highway were HIV-positive, as were 35 percent of the truckers. Each of the seven main truck stops in Tanzania averaged about 700 commercial sex workers. One of this book's authors (Rogers) visited a truck stop near Dar es Salaam in the mid-1990s. Bowls of free condoms were placed in restaurants, bathrooms, and hotel rooms. The truck stop seemed almost to be drowning in condoms. Making condoms available, of course, is quite a different matter from getting them used. In East Africa, truckers commonly pay a higher price to commercial sex workers for condomless sex.

A recent report from the South African Medical Research Council indicates that 95 percent of the truck drivers stopping at Newcastle, a truck stop in KwaZulu Natal Province, are HIV-positive. Some 64 percent of the commercial sex workers at Newcastle have HIV (Lamont, 2001). India has 3.5 million truck drivers; they were identified as a high-risk target group in spreading the epidemic (Plate 1.3). In Thailand, the government encouraged long-distance truck drivers to take their female partners along on their trips (Steinfatt, 2002, p. 213).

Thus, during the second era of the epidemic, HIV got its "legs" by moving along lines of ground transportation. It broke out of its initial nodes among high-risk populations, and spread into the general population. Thereafter, the population is at risk; containment within particular groups becomes a lost opportunity. Now the epidemic is "out of the bag." Senegal is one of very few developing nations that moved immediately, once the first six AIDS cases were identified in 1986, to establish a national AIDS control program. Thanks to strong political commitment and to speedy action, Senegal did not allow the epidemic to break out of the initial high-risk groups (Pisani, 1999).

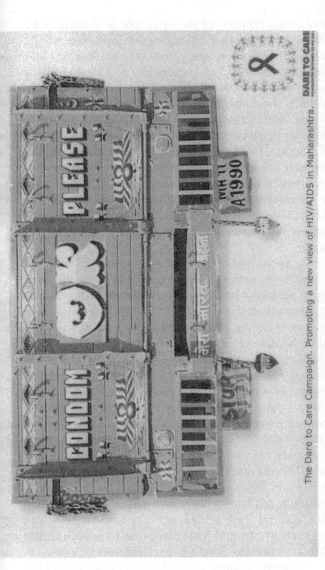

The Dare to Care Campaign. Promoting a new view of HIV/AIDS in Maharashtra.

DARE TO CARE

Plate 1.3 This "Condom OK Please" Message on the Back of a Truck in India Signifies the High-risk Audience for HIV Infection Represented by Truck Drivers

Trucks in India are colorfully decorated with one-liners, slogans, and sayings. Most trucks have the message "Horn OK Please" on the back. This standard message has been modified to promote safer sex on the highways. In India, and in many other countries, truckers played a key role in the interiorization of the epidemic.

Source : AVERT Project of the U.S. Agency for International Development (in the state of Maharashtra).

Era 3: Interiorization

The process of interiorization of the epidemic is illustrated by
Figure 1.3, which shows the spread of registered AIDS cases among
municípios in Brazil. In Era 1, roughly from 1980 to 1986, the black
dots were concentrated in urban centers like São Paulo (on the
Atlantic coast in southern Brazil). During Era 2, approximately
from 1987 to 1993, the epidemic spread rapidly along the entire
Atlantic seacoast, with large concentrations in and around São
Paulo, Rio de Janeiro, and Recife (located in the poverty-stricken
north-east of Brazil). The black dots then begin to move into the
interior of this vast nation, whose land area represents about half
of all of Latin America. During Era 3, from 1994 to 2000, however,
the epidemic spread more widely throughout the nation, including
to the sparsely populated interior of Brazil. Note the line of black
dots that outlines the Amazon river, an important travelway in
northern Brazil.

By 2000, only about half of Brazil's *municípios* had reported
AIDS cases, in part due to the lag of several years while the virus
is incubating in an individual (there may also be a lag due to
inadequate testing sites in rural areas). While interiorization was
well underway in Brazil by 2002, half of all HIV cases were still
concentrated in the state of São Paulo. The city of São Paulo has a
population of 12 million, and is one of the largest cities in the
world. It is the major center for the AIDS epidemic in Latin America.

An illustration of the interiorization process in the United States
is provided by a young medical doctor, Dr. Abraham Verghese
(1995), who was employed in a hospital in Johnson City, Tennessee,
in the mid-1980s.[1] Johnson City is a rural and remote location,
deep in the Appalachian region. Local people in Johnson City
believed that AIDS was an epidemic that only affected people in
distant cities like San Francisco and New York. One day in 1986,
a man suffering from AIDS presented himself to Dr. Verghese at his
hospital. This patient had contracted *Pneumocystis carinii*
pneumonia in a far-off city, and had come home to be with family
members who cared for him. Soon a gay couple with HIV came to
Dr. Verghese, and soon thereafter arrived another gay couple, both
HIV-positive. Verghese was becoming known in the local gay
community as a doctor who was willing to treat AIDS patients.

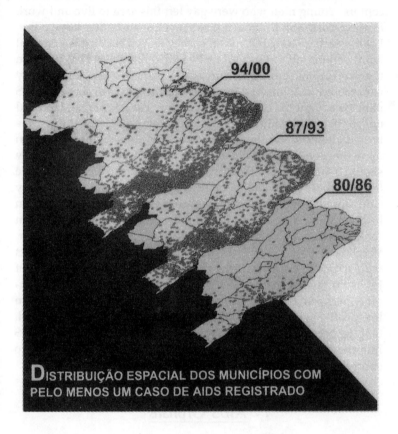

Figure 1.3   Interiorization of the Epidemic in Brazil from 1980 to 2000

Initially, in 1980–86, reported AIDS cases were concentrated in urban centers like São Paulo. Then in 1987–93, the epidemic spread along the Atlantic coast, forming concentrations in São Paulo, Rio de Janeiro, and Recife. After 1994, AIDS cases were reported in the interior of Brazil. The interiorization process occurs after HIV infection has broken out of high-risk populations like injecting drug users and commercial sex workers.

Source: Brazilian Ministry of Health.

The epidemic was introduced to eastern Tennessee from urban centers. Young men who were gay left this area to live and work in New York, San Francisco, Los Angeles, and other large cities. Later, after becoming HIV-positive, they moved back to their original home community to be cared for by family members. HIV infection then spread locally. To his surprise, Verghese learned that a gay bar existed in Johnson City. One reason why Verghese's AIDS patients sought his care was because he was a foreigner, and did not share local prejudices. The strong degree of local stigma was brought home to Verghese when one of his nurses, who had grown up in Johnson City, angrily questioned the doctor about why they should treat gay AIDS patients, who were going to die anyway. She felt that these patients had sinned, and were being punished by God. Because of the strong local anti-gay and anti-AIDS stigma in Johnson City, each of Verghese's AIDS patients approached him for health care in a very surreptitious manner. After four years, Dr. Verghese (1995) counted the number of his present or former patients with AIDS. There were more than 80! Yet the average citizen of Johnson City still insisted that the epidemic was found only in far-off American cities. Here we see how stigma keeps the epidemic in low profile, with the result that little is done to control its spread. Only by breaking the silence about the epidemic, and moving AIDS into the public sphere, was the United States eventually able to control the spread of HIV/AIDS.

AIDS Orphans

As mentioned previously, the commonly used indicator for marking the point at which the HIV epidemic begins to break into the general population is the percentage of HIV-positive mothers who visit antenatal clinics. This indicator is convenient, especially if the mothers are given a blood test, because even in very poor countries, large numbers of pregnant women seek clinic check-ups. The indicator is often biased, however, because urban women of lower socioeconomic status (who generally have higher rates of HIV infection) are less likely to seek care at antenatal clinics. The argument for this indicator is that when a certain percentage of pregnant women are seropositive (they are usually infected by their husbands), the epidemic is beginning to reach the general population.

HIV-positive mothers lead to one of the saddest aspects of the AIDS epidemic: babies born to mothers who will succumb, and who are going to have an abbreviated and painful life themselves. AIDS orphans, 14 million of them, are one of the most heart-tugging tragedies of the worldwide epidemic. Each orphan typically has lost one or both parents to the epidemic. By 2010, 44 million children will have lost one or both parents to AIDS. Most AIDS orphans are born HIV-positive. They were infected by their mothers, who in turn were probably infected by their husbands, who got the virus from someone else. In Zimbabwe, 45 percent of children under the age of five are HIV-positive. Sadly, few of these children will live to see their tenth birthdays, given the usual incubation period of the disease. Among orphans, the girl child is usually the hardest hit, often dropping out of school and taking on family responsibilities when her mother dies. In Zambia, where one in four children is an AIDS orphan, about 10 percent of all households are headed by children less than 14 years of age (Singhal & Howard, in press). Figure 1.4 shows how the number of AIDS orphans in KwaZulu Natal Province in South Africa, 125,000 in 2002, will shoot up to half a million in the following years.

In AIDS orphanages, a spoon is a subtle symbol of the presence of AIDS. A fork can be dangerous in case the children poke themselves and bleed infectious blood (Pang, 1998). Staff members in AIDS orphanages hug and kiss the children on their cheeks. Nursery staff wear plastic gloves when washing the children. In most other ways, the typical AIDS orphanage seems much like any other nursery school or daycare center.

The ABC Orphanage

The AIDS Babies' Center (ABC) in Chiang Mai, Thailand, is fairly typical of the many AIDS orphanages around the world. Seven children, HIV-positive, live in ABC, along with 70 other AIDS orphans, and a staff of eight caregivers who look after their tiny charges and give them their medications. The ABC was established in 1995 by Ricky Tan, a young Christian minister from Malaysia, and his Singaporean wife, Lay Hwa. With initial support from

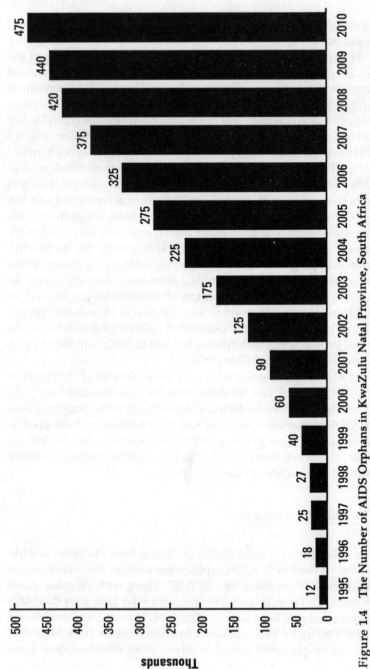

Figure 1.4 The Number of AIDS Orphans in KwaZulu Natal Province, South Africa

A particularly sad aspect of the worldwide epidemic is the rapidly increasing number of children who have lost one or both parents to AIDS, and who may be HIV-positive, infected at birth through mother-to-child transmission of the virus.

religious organizations in Singapore, Ricky Tan and his wife obtained a 5-acre plot some 18 miles south of Chiang Mai, and built the Care Corner Orphanage, of which the ABC nursery is the component for HIV-positive children. This AIDS orphanage is located in the district with the highest rate of HIV infection in Chiang Mai Province, which is the center of the epidemic in Thailand (half of all the reported AIDS cases in Thailand are in the nation's northern region, of which the city of Chiang Mai is the hub). The villages surrounding the orphanage supply commercial sex workers, including child prostitutes, to nearby Chiang Mai and to Bangkok. Many of the children in Ricky Tan's orphanage are members of northern Thailand's hill tribes, and come from families with low socioeconomic status. Some of the children are referred to the orphanage via informal networks; others come through the government's Department of Public Welfare. Most children have lost both parents to the epidemic. The family members of other orphans are unable, or unwilling, to care for them.

The ABC orphanage faced a crisis in 1997, when financial support from Singapore ended suddenly. Ricky Tan and his wife prayed for a solution. After several months, they decided to develop a handicrafts business, fabricating products out of mulberry tree bark, which is plentiful in the Chiang Mai area. The handicrafts are sold in Singapore, the United States, and Japan through churches and other outlets. The sale of handicrafts, along with the poultry, fruit, and fish produced on the 5-acre grounds, has made the orphanage almost self-sufficient. The orphans hurry home from school each day to their duties of making handicrafts or carrying for the farm enterprises. Ricky Tan plans to expand the sale of handicrafts through the orphanage's website (www.CareCornerOrphanage.com).

Plate 1.4 shows the ABC children in early 1998. By mid-year, the staff noticed that one child, Fon, 5 years old, was acting differently from the other children. Her father had died from AIDS-related causes, and she had been hospitalized along with her 24-year-old mother and her 7-year-old brother. Out of desperation, Fon's mother had attempted to cut her children's throats and to commit suicide herself. The hospital asked Ricky Tan to take in the three family members. Fon's mother and brother had AIDS symptoms, and Fon was expected to be next. But the ABC staff observed that Fon seldom caught the colds, fevers, and opportunistic diseases of her peers.

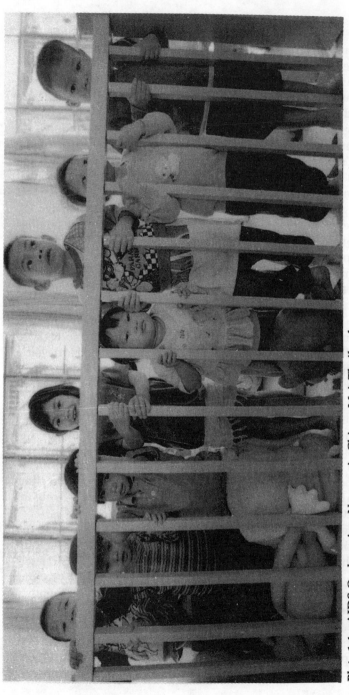

Plate 1.4 AIDS Orphans in a Nursery in Chiang Mai, Thailand

One of these seven children, a little girl named Fon (left centre), photographed in 1998, was later found to be HIV-negative. The other six AIDS orphans had died by late 2001 because the cost of anti-retroviral drugs was unaffordable.

Source: *The New Paper*, Singapore. Photograph by Philip Lim.

Further, Fon had a healthy appetite and was full of energy. Ricky Tan ordered a blood test for Fon, which came back negative. This surprising result was confirmed by a second blood test: also negative. Fon had not been infected by her mother at birth.

When Ricky Tan told Fon's mother the good news, she jumped up, hugged him, and said with elation, "Now she can go to school!" Fon's mother converted to Christianity, and asked Ricky Tan to adopt her daughter after her death. Ricky Tan and his wife raised Fon as an addition to their family of three children. A year later, however, Fon's grandmother expressed a desire to raise Fon, and Ricky Tan and his wife returned Fon to her village. The strength of anti-AIDS stigma in Thailand is demonstrated by her grandmother's rejection of Fon when she was thought to be HIV-positive, but her acceptance when Fon was found to be seronegative.

Fon does not know that she had been classified as HIV-positive by the hospital that sent her to the orphanage, so she does not understand the miracle that happened in 1998. For Fon, life goes on. Unfortunately, for most AIDS orphans, the future is bleak and short. Their lives could be saved, or at least prolonged indefinitely, by anti-retrovirals. But the drugs are too expensive for the orphanage to afford.

In late 2001 when we visited the ABC nursery, all seven of the children in the 1998 photograph, except Fon, had died.

My Name is Non*

"Hello, my name is 'Non.' I am seven years old and I have AIDS. I was born in Chiang Dao, Thailand, and my family still lives there. My parents are dead; my father died three years ago from malaria, and my mother died two months ago from AIDS. My grandparents cared for me, but my grandpa has leprosy. So my uncle brought me to the ABC Orphanage. I miss my parents and relatives, but I have adjusted to my new home.

I am just getting over a large, open viral rash [Herpes Zoster]. I also had a bad stomach ache [Cystitus], but the doctor gave me medications and I feel better now. I weigh 18 kilograms [about 40 pounds]. I am developing a little soreness on my tongue [a fungal infection]. I am losing weight because I throw up frequently, but I still love to eat. My sickness does not slow me down. I get two baths a day, three good meals, and two snacks a day. I get plenty of rest, and I have time to play with toys and with my friends here at ABC."

*This message from Non was written with the help of a volunteer at the ABC orphanage a year before Non passed away on 25 November 1999.

Commercial Sex Workers

It is no accident that countries with a booming sex industry, like India, South Africa, Kenya, and Thailand, have, or have had, a major AIDS epidemic. Poverty and commercial sex work go hand in hand. Commercial sex workers play an important role, especially in the early stages of the epidemic, in every country.

The sex industry in Thailand expanded greatly during the Vietnam War, especially in Bangkok, which was a popular site for U.S. military personnel on rest and recreation leave. The Thai sex industry was also amplified by international tourism. The typical Thai commercial sex worker is a young girl, with less than a high school education, often from a rural area, who sends remittances home to support her family (Bond et al., 1997). Perhaps she is from northern Thailand and was recruited by an agent in her village who knew that her father was desperate for money to pay off a loan. Perhaps the father received several hundred dollars (U.S. equivalent) from the recruiting agent when she was sold to a brothel owner in Bangkok or in Chiang Mai. She probably lives in a room in the brothel, under the complete control of the owner. She can only leave the brothel with the owner's permission.

Not all of the approximately 200,000 commercial sex workers (out of the total Thai population of 63 million people) are Thai.[2] Also well represented are sex workers from China, Burma, Vietnam, Cambodia, Russia, Poland, and other countries. One brothel arrangement consists of a glass-encased room with several levels of carpeted steps. The glass is dark on the inside and lighter on the outside, so that the women can be seen by, but cannot see, their potential customers. Each woman wears a number pinned to her dress, so that customers can specify their choice (Bond et al., 1996). Under such dehumanizing conditions, it is no wonder that many commercial sex workers feel a loss of self-efficacy (a belief that they can control their lives). Some commercial sex workers do not work in a brothel, but rather in a restaurant or bar where they meet their customers. These women are called "informal" sex workers in Thailand, and it is difficult for public health programs to reach them with prevention messages.

In preparing this book, we met with commercial sex workers in Thailand, such as leaders in the EMPOWER Foundation, an NGO that seeks to assist its members in learning languages (classes in English, German, and Japanese are the most popular), in gaining a feeling of collective efficacy (a belief that they can control the events in their lives through group actions), and in simply having fun. EMPOWER trains all police recruits in Bangkok during a two-week course in what it is like to be a commercial sex worker. EMPOWER does not try to get women out of commercial sex work. After visiting with the EMPOWER Foundation leaders in Patpong, the famous red-light district in Bangkok, one afternoon in August 2001, Rogers and his wife excused themselves from the discussions when the sex workers politely hinted that they had to change clothes and go to work.

What is the future for a commercial sex worker in Thailand? Most women work an average of only three years, about the same tenure as a professional football player in America's National Football League. A few save some of their earnings, and use these savings to leave the sex industry for other work. Sex workers may contract HIV/AIDS, the disease that represents another exit route from their occupation.

Conclusions

HIV is not a common everyday infectious disease. It cannot be transmitted in contaminated water and food, like cholera or typhoid. The virus cannot be transmitted by an insect, as are plague and malaria. HIV is not transmitted through the air, like influenza and tuberculosis, nor through physical touch, like fungal infections. HIV transmission usually requires the active participation of an individual in activities in which bodily fluids (semen or blood) are exchanged. Theoretically, HIV's spread can thus be controlled.

Why have a few developing countries been relatively successful in controlling the AIDS epidemic, while most have not? This chapter suggests the importance of political will on the part of top government leaders. One key indicator of such political will is whether the chief government leader heads the national AIDS control program. If so, HIV/AIDS prevention becomes the responsibility of *every* government official, not just of those in the AIDS control section of the ministry of health. A key question, addressed in the following chapter, is how advocates and champions can secure government policies to combat the epidemic. HIV/AIDS still does not have a high priority in most Latin American, African, and Asian nations. Barring very few exceptions, national government leaders do not head AIDS control programs.

Prevention activities and providing free anti-retroviral drugs can play crucial roles in controlling the AIDS epidemic, but unless these interventions are implemented in an effective way, little benefit results (Pang, 1999). The anti-retrovirals are still prohibitively expensive (although the cost is dropping), far beyond what people in developing nations can afford. Most HIV-positive people, perhaps 95 percent of all PWAs, are doomed to an early death, except in Brazil where people living with HIV/AIDS receive free anti-retroviral drugs.

What can a relatively poor developing nation do to control the epidemic?

1. Move immediately to mount prevention interventions when the epidemic is first detected (as Senegal did). Launch prevention programs encouraging condom use and other safe sex behaviors that are targeted at high-risk audiences (such as commercial sex workers and injecting drug users), in the early years of the epidemic. Provide free condoms. Condom use can dramatically reduce the rate of HIV infection. Motivation to use condoms is the problem. Utilize an opinion leadership strategy through peer educators to leverage social networks for HIV prevention.

2. Provide anti-retroviral drugs free or at a reduced price, if the funding can somehow be found. Begin by targeting

pregnant women who are seropositive, so as to prevent children being born HIV-positive, who will become AIDS orphans. If anti-retrovirals are available and affordable, offer free testing and counseling.

3. Seek to remove the stigma of HIV/AIDS, so that people living with HIV/AIDS can live with dignity. Encourage the organizing of people with HIV/AIDS (PWAs) so they can gain political power, lobby for favorable policies, and fight stigma.

4. Address the social problems of poverty and gender inequality, which are linked to vulnerability to HIV infection.

Some nations tried other approaches. For example, Cuba mounted a massive blood testing program early in the epidemic to identify people who were HIV-positive, and then isolated these individuals in *sidatorios*, internment camps (SIDA is the Spanish name for AIDS). Most other countries would not allow this violation of individual rights. Cuba has a relatively low level of HIV infection today, in part as a result of the *sidatorios*.

This chapter showed that the epidemic is the world's problem, not just a problem of individual nations. In a globalized world of relatively easy travel and rapid transportation, sexual tourism, and migrant workers and commercial sex workers who move across national borders, no single nation can prevent the epidemic from entering its borders. During the 1980s, AIDS started in one or a few countries and then spread fairly rapidly throughout the world, transported by airline personnel, truck drivers, sex tourists, and others. In one sense, "We all have AIDS."

The epidemic is everywhere in today's world. In the Ukraine, a nation previously part of the Soviet Union, the disease was virtually unknown until 1994, when 187 cases were reported. By 2002, 300,000 to 400,000 individuals were HIV+, mainly injecting drug users. The Chinese government estimated that 600,000 people were living with HIV/AIDS in 2000, and that this number may have climbed to one million by 2001. The epidemic is concentrated in certain areas, such as Yunnan Province, where many injecting drug users are infected, and in villages in Henan Province where villagers sell their blood to collection centers that use unclean needles. Similar HIV epidemics related to blood donation have been reported in Hebei, Anhui, Shaanxi, and Guizhou Provinces. HIV is also spreading in certain cities among commercial sex workers. By 2002, all 31 provinces in China reported HIV/AIDS individuals.

We have seen that sexual networks may include individuals who are distanced by many miles. For example, the CDC analysis of the first 40 men to contract AIDS in the United States showed that they were located in three widely separated cities (Klovdahl, 1985). The interconnectedness of people who are seropositive suggests that using network-based strategies (such as the opinion leadership approach) to combat the epidemic can be particularly effective.

Much is yet to be learned about how to control the AIDS epidemic. The world is doing a rather poor job of utilizing known communication strategies to control the spread of HIV. We must do much better in the future.

Notes

1. Dr. Verghese practiced in a Veterans' Hospital in Johnson City. All of the buildings of the hospital campus face south, just as General Ulysses S. Grant's Union Army did in 1863 when it invaded the South, thus indicating the strongly anti-secessionist sentiments of eastern Tennessee during the Civil War.

2. Dr. Tom Steinfatt (2002, p. 348), on the basis of his past decade of research in Thailand, estimated the total number of commercial sex workers at about 200,000, with another 330,000 people employed in the sex industry as owners and managers of bars, restaurants, and brothel employees, etc. If each of these individuals supports a family of four additional members, about 1.65 million Thais are supported by the sex industry.

2

AIDS Advocacy and Policies

■

We are sitting on top of a volcano. How can one keep quiet?

> Ms. Usha Bhasin, an official of the Prasar
> Bharati (Broadcasting) Corporation, at a
> December 2001 AIDS workshop in New
> Delhi.

If my work can prevent just one child from contracting
HIV/AIDS, it is all worthwhile.

> Pieter-Dirk Uys, a leading satirist in South
> Africa and advocate for children with HIV
> (quoted in Bergman, 2002, p. 41).

In December 2001, while in India, the present authors were invited
to participate in a panel on communication strategies for AIDS
control at the India International Center in New Delhi. Also on the
panel were both the official in charge of communication for the
National AIDS Control Organization (NACO), and a senior
television broadcasting official involved in AIDS communication
programs. Several dozen NGOs were represented in the audience.
After the panelists' presentations, the discussion became unruly as
various organizations criticized each other, and the presenters, for
implying that one segment or another (gays, PWAs, female CSWs,
etc.) was to blame for the epidemic. Strategies like using fear appeals

for HIV prevention were attacked by various NGO leaders. Other NGO leaders resented the military metaphor of "combating" AIDS, and of "targeting" certain audiences for prevention activities. Several individuals stalked out of the meeting in anger. The politics of the AIDS epidemic are an interesting arena, although one that has been little analyzed by communication or other scholars.

The purpose of this chapter is to analyze the evolution of AIDS policies and programs, focusing on the responses to the epidemic by national governments, international agencies, non-governmental organizations (NGOs), and advocacy groups. Our conceptual framework for analyzing the AIDS policy process is *agenda-setting*, the process through which an issue climbs to a higher priority in a system.

The Unruly Policy Agenda for AIDS

When the epidemic initially burst upon the world scene after 1981, no AIDS policies or programs existed in any nation. Efforts to control the epidemic had to force their way onto an already crowded agenda of social problems, pushing out other problems and programs in jostling for public attention, funding, and other scarce resources. This agenda-setting process required several years in most nations, and the struggle for full recognition of AIDS as a major world problem is currently far from completed. Here we focus on visionaries, champions, and activists, brave individuals who advocate for AIDS policies and programs. They represent some of the true heroes of the worldwide movement to control the epidemic. We also tell about politicians and others who deny that the epidemic exists, who even question the causes of AIDS, and who generally block progress toward combating the epidemic.

The struggle by AIDS activists to gain a toehold on national agendas is a very political process, and usually a very messy one. One conflict is between government AIDS control agencies, usually located within a ministry of health, and non-governmental organizations, who typically receive much of their funding from the government, and carry out specialized program functions that a government agency could not implement as efficiently. Yet the NGOs are often highly critical of the national AIDS control agency, as the two systems have very different organizational cultures.

Usually, government agencies move more slowly than NGOs feel is necessary. Often, the NGOs serve different constituents, and disagree about how best to combat the epidemic.

Women's groups complain that too much emphasis is placed on changing the behavior of female commercial sex workers, and resent the inference that female CSWs are to be blamed for the epidemic. Gay NGOs feel that homosexuality is being stigmatized by the government AIDS control agency through labeling them as a "high-risk group." Non-governmental organizations representing people living with HIV/AIDS (PWAs) feel that not enough funding is allocated to treatment and care; they protest against being called "patients," a medical term. Many PWAs lose their jobs when identified as HIV-positive, and so they are understandably concerned about privacy issues.

In India, a rather moralistic society, "high-risk groups" resist being designated as such by the Indian government, which they feel is vilifying them. So there is anything but unity in how the epidemic is defined, how it should be dealt with, and even what it should be called. Obviously, controlling the epidemic is difficult when key actors cannot agree on basic terms.

Nkosi Johnson at the 2000 Durban Conference

The highlight of the 2000 International AIDS Conference in Durban, South Africa, was a speech by the late Nkosi Johnson, a diminutive, personable man-child who served during his short life as a powerful AIDS activist. Nkosi began his speech at the Durban Conference by saying: "Hi, my name is Nkosi Johnson. I live in Melville, Johannesburg, South Africa. I am 11 years old and I have full-blown AIDS. I was born HIV-positive." Clutching a microphone that seemed almost as big as he was (Plate 2.1), Nkosi went on to explain that he had been abandoned by his mother because she feared her neighbors' prejudice when they learned of her son's health condition.

Nkosi was the only black person among the white, homosexual South African men in a Johannesburg hospice directed by an activist named Gail Johnson. Eventually, the hospice closed because of a lack of funds, and Gail Johnson adopted the adorable child. She was white, and outspoken, and knew how to use the media. When

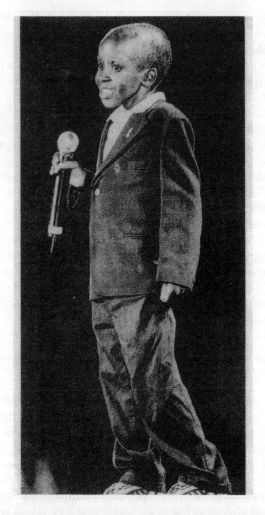

Plate 2.1   Nkosi Johnson, Diminutive AIDS Activist, Addressing the 13th International AIDS Conference in Durban, South Africa, in 2000

Nkosi concluded his address to the Conference: "Care for us and accept us— we are all human beings . . . . We can walk, we can talk, we have needs just like everyone else—don't be afraid of us—we are all the same." When Nkosi died on 1 June 2001, he was 12 years old and weighed just 22 pounds. United Nations Secretary General Kofi Annan said: "We have lost a voice."

Source: United Nations.

she tried to enroll Nkosi at a predominantly white school in the elegant Johannesburg suburb of Melville, he was turned away because of fear that he would infect the other children. The feisty Johnson promptly called in the media for interviews with Nkosi. The ensuing high-profile battle led to his acceptance in the school, Newpark Primary, and to a government policy forbidding schools to discriminate against HIV-positive children. As a result of his extraordinary natural charm, Nkosi soon became one of the most popular children in the school.

In 1999, the charismatic Nkosi raised sufficient funding to found Nkosi's Haven, a Johannesburg shelter for HIV-positive women and their children. Some 200 HIV-positive babies are born every day in South Africa. Nkosi agitated for making AZT available to pregnant HIV-positive mothers, so that their babies would not be born HIV-infected.

While thousands of scientists, health ministers, and AIDS advocates at the Durban Conference were held spellbound, Nkosi attacked the South African government's failure to supply the anti-AIDS drugs to pregnant mothers. Nkosi told the Durban Conference: "I just wish that the government can start giving AZT to pregnant HIV mothers to help stop the virus being passed on to their babies." South African President Thabo Mbeki walked out of the Conference in the middle of Nkosi's speech. His aides said that Mbeki had a busy schedule, and was pressed for time.

Later, Mbeki's wife, Zanele, visited Nkosi at his deathbed. The adorable child said he wanted to meet Mbeki himself, but the president never came. Nkosi died in his sleep on 1 June 2001, a few days before we arrived in South Africa. As former South African President Nelson Mandela remarked, Nkosi Johnson was an icon for the struggle for life itself.

Agenda-Setting for the Issue of AIDS

Why did the tragedy involving cyanide-laced Tylenol in the United States, which claimed seven lives in 1982, get front-page, top-of-the-news coverage, while the issue of AIDS languished in the U.S. media? *The New York Times* ran four front-page articles on the Tylenol tragedy, and printed over 50 articles in a three-month period (Kinsella, 1989). It took four years and 20,000 AIDS deaths before the media, including *The New York Times*, began to give news coverage to the issue of AIDS. How does a new issue like the AIDS epidemic come to public attention, gain followers who believe that it is an important social problem, and climb to prominence on the national agenda? Communication scholars and political scientists have been studying this agenda-setting process for several decades, and the agenda-setting process is well understood today (Dearing & Rogers, 1996).

The Media Agenda

Figure 2.1 shows the usual steps in this process, beginning with an issue getting on the *media agenda*, which consists of the hierarchy

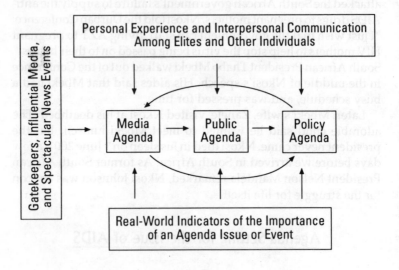

Figure 2.1   Stages in the Agenda-setting Process

The media agenda, indexed by the amount of news coverage given to an issue, influences the public agenda (the degree to which the public thinks the issue is important), which in turn influences the policy agenda.

Source: Dearing & Rogers (1996, p. 5).

of news issues ranked according to the degree of news coverage they receive. What puts an issue on the media agenda? Often this process begins with a tragic event or figure, like Nkosi Johnson in South Africa. Seldom does an issue climb the media agenda due to indicators of the severity of a social problem. A *real-world indicator* is a variable that measures more or less objectively the degree of severity or risk of a social problem. In the early years of the epidemic, the weekly reports by the CDC on the number of HIV infections and the number of AIDS deaths did not put the issue of AIDS on the media agenda in the United States (Rogers et al., 1991). The media reported these data, but the issue of AIDS did not yet have a human face. The mass media prefer to describe an abstract issue like the epidemic in terms of one or a few individuals who are suffering from HIV/AIDS, rather than in aggregate numbers or trends. So the abstract numbers of people living with HIV/AIDS, or dying from AIDS, provided regularly by the CDC, did not attract much media attention.

Research on the agenda-setting process in the United States shows that two factors often put an issue on the national agenda: (*a*) when a news article about the issue appears on the front page of *The New York Times*; and (*b*) when the U.S. president gives a talk about the issue. *The New York Times* is the most respected U.S. news medium. Other media follow its lead in judging the news value of various issues. In the case of AIDS in the 1980s, a news article about the epidemic did not appear on the front page of *The New York Times* until 25 May 1983, two years into the epidemic, 12 months later than *The Los Angeles Times*, and 10 months later than *The Washington Post*. So *The New York Times* lagged behind, rather than led, in providing media attention about the epidemic.

American President Ronald Reagan did not give a speech about AIDS until May 1987, an unbelievable six years into the epidemic, a time when 35,121 AIDS cases had been reported by the CDC. For the first four years of the epidemic, the U.S. media were strangely muted about AIDS. In mid-1985, the average number of news stories about AIDS in the six most important U.S. media (the three national television networks and the three most prestigious newspapers) suddenly increased tenfold, from a previous average of 14 stories per month, to 143 stories per month (about five a day). Finally, the issue of AIDS was on the media agenda! As detailed later, two important tragic figures, actor Rock Hudson and schoolboy Ryan White, helped put it there.

Not only did the world's mass media begin to give much greater news coverage to the epidemic beginning in the mid-1980s, but the issue of AIDS was also framed differently. The idea of "framing" a news story comes from the late sociologist Erving Goffman, who observed that communication media are like a window to the world. The view that is provided may be opaque or clear, large or small, depending upon the nature of the window, including whether it looks out on the street or on a backyard. Gradually, the media put a human face on the epidemic by telling the stories of individuals living with AIDS.

The media draw "the pictures in our heads" (Lippmann, 1922). They tell us not *what* to think, but rather what to think *about* (Cohen, 1963). That is, the mass media give us the relative importance of a set of issues, conveyed to us by the amount of news coverage that each issue receives. So when the media finally began to give considerable attention to the issue of AIDS, it climbed the public agenda, and began to command an emphasis from policy-makers.

Here we see the power of the press in helping members of the public socially construct the meaning of a news issue like the AIDS epidemic. First, of course, journalists themselves must decide how they will frame an issue. Kinsella (1989) shows how a small number of brave newspeople took the lead in framing the AIDS issue as an important social problem in the United States. Initially, the media were squeamish about reporting on AIDS. Reporters could not use terms like "anal intercourse," "swallowing semen," "fisting," or "rimming." Abe Rosenthal, then managing editor of *The New York Times*, insisted that his reporters use the word "homosexual," rather than "gay." When the news media first used general terms like "the exchange of bodily fluids" to describe how the virus was transmitted, the public was confused. Marlene Cimons, a reporter at *The Los Angeles Times*, protested against such editorial practices, saying: "Words don't kill . . . but can save lives" (quoted in Netter, 1992, p. 249). Many of the newspeople who first reported the AIDS epidemic were shunned and criticized by their colleagues, and their careers suffered accordingly. But they persevered in reporting on the epidemic, because they realized the news value of the epidemic, and that human lives were involved.

Randy Shilts: Chronicler of the Castro

One of these several brave journalists was the late Randy Shilts in San Francisco, who was gay himself. Shilts was hired by *The San Francisco Chronicle* in 1981, when its editors decided to recruit a reporter to cover the city's gay community (the *Chronicle* was the first newspaper in the world to do so). In the early years of the epidemic, the five gay newspapers in San Francisco regularly scooped the *Chronicle* and *The San Francisco Examiner* in covering the epidemic. But after Shilts joined the *Chronicle*, he convinced its gatekeepers to publish almost daily articles about HIV/AIDS. Often his stories were about individuals living with AIDS, or he wrote investigative reports about the role of the gay bathhouses in spreading HIV. Shilts also wrote about the STOP AIDS campaign, and about Gaetan Dugas, Patient Zero.

Shilts penned words that others dared not. Once, Shilts took *Chronicle* readers on a tour of a gay bathhouse in the Castro district, describing its raunchy "sling rooms," spaces where men strapped themselves to devices that suspended them in mid-air, while others performed anal sex or engaged in fisting. His columns argued for closing down these bathhouses: "You can't open a candy store to show people how to diet" (quoted in Kinsella, 1989, p. 175). The city health department attempted to close the bathhouses, but this effort was unsuccessful.

The San Francisco Chronicle was the first U.S. newspaper to cover the epidemic in the early 1980s. Unfortunately, the *Chronicle*'s extensive coverage did not put the issue of AIDS on the national media agenda (this was not to happen until late 1985). Randy Shilts wrote an important book, *And the Band Played On* (1987), about the epidemic's initial era. As noted previously, this title is a metaphor drawn from the sinking of the *Titanic*, whose captain ordered the ship's musicians to continue performing as the luxury liner settled deeper in the water, so as to keep the passengers from panicking. Denial characterized many nations in the initial phases of the AIDS epidemic.

> Shilts died of AIDS-related complications in 1994 at age 42. He did more single-handedly to draw attention to the AIDS epidemic in San Francisco than any other news reporter in the United States.

The Public Agenda

After the media agenda is set, an issue like AIDS climbs the *public agenda*, defined as the priority accorded to issues that the public perceives as important. The public's agenda of issues is usually indexed by questions asked in public opinion polls, such as "What is the most important problem facing the nation?" Not until late 1985, soon after AIDS climbed the media agenda, did sizeable numbers of the American public begin to identify AIDS as an important social problem. Eventually, in early 1986, the AIDS issue was rated in national polls as the most important health problem facing the nation.

Each month for the past 50 years, the Gallup polling organization has asked a national sample of the U.S. public, "What is the most important problem facing the nation?" These "most important problem" (MIP) data collected over many years show that four or five issues are on the national agenda at any given time. When a new issue climbs the agenda, it pushes one of the previous issues off the agenda. So the national agenda is a zero-sum game in which all issues compete for attention. An issue typically remains on the national agenda for six months to a year, although the AIDS issue in the United States has stayed on the agenda for a longer period.

The Policy Agenda

Finally, an issue like AIDS climbs the *policy agenda*, the set of issues that public officials consider as they allocate funding, pass laws, and make policies. Despite the resistance of the White House and *The New York Times*, once the media started giving heavy news coverage to the epidemic after the mid-1980s, the public began expressing concern about AIDS, and policy-makers began to increase appropriations sharply for HIV/AIDS prevention, treatment, and research. This third step in the agenda-setting process is really the bottom line, when policies are implemented, budgets are determined, and programs are put into practice. Total spending on AIDS prevention, treatment, and research, after a slow start in the early 1980s, climbed rapidly to almost $10 billion by 2000 (Sepkowitz, 2001).

These actions do not necessarily mean that the original social problem is solved by the new policies and programs. Instead, after some months or years, the issue may simply be pushed off the national agenda, and the social problem is gradually forgotten. Then attention shifts to a new social problem.

We can wonder how different the path of the epidemic in the world might have been had the United States moved quickly to control the AIDS outbreak. The first cases of AIDS were identified in the United States in mid-1981. What if the American government had moved immediately to mount effective prevention programs targeting high-risk groups when only a few hundred individuals were HIV-positive? Perhaps the world could have been spared the catastrophe with which it currently faces. In retrospect, the four years from 1981 to 1985, during which the agenda-setting process was held up by the inaction of the United States government and the inattention of *The New York Times*, have been very costly.

The Role of Tragic Figures

The agenda-setting process begins with the media agenda (see Figure 2.1). So when and how the media agenda was set for the AIDS issue in the United States is an important matter. Two tragic figures played key roles in putting the epidemic on the media agenda. One was Rock Hudson, the masculine, handsome, clean-cut Hollywood actor who was diagnosed with AIDS and who died in October 1985. Although he played heterosexual roles in the movies (often opposite Elizabeth Taylor or Doris Day), he was gay and contracted HIV while visiting San Francisco. Ten weeks before his death in 1985, a pale, hollow-cheeked Hudson collapsed in the lobby of the Hotel Ritz in Paris, spurring the paparazzi to action. Hudson was in Paris for AIDS treatment at the Pasteur Institute. He returned to Los Angeles, and then died in the UCLA Medical Hospital.

At about the same time as Hudson's death, Ryan White, a 13-year-old boy in Kokomo, Indiana, who had become HIV-positive through transfusions of a blood clotting factor, was barred from attending his junior high school by local authorities. Stigmatized by neighbors, White's family lived with hostility for several months, before moving to Arcadia, another town in Indiana. White was a hemophiliac, and had to have regular blood clotting transfusions (at this point, the U.S. blood supply was contaminated by donors who were HIV-positive). In an 18-month period, White was on national network television 40 times, becoming the public face of AIDS in the U.S. News coverage showed him as the paperboy for the *Kokomo Times*, zipping from house to house, and tossing the newspaper on people's front lawns (Kinsella, 1989). Ryan White died in 1990, and became a focal point for public sympathy. Elton John wrote a popular song about White.

Major news attention was given to both Rock Hudson and Ryan White as tragic figures, which raised public awareness-knowledge about HIV/AIDS, and put a human face on the epidemic. Thereafter, U.S. news media like *The New York Times*, *The Los Angeles Times*, *The Washington Post*, and the ABC, NBC, and CBS television networks gave very heavy attention to AIDS (Rogers et al., 1991). Their coverage increased tenfold within a month. So Hudson's death and White's expulsion from his school represented a turning point in the agenda-setting process for the AIDS issue in the United States. These tragic events helped the media begin to frame the issue as a human problem. The public began to think that HIV/AIDS was something that could happen to them.

As mentioned previously, real-world indicators like rates of HIV infection and the number of AIDS deaths did *not* play an important role in setting the media agenda in the United States. Tragic figures like Nkosi Johnson, in contrast, are newsworthy in that they appeal to media audiences by converting an abstract issue into very human terms. Thereafter, news coverage of the epidemic helped boost newspaper circulation and television audience ratings. And the public began to realize, "Hey, this is a problem that affects all of us!" Also, especially in the initial stages of the epidemic, homophobia on the part of newspeople and the public kept HIV/AIDS from getting the news attention that it deserved.

Real-world indicators in some countries and under some circumstances played a crucial role in putting the AIDS issue on the national agenda. Later in this chapter we shall describe how the percentage of commercial sex workers who were found to be HIV+ served as a wake-up call, leading to the launching of national AIDS control programs in Thailand and in Cambodia. The epidemic in Thailand was becoming very serious but government action was not forthcoming until 1989, when a survey in Chiang Mai showed that 44 percent of the CSWs in that city were HIV-positive, and that HIV infection was spreading into the general population. No longer could the epidemic be perceived as a foreigners' disease. Forces were set in motion that eventually led to a national program, energized by Mechai Viravaidya in 1991–92.

In Cambodia in 1995, a similar survey found that 38 percent of commercial sex workers were HIV-positive. Health officials arranged for national leaders to talk with several people living with AIDS, who were hospitalized in a government hospital in Phnom Penh. In these two cases, it was the combination of real-world indicators with an influential, daring activist (Mechai in Thailand) or an emotional confrontation (in Cambodia) that served as a trigger event in the agenda-setting process.

In 2000, Ashok Pillai, an attractive young man, became the "poster boy" for people living with AIDS in India. When we met Pillai in Chennai in December 2001 (four months before he passed away), he told us he had been discharged by the Indian Navy when he tested HIV-positive during a routine exam. In 1997, Pillai, with 11 other HIV+ people, took the lead in forming INP+, the Indian Network for People Living with HIV/AIDS, an NGO. Pillai tried to convince a movie star or some other celebrity to disclose publicly their HIV status, but all refused out of fear that the stigma attached to HIV/AIDS in India would harm their careers. Finally, Pillai reluctantly agreed to put his own photograph on the poster, above the statement: "I am 31. I have a successful career. I enjoy music. I like to work out at the gym. I miss my flights sometimes. I am also HIV Positive for the last 11 years." The image conveyed by the poster is of a modern young individual, a member of the rapidly growing upper middle class in India (Singhal & Rogers, 2001a). In other words, the preppie young individual with HIV could be you. Pillai's poster may have helped change the meaning of HIV/AIDS in India by giving the epidemic a human face, and thus boosted the issue, at least to some degree, up the agenda.

The Role of Champions

A *champion* is a charismatic individual who puts his/her weight behind an issue, thus helping it to gain acceptance. Different types of champions played their role as the issue of AIDS climbed the agenda in various countries.

Some champions for the issue of AIDS were national politicians like Presidents Jose Sarney, Fernando Henrique Cardoso, and Itamar Franco in Brazil, and Minister Mechai Viravaidya in Thailand. Certain other champions, like Judge Edwin Cameron and Zachie Achmat in South Africa, and Betinho and Jorge Biloqi in Brazil, have been citizen activists. President Mbeki of South Africa is a champion opposing certain interventions to control the AIDS epidemic. Some champions are technocratic experts, like Dr. Abraham Verghese, formerly of Johnson City, Tennessee (and now at Texas Tech Health Sciences Center, in El Paso, Texas); the late Dr. Jonathan Mann, formerly director of the Global Program on AIDS in the World Health Organization; and Dr. Garth Japhet and Shereen Usdin, co-founders of Soul City, the highly effective entertainment-education intervention in South Africa. Children with AIDS have played an agenda-setting role: Ryan White in the United States, Nkosi Johnson in South Africa, and Sheila Cortopassi de Oliveira in Brazil, a 4-year-old who was banned from attending school in São Paulo because she was HIV-positive. Finally, some AIDS champions are celebrities like movie stars (for example, Elizabeth Taylor) or sports heroes (for example, Magic Johnson) who use their fame to draw public attention to preventing the epidemic. Here we profile six key champions for HIV and AIDS.

Magic Johnson: Basketball superstar Earvin "Magic" Johnson originally represented a role model for irresponsible sexual behavior in the era of AIDS. At the time of his public disclosure that he was HIV-positive and was retiring immediately from the Los Angeles Lakers basketball team, Johnson acknowledged that he had slept with hundreds of women while on NBA road trips. His disclosure that he was seropositive on 7 November 1991 stunned the world. Johnson was the first African American celebrity to disclose his HIV-positive status. At the time, he was one of the most famous athletes in the world. *The New York Times* devoted 300 column inches of news space to the Magic Johnson story from 8 to 10 November 1991. Within a few days, almost every American knew about Magic Johnson's HIV status, as did many people around the world. A hand-lettered sign in the window of a Baptist church in a Baltimore ghetto said: "We love you, Magic."

Eight years earlier, the U.S. government had established the National AIDS Hotline, which provided a toll-free telephone system to answer callers' questions about HIV/AIDS. Immediately after the Magic Johnson announcement, the National AIDS Hotline was deluged with telephone calls. Some 118,124 call-attempts were made on 8 November 1991, 19 times the number of calls received on a usual day. During the 60 days immediately following Johnson's disclosure, 1.7 million calls were attempted, four times the usual rate. Many of these inquiries were about where to obtain an HIV blood test. An analysis of individuals who sought such tests in Orange County, California, showed they were young males and many were African Americans. Their personal and social characteristics were much like Magic Johnson's (Gellert et al., 1992).

Figure 2.2 shows how the National AIDS Hotline was completely inundated by the large volume of calls following Magic Johnson's announcement, with the Hotline only able to answer a fraction of the calls. Here we see how a celebrity, through disclosure of his personal life-experiences, can influence the agenda-setting process. Magic Johnson became a dedicated champion for the AIDS issue, serving as a public spokesperson for the issue, appearing on late-night talk shows, and distributing a video about HIV/AIDS prevention that he narrated.[1] Did this celebrity announcement have any effect on increasing knowledge and raising concern about HIV/AIDS?

A study by communication scholars William Brown and Michael Basil (1995) found that individuals who were emotionally connected with Magic Johnson, such as those who thought of him as a friend or as a personal role model, were led by his announcement (*a*) to an increased personal concern about AIDS, and (*b*) to an intention to reduce their own high-risk sexual behaviors. *Parasocial interaction* is the tendency of individuals to perceive themselves as having a personal relationship with a media or public personality (Sood & Rogers, 2000). Had Magic not been so popular and so well liked, the public's involvement with him would have been much less, and his potential for inducing such behaviors as information-seeking and reducing risk would not have been so great.

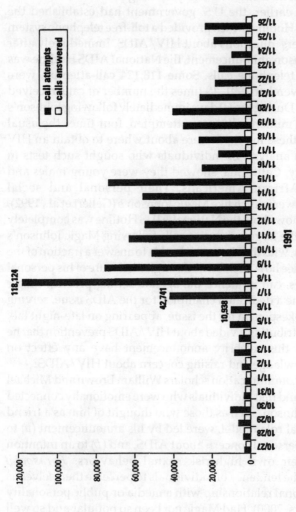

Figure 2.2 The Effects of Magic Johnson's Disclosure of his Seropositivity on 7 November 1991 on the Number of Call-attempts to the National AIDS Hotline in the United States

The Hotline was completely swamped by the huge increase in telephone calls following Magic's surprise announcement.

Source: CDC National AIDS Hotline.

Because of their position in the public eye, celebrities have the power to promote preventive health behavior. But relatively few have done so. Of the famous Americans who have died from AIDS, like Liberace, Arthur Ashe, Perry Ellis, and many others, only Magic Johnson has been an outspoken champion for the issue of AIDS. He helped Americans understand the difference between HIV and AIDS, and that the virus could be transmitted hetero-sexually. Magic disclosed intimate details about his personal sexual behavior to emphasize these crucial points.

Philly Lutaaya: In Africa, the first celebrity to disclose that he had AIDS was the Ugandan singer, Philly Bongoley Lutaaya. A political exile, Lutaaya returned to Uganda in 1988 as a national hero, with sold-out public concerts. His song, "Born in Africa," became the unofficial "national anthem" in Uganda, and topped the charts in several African nations. In 1989, Lutaaya shocked his fans by announcing that he was dying of AIDS, contracted through heterosexual sex. Lutaaya's candid admission helped the media spotlight the AIDS issue, hitherto taboo in Uganda (UNAIDS, 1998a). In the last few months of his life, his body ravaged by opportunistic infections, Lutaaya traveled across Uganda crusading for HIV prevention. His fans witnessed Lutaaya's body succumbing to AIDS on a daily basis, as he was featured prominently on national television and in other news media.

Akin to the role played by Rock Hudson and Magic Johnson in the United States, Lutaaya's disclosure helped put the issue of AIDS on the media, public, and policy agendas in Uganda. Guided by the political leadership of President Yoweri Museveni, swift political action followed, making Uganda one of the first countries in Africa to effectively stem the tide of AIDS.

Cazusa: During our visit to Brazil in March 2001, we heard a great deal about the role of Brazilian singer Cazusa in stimulating mass media coverage of AIDS. Cazusa disclosed that he had AIDS in 1989, and died in 1990. Much like Lutaaya, Cazusa, in the last year of his life, campaigned tirelessly in Brazil for AIDS prevention, care, and support, and the public literally saw him "dying on television" (personal interview, Veriano Terto, 15 March 2001). Media coverage of Cazusa's disclosure was highly sensational, given that Cazusa was gay and a drug user. While Cazusa undoubtedly helped stimulate public discourse on HIV because of his celebrity status, some feared that his gay and drug user status may have reinforced prejudice against already stigmatized groups. Cazusa's mother founded Viva Cazusa, a foundation that supports AIDS orphans in Brazil.

Betinho: Herbert de Souza, nicknamed "Betinho," was a sociologist and AIDS activist in Brazil who died in 1997 (Plate 2.2). A hemophiliac who contracted HIV through a blood transfusion, Betinho fought against hunger, promoted citizens' rights, and worked tirelessly to reduce poverty in Brazil. He advocated for a civil society, calling for the return of his country by its military rulers to a popularly elected government. This activism led to his being exiled from Brazil. Eventually, he returned from exile, started an NGO, and led the civil society movement in Brazil.

In 1986, partnering with Dr. Walter Almeida, a medical doctor, Betinho established Associação Brasileira Interdisciplinar de AIDS (ABIA), one of the most influential of some 600 NGOs currently involved in combating the epidemic in Brazil. The ABIA mobilized educational, business, medical, government, and other civil society institutions to create an advocacy-driven social movement for AIDS. Betinho influenced ABIA to give attention to "the criminal situations in the blood service system in Brazil, to the lack of quality information on HIV/AIDS, and to the violation of civil rights of people living with HIV/AIDS" (Parker & Terto, 2001, p. 16). Betinho worked with pastors of several Catholic churches in Brazil, reinforcing the notion of liberation theology. When we met Dr. Veriano Terto, executive director of ABIA, in his Rio de Janeiro office, he noted that ABIA was in the business of "breaking the silence" on AIDS by creating a "vocal, multidisciplinary, and complex response to AIDS" (personal interview, 15 March 2001).

The ABIA currently employs 20 paid staff and hundreds of volunteers. This NGO receives one-third of its annual budget from the Brazilian government's AIDS control program, and the remainder of its funding from the Ford Foundation, the McArthur Foundation, German churches, and from other contributors. Financial stability helps ABIA maintain its independence from the government of Brazil, allowing it to perform a watchdog function.

When we visited the ABIA offices, we found a beehive of activity, with a training course on reporting the epidemic underway for

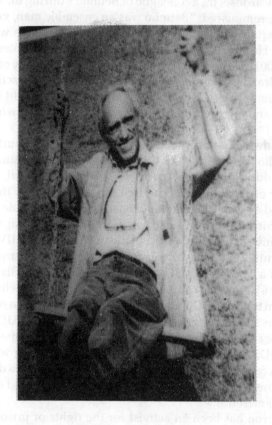

Plate 2.2 The Late AIDS Activist Betinho of Brazil

Herbert de Souza ("Betinho") was infected through the blood supply and became a leading AIDS activist in Brazil until his death in 1997.

Source: Personal files of the authors.

media personnel, sponsorship of an art show about AIDS, and an active program of counseling people living with HIV/AIDS. The main contribution of ABIA, however, is its advocacy work. The ABIA's background publications about the epidemic are particularly influential.

Betinho, and his two well-known brothers, Henfil and Chico Mario, all contracted HIV, and died from AIDS-related complications.

Ranulfo Cardoso, Jr., a colleague of Betinho's during the founding of ABIA, reminisced: "Betinho was an ensemble man, very calm, and tranquil. He was thin and fragile, but he spoke with great passion. He spoke many truths directly" (personal interview, 13 March 2001). During our two-week visit to Brazil, many others told us that Brazil was fortunate to have had Betinho, the activist, and Paulo Freire, the educator, individuals who brought ethics to politics, and engaged the Brazilian citizens in their own welfare.

Judge Edwin Cameron: Edwin Cameron is a gay South African judge who lives with AIDS. Cameron was a tireless human rights activist during the anti-Apartheid struggle (de Waal, 1999). A member of the South Africa High (Supreme) Court, this highly respected 47-year-old public official says that he is a triple minority: gay, white, and HIV-positive. Cameron was diagnosed as seropositive in the mid-1980s, but did not disclose his HIV-positive status until 1998. The trigger for his public disclosure was the death of a 36-year-old HIV-positive woman, Gugu Dlamini (see Chapter 6). A public campaigner for HIV and AIDS who lived in a Durban township, Dlamini made a public declaration of her HIV status on a Zulu language radio station on World AIDS Day, 1 December 1998. Dlamini's intention was to overcome the stigma of HIV/AIDS and to foster acceptance of people living with HIV/AIDS. A few days later, she was stoned and stabbed to death by a gang of neighborhood boys. Her death had a profound impact on Judge Cameron.

Cameron has been an activist for the rights of prisoners who were stigmatized because they were HIV-positive or had AIDS, and for a patient's right to confidentiality about his/her HIV/AIDS status. Cameron also sought to protect gays against discrimination. Earlier, before he became a judge, he had been a civil rights activist defending anti-Apartheid leaders and African National Congress (ANC) guerillas (the ANC, led by Nelson Mandela, played the key role in demanding public elections and in ending Apartheid in South Africa).

Cameron was born in poverty in Pretoria, but soon demonstrated great intellectual promise. A Rhodes scholar at Oxford University, he married, and then came out of the closet in the early 1980s. Cameron is open about his own homosexuality, uses gay slang, and has co-edited a book about the gay experience in South Africa.

In the mid-1990s, Cameron nearly died, but his life was prolonged by the triple cocktail of AIDS drugs. He is very aware of his advantage over most South Africans in being able to afford these expensive drugs. Only an estimated 10,000 of the 4.7 million South Africans who are HIV-positive can afford the high cost of the anti-retroviral drugs. He is outspokenly critical of the international drug companies and of South African president Thabo Mbeki for his do-nothing policy regarding the anti-retrovirals, which Cameron calls a policy of "AIDS Apartheid." South Africa is now divided into the few (mainly white and wealthy) who can afford the AIDS drugs, versus the many who will die for lack of the anti-retrovirals. Forty percent of all adult deaths in South Africa in 2000 were caused by AIDS-related illnesses. Over the next decade, AIDS will kill from five to seven million South Africans. Yet, in 2000, $6.2 million of South Africa's $17 million AIDS control budget went unspent!

In his keynote speech at the 2000 International AIDS Conference in Durban, Judge Cameron berated President Mbeki for having created "disbelief," "confusion," and "consternation" through his bizarre beliefs about the causes of AIDS.

President Thabo Mbeki: Opponent: In contrast to the advocates and champions who are combating the epidemic, a countervailing set of opponents exists in many nations. One of the most noted negative champions is President Thabo Mbeki of South Africa (Plate 2.3). He leads a nation of 43 million people, of whom 4.7 million are HIV-positive. Mbeki challenges these infection rates, even though they are compiled by his own government's ministry of health. In October 2001, Mbeki charged whites and their unwitting black allies with deliberately overplaying the AIDS epidemic in order to perpetuate stereotypes of Africans as "promiscuous carriers of germs" (Swarms, 2001). Finally, after setting off several public firestorms of controversy, Mbeki decided to stop discussing AIDS publicly. That decision, of course, did not make the controversy go away.

Mbeki is most noted for his opposition to providing anti-retroviral drugs to HIV-positive individuals in South Africa. He questions whether HIV actually causes AIDS, a point on which there is overwhelming evidence. However, Mbeki supports the bizarre views of Dr. Peter Duesberg, a scientist at the University of California at Berkeley who claims that sufficient evidence has not been presented.

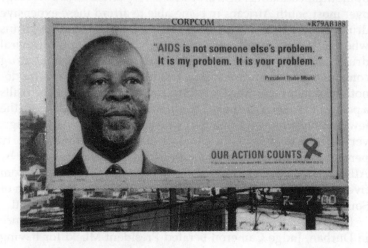

Plate 2.3   President Thabo Mbeki of South Africa on a Billboard near Soweto Township, Johannesburg

Despite the claim stated on this billboard, Mbeki's "confused" stance on the epidemic has impeded South Africa's response to HIV/AIDS.

Source: Personal files of the authors.

Duesberg opposes anti-retroviral therapies and urges HIV+ people not to take AZT.

Further, Mbeki argues that anti-retrovirals are toxic. He especially opposes the provision of Nevirapine, which limits mother-to-child transmission of HIV. Even though the drug costs only a few dollars for each pregnant mother, and despite the December 2001 ruling by South Africa's High Court allowing widespread provision of Nevirapine, Mbeki refuses to comply. He insists on waiting until South Africa's trial of Nevirapine, underway at 18 sites in 2002, is completed, despite the results of similar, completed trials of the drug in Uganda. In March 2002, 22 of South Africa's leading scientists published a letter in *Lancet*, the British medical journal, complaining that Mbeki's government was disregarding research-based evidence on Nevirapine.

Many had hoped that President Mbeki, in his opening address to the International AIDS Conference in Durban, South Africa, in July 2000, might state that HIV did cause AIDS, but he did not. Former president Nelson Mandela, in his closing address at the Durban Conference, said:

> It is never my custom to use words lightly. If 27 years in prison have done anything to us, it was to use the silence of solitude to make us understand how precious words are and how real speech is in its impact upon the way people live or die. (Bartholemew, 2002a)

Each time that Mandela said "HIV/AIDS" in his speech, obviously linking the two, he received deafening applause from the audience. Mandela concluded: "A constant theme in all our messages has been that in this interdependent and globalized world, we have again become the keepers of our brother and sister. That cannot be more graphically the case than in the common fight against HIV/AIDS." The applause was prolonged.

Thailand: Success!

An effective model of AIDS control is provided by Thailand. This nation's efforts to combat the epidemic present something of a contrast to those of South Africa. The 1996 Vancouver Conference was an upbeat affair, not only because of the public announcement about the triple cocktail of anti-retrovirals, but also because on this occasion, Thailand and Uganda were identified as the two nations (of some 200 countries in the world, of which about half had serious AIDS epidemics underway at the time) that had implemented successful AIDS control programs. At the 1998 International AIDS Conference in Geneva, Senegal was added to this list of successes, and at the 2000 Durban Conference, a fourth country, Cambodia, was identified as having effectively stabilized its rate of HIV infection. The Durban Conference also celebrated the role of Brazil in providing free anti-retroviral drugs to people living with HIV/AIDS.

All the developing nations classified as having been successful in combating the epidemic have accomplished this via somewhat different routes. Uganda's HIV infection rate peaked in 1992, and has since fallen by half as the result of educational efforts, extensive

HIV testing and counseling, and very active condom promotion. Thailand focused on its sex industry, and Cambodia generally followed its neighbor's lead, also promoting 100 percent condom use by CSWs, although in a modified approach. Senegal emphasized sex education, a clean blood supply, and condom promotion. All four nations have had certain factors in common: a focus on prevention, and national governments with a firm resolve to control the epidemic.

Perhaps the most spectacular success occurred in Thailand, particularly because it was the first developing nation to effectively combat the epidemic. A World Bank assessment of AIDS in Thailand concluded:

> There are very few developing countries in the world where public policy has been effective in preventing the spread of HIV/AIDS on a national scale. Thailand—where a massive program to control HIV has reduced visits to commercial sex workers by half, raised condom usage, curtailed STDs dramatically, and achieved substantial reductions in new HIV infections—is an exception. (Ainsworth et al., 2000, p. 1)

How did Thailand accomplish this admirable feat? Fortunately, "the epidemic in Thailand is among the best documented in the world" (Steinfatt, 2002, p. 186).

Minister Mechai

Thailand was the first Asian nation to recognize that it had a major HIV/AIDS problem. Nevertheless, Thailand had a late start in controlling the epidemic. After a seven-year period of denial and do-nothing, the Thai government finally, in a short period of less than two years, launched an all-out AIDS control program in 1991–92, led by a dynamic activist, Mechai Viravaidya. Prime Minister Anand Panyarachun had appointed him to the Tourism, Public Information, and Mass Communication portfolios. These multiple duties included responsibility for the National Zoo, overseeing radio and television broadcasting, and a myriad other tasks. Mechai said he would accept the Cabinet appointment offered to him by the prime minister if he could also lead the National AIDS Prevention and Control Program.

The prime minister readily agreed, and what has been called the "Prague Spring" for HIV/AIDS control in Thailand quickly began. The period was very brief, lasting only from February 1991 to October 1992, a total of 20 months. The Anand government was set up following a military coup d'état and was intentionally interim in nature, appointed only to fill in until the country could be returned to a democratically elected government. As an interim government, the Anand administration was not concerned with its political popularity or with being re-elected.

Condom King

Mechai is the son of medical doctor parents, his mother a Scot and his father a Thai. His mother encouraged Mechai to devote his life to helping poor people, and he has not wavered from this commitment to the underprivileged of society. Educated in Australia, Mechai became known worldwide in the 1970s and 1980s as an audacious family planning advocate (Plate 2.4). In Thailand, Mechai is called the "Condom King" or "Mr. Condom," and a condom is commonly called a *mechai*. He pushed the envelope to desensitize the condom in Thailand, such as by leading condom-blowing contests, by his Cops and Rubbers program (in which police distribute condoms in Bangkok's red-light districts), and his Cabbages & Condoms Restaurant in Bangkok (in which condoms, instead of mints, come with the change when the dinner bill is paid).

Partly as a result of Mechai's activities, Thailand achieved a remarkably successful family planning program, with 78 percent of eligible couples using contraception in 2001. The annual population growth rate dropped from 3.3 percent in the early 1970s to 1.8 percent by 1982, to 1.2 percent in 1994, and to 0.9 by 2001. Compared to other Asian nations like India and Pakistan, such a successful national family planning program is almost miraculous. Mechai learned important lessons about communication strategies for changing sexually related human behavior. These strategies, gained in the national family planning effort, were carried

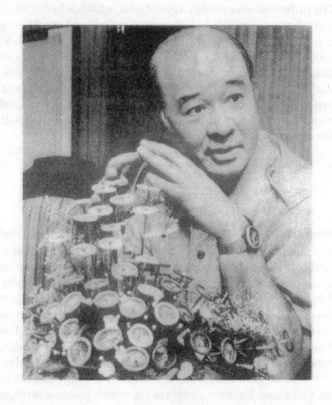

Plate 2.4   Mechai Viravaidya, "Condom King," led Thailand's
AIDS Control Program in 1991–92

Source: United Nations.

over, with appropriate modifications, to HIV/AIDS
prevention.

The Epidemic in Thailand

The first case of AIDS in Thailand was diagnosed in 1984. The
patient was a gay man who had returned to Thailand after the
death of his long-term partner, a Westerner. Then, in 1985, a

20-year-old Thai man who had not lived abroad was diagnosed with AIDS. This individual was employed in a gay bar in Bangkok. He had had multiple sexual partners of both sexes, including both Thais and Europeans (Beyrer, 1998). Surprisingly, the center of the epidemic soon developed, not in Bangkok, the capital and largest city in Thailand, but in Chiang Mai, located in the north of Thailand.[2] Poverty, injection drug use, and a flourishing sex industry provided fertile conditions for the rapid spread of the virus. Initially, the epidemic was perceived as a foreign (*farang*) disease, one that was not a threat in a society with strong family values. This type of denial did not last for long.

The epidemic passed through six waves in Thailand. The first wave consisted of infected male homosexuals, followed over time by injecting drug users, female prostitutes, the male clients of these commercial sex workers, the wives and partners of these males, and finally by the children of these infected females. An estimated 200,000 of Thailand's 63 million people are commercial sex workers, so the third and fourth waves of the epidemic occurred with startling rapidity (Figure 2.3). From 1989 to 1995, at least 600,000 Thai men became HIV-positive, "the fastest spread ever documented" (Beyrer, 1998, p. 28). By 2002, 984,000 Thais had been infected with HIV.

During the 1980s, Mechai became an outspoken advocate for action to control the AIDS epidemic. He criticized the then prime minister Chatichai Choonhaven for being "more interested in golf than in AIDS" (D'Agnes, 2001, p. 332), and deplored government inaction. Mechai became an enthusiastic advocate in the fight against AIDS. In 1989, after returning from a year at Harvard University (where he studied the nature of the HIV/AIDS epidemic and its impacts on economic development), Mechai began to hold "Condom Nights with Mechai" in the Patpong red-light area, a main center for commercial sex work in Bangkok. Attracting a large crowd by using loudspeakers, Mechai invited passersby to blow up a condom and win a T-shirt. Captain Condom, a Harvard MBA student dressed in a Superman costume, toured Patpong bars, encouraging safe sex. Mechai handed out condoms to the girls in nightclubs, telling them to practice safe sex with their customers. A Miss Condom Beauty Contest was held.

Gradually, the issue of AIDS began to climb the Thai national agenda. A tragic figure emerged, Cha-on Suesom, a factory guard

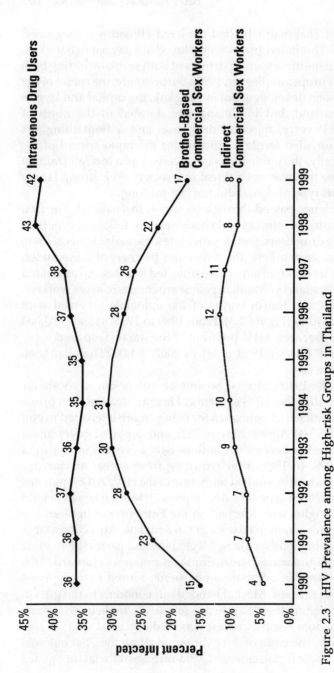

Figure 2.3 HIV Prevalence among High-risk Groups in Thailand

"Indirect commercial sex workers" are employed in bars, go-go clubs, massage parlors, hotels, and restaurants, and often do not self-identify as commercial sex workers, although they engage in sex work for pay.

Source: Ainsworth et al. (2000, p. 6).

infected through a blood transfusion. Suesom began to talk to news reporters, appeared on television talk shows, and discussed his experiences with AIDS and the stigma surrounding the disease at public occasions. The Thai public avidly followed television reports of Suesom's rapid decline in health. His death helped put the issue on the agenda, as did awareness of the surprisingly high incidence of HIV infection (44 percent) among CSWs in Chiang Mai in 1989.

Total Mobilization

In December 1990, Mechai was invited to brief the Thai Cabinet of Prime Minister Chatichai Choonhaven on Thailand's AIDS epidemic. He called for total mobilization: "If AIDS prevention and control is to work, it must be multisectoral. It is not a medical problem. It is a behavioral problem and any institution that can affect behavioral change must be involved" (D'Agnes, 2001, p. 336). Mechai demanded that the prime minister become chairman of the National AIDS Committee. But nothing was done to provide top leadership to halt the epidemic. Political will was lacking. The epidemic continued to spread.

Finally, when he was appointed as a Cabinet minister in the Anand government in 1991, Mechai had the opportunity he had been eagerly waiting for. Mechai's first step was to encourage Prime Minister Anand to serve as chair of the National AIDS Committee, with the minister of public health as the committee's deputy chairman. This structure ensured that all government ministries would participate in the campaign against the epidemic. At the time, Uganda was the only other country in the world in which the head of government chaired the national AIDS committee (and Uganda was the other country in the world, along with Thailand, to achieve a successful AIDS control program, by 1996). High-level leadership provides a strong statement about the degree of political will assigned to the AIDS epidemic.

Mechai increased the AIDS budget in Thailand from U.S.$2.5 million in 1991, to $48 million in 1992 (funding increased further to $100 million in 1997). The major part of the AIDS budget (96 percent) came from the Thai government, rather than from international donors. A substantial share of the budget went to prevention, in the realization that AIDS was a behavioral problem without a medical solution. Minister Mechai ordered the 488 radio stations and the 15 television stations in Thailand to provide free air time to broadcast 30-second AIDS spots, one every hour. Ogilvy-Mather created the prevention spots and other messages pro bono. One television spot asked viewers, "Do you want to go to your kid's college graduation, or to his/her funeral?" The broadcasting stations were also allowed to sell an additional 30 seconds of air time for commercial advertising each hour, to repay them for donating their HIV prevention activities. This massive AIDS communication activity amounted to 73 hours of radio time and two hours of television time *per day*! The public was literally deluged with information, as the issue of AIDS rose rapidly on the media and public agendas.[3]

Government employees in all ministries were given HIV/AIDS training. Teachers incorporated AIDS education into the curriculum for primary and high school students. Even first graders were exposed to AIDS education (Phoolcharoen, 1998). A version of a popular game, Snakes and Ladders, was created to teach about the epidemic. Under Mechai's dynamic leadership, every effort was given to AIDS prevention. It was an all-out communication campaign intended to blunt the force of the epidemic.

Also during this period, repressive policies were repealed. For example, the mandatory reporting of the names and addresses of AIDS patients was abolished. A draft bill enabling the police to incarcerate a PWA was repealed under Mechai's leadership. So the rights of people living with AIDS were given attention. Anti-AIDS stigma was attacked and greatly diminished in Thailand. Some critics feared that the AIDS control program would scare away international tourists. Instead, the number of tourists increased from 2.5 million to 10 million under Mechai's watch.

The 100 Percent Condom Program

One key element in the successful anti-AIDS campaign in Thailand was the 100 Percent Condom Program, led by the Ministry of Public Health. As 83 percent of all HIV infections in Thailand resulted from sexual contact, it was really a no-brainer to focus special efforts on commercial sex workers. The typical CSW at this time had a risk factor for HIV that was 1,000 times that of the average

Thai citizen (personal interview, Dr. Wiwat Rojanapithayakorn, former director, AIDS Control Program, Ministry of Public Health, Bangkok, 2 August 2001).

In 1989, a pilot project was launched in Ratchaburi Province in the west of Thailand. All sex work establishments were required by health inspectors to insist that their sex workers demand that their customers use condoms. The logic was that if all sex establishments adopted the 100 Percent Condom Program, none of them would lose business volume due to customers who objected to using condoms. The Ministry of Public Health provided free condoms to sex establishments. By mid-1992, when the 100 Percent Condom Program was expanded to all provinces, 60 million condoms were being provided to 6,000 sex establishments by the ministry per year.

By 1992, condom use in brothels had climbed to 90 percent. Figure 2.4 shows that as condom use increased, the rate of increase of sexually transmitted diseases (STDs) among males dropped. The results of the 100 Percent Condom Program were spectacular, although some of the drop in infection rates might have been due to the effects of contemporaneous factors. For instance, in some

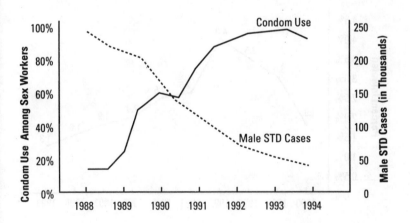

Figure 2.4   Rising Condom use and Declining STDs in Thailand, 1988–94

Source: Ainsworth et al. (2000, p. 11).

countries, the number of people living with HIV/AIDS decreased because some of these people died.

HIV transmission occurred in Thailand mostly via heterosexual sex, much of it between commercial sex workers and their customers. Thus it made sense to target sex workers (Celentano et al., 2000) in the 100 Percent Condom Program. Ministry of Public Health personnel found it rather difficult to force sex establishments to follow the 100 percent condom policy. But accompanied by the provision of free condoms, and with public awareness of the AIDS epidemic at a high level (partly as a result of Mechai's efforts with radio and television broadcasters), condom use by commercial sex workers increased rapidly.

This massive public campaign yielded strong results. Infection rates among conscripts in the Royal Thai Army dropped from 4 percent in 1993 to half that in four years (Figure 2.5). From 1991 to 1993, a tenfold reduction in STD incidence occurred among Army recruits, along with a drop in the number of visits they paid to sex workers. Condom use in brothels rose to more than 90 percent, and STD rates dropped by 90 percent (Ainsworth et al., 2000). Despite

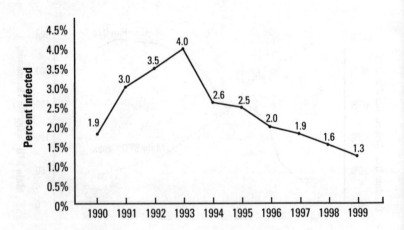

Figure 2.5 Decline in HIV Prevalence among Thai Military Conscripts

Source: Ainsworth et al. (2000, p. 6).

these impressive accomplishments, critics of STD testing and the 100 Percent Condom Program pointed out that one of its consequences may have been to drive some prostitution out of brothels into "informal" sites like bars, restaurants, and go-go clubs. During STD check-ups, if a commercial sex worker in Bangkok tested positive, she was usually fired by the employer and her name and photograph were posted in nearby bars and brothels. Thus, testing seropositive meant that a CSW had to relocate (Steinfatt, 2002). Further, condom use was not necessarily the best means of HIV prevention, due to problems of adequate supply and the sustained use of condoms by individuals over time.

Sustainability of the Mechai Initiatives

In October 1992, the Anand government turned the nation over to its elected replacement, and Mechai Viravaidya left the Cabinet. He did continue as a national spokesperson for AIDS. Further, the policies and structures that he had introduced remained in place in the years that followed. The prime minister of Thailand still serves as chair of the National AIDS Committee. Thailand's AIDS budget continued to rise, reaching $100 million in 1997, after which the funding level dropped somewhat as a result of the Asian economic crisis. However, without a communication enthusiast in charge, "prevention has been put on the back burner," says Mechai (personal interview, Bangkok, 2 August 2001). Prevention dropped to only 8 percent of the national AIDS budget (of which 6 percent goes toward the cost of supplying condoms). Only 5 cents (U.S.) is spent for prevention per capita. Mechai advocates an ideal formula of 75 percent of the prevention budget for communication and 25 percent for providing condoms.

Overall, the Thai AIDS control program reduced the number of new HIV infections each year from 143,000 in 1991 to 29,000 in 2000, a drop that represents a huge behavior change. Unfortunately, however, about 1.9 percent of the adult population (of 63 million people) was HIV+ in 2001. This rate is higher than in the United States, but much lower than in nations like South Africa, with more than a 22 percent infection rate. The turning point in Thailand's successful campaign occurred in the 1991–92 Mechai era. These years created a programmatic momentum that has carried over through later Thai government administrations.

Despite the successful AIDS control program launched in 1991–92, Thailand has suffered terribly from the epidemic. Nearly one million Thais have been infected, and 290,000 have already died of AIDS. Nevertheless, an estimated 200,000 HIV infections would have occurred from 1993 to 2000 had it not been for the national prevention campaign initiated by Mechai. This impact, while important, would have been much greater, of course, if an effective AIDS control program had been launched five years earlier. Nevertheless, these 200,000 Thais owe their lives to effective communication. And to an effective communicator, Mechai Viravaidya. He was in a position of political power. He had experience in, and an understanding of, behavior change communication strategies, gained previously in the family planning and rural development field. Perhaps most importantly of all, Mechai was able to institutionalize the AIDS control program by building political will and a continuing commitment to combating the epidemic. Mechai's role as a leader and coordinator of Thailand's prevention activities cannot be overemphasized. But Thailand's success entailed much more, including the participation of countless other government officials, key NGOs, and an entire nation that was willing to act.

Cambodia

Historically, the gathering and presenting of data have led to the solution of various public health problems. For example, in 1854, Dr. John Snow, a medical doctor in London, plotted the locations of cholera deaths on a spot-map of the crowded center of the city. Snow observed that the cholera deaths were concentrated around the Broad Street water pump in London. Snow's analysis led him to suspect that the disease was waterborne, and that the well was contaminated. Dr. Snow removed the pump handle, promptly halting the epidemic. His analytical role in the London cholera outbreak, based on plotting the cholera-related deaths, led to the evolution of today's academic specialty of epidemiology.

Coincidentally, also in 1854, Florence Nightingale was serving as a British Army nurse during the Crimean War. She maintained careful records of her hospital patients, with some 10,000 wounded soldiers under her care. Nightingale concluded that grossly inadequate sanitation was killing more British soldiers than enemy bullets were. When Nightingale's report was published in English newspapers, the public demanded a cleanup of British Army hospitals. The death rate among hospital patients immediately dropped.

In these two famous cases, epidemiological data led to action. In the case of the AIDS epidemic, data alone (the so-called real-world indicators) have seldom led to a response, at least immediately. However, after the first HIV-positive individual was identified in 1991 (a blood donor in the capital city of Phnom Penh), Cambodian health officials gathered data on the growing number of HIV-positive people, and presented their analysis to the minister of health and to the two co-acting prime ministers.[4] Then they took these high officials to meet personally with AIDS patients in a government hospital in Phnom Penh. As a result, the Cambodian response to the epidemic was swift, and political commitment was ensured (WHO, 2001).

In 1993, the prime minister of Cambodia became chair of the national AIDS control program, and King Sihanouk also supported the program. The first of several media campaigns for HIV/AIDS awareness was launched. A survey of female commercial sex workers in 1995 showed that 38 percent were HIV-positive. In 1998, Cambodia borrowed the idea of a 100 Percent Condom Program, aimed at the nation's 20,000 or so CSWs, from neighboring Thailand. However, Cambodia implemented this program with several important modifications. First, starting in 1995, the AIDS control program provided knowledge about the epidemic and about the means of HIV transmission to commercial sex workers, along with training in negotiating condom use with customers. However, condom use did not become widespread because of the abuse of CSWs by brothel owners and by clients. A census to identify sex establishments was conducted. Brothels, bars, karaoke, and other sex-related businesses were mapped. Some 757 brothels were identified, employing 3,872 CSWs. A total of 20,000 commercial sex workers of all types were identified. About 30 percent of the commercial sex workers were migrants from neighboring Vietnam. A nationwide mass media campaign, supplemented by outreach contacts with CSWs, was devoted to making condom use the national norm. As in Bangkok, motorcycle taxi drivers, mainly young unmarried men recently migrated from the countryside, were identified as a high-risk group who frequently visited CSWs.

At this point, in 1998, a pilot project for the 100 Percent Condom Use Program was launched in Sihanoukville, a seaport city in Cambodia. The provincial governor invited brothel owners to a meeting in order to urge them to support the program. A special health clinic was established for CSWs that was designed to be "sex worker friendly." The CSWs perceived the clinic as theirs. Regular monthly check-ups of every CSW were initiated. "Mystery clients" were used to check on each brothel at six-month intervals. Pressure was applied on brothels that did not comply with the 100 Percent Condom Use Program. The first offense resulted in a written warning, the second offense called for closing the brothel for one week, the third offense led to closure of the brothel for one month, and a fourth offense resulted in permanent closure of the brothel. Two brothels in Sihanoukville were permanently closed down, after repeated warnings.

The results of the pilot project were spectacular. Condom use by brothel-based CSWs increased from 53 percent in 1998 to 78 percent in 1999. Syphilis rates dropped from 9 percent of CSWs in 1998 to 1.2 percent in 2000. In 1999, the pilot project was expanded to the other 23 provinces in Cambodia.

By 2001, an estimated 80 percent of CSWs were using condoms with their customers (personal interview, Dr. Hor Bun Leng, deputy director, National Center for HIV/AIDS, Dermatology and STDs, 15 December 2001). The percentage of HIV prevalence among antenatal women in Cambodia dropped from 3.2 in 1997 to 2.2 in 2000, a drop of one-third. At that time, the AIDS control program in Cambodia was declared a success.

India

At least four million Indians were living with HIV in late 2001 when we visited India in the process of writing this book. There was little consensus about this estimate, however, with some observers arguing that the number of HIV-positive people might actually be as high as 10 million. The Indian minister of health and the UNAIDS representative publicly disagreed about the number of people living with HIV/AIDS in India, and this in front of 150 media newspeople at a conference in New Delhi in 2000. While the estimate of four million PWAs works out to less than one half of 1 percent of all Indian adults, the number is surpassed only by South Africa (and it may have already surpassed South Africa's), given India's huge total population of more than one billion people. During recent years, the epidemic in several Indian states moved out from high-risk groups like injecting drug users, commercial sex workers, and truck drivers, into the general population. HIV infection has now been detected in all Indian states. The World Bank warns that by 2005, unless strong action is taken, 20 million Indians will be HIV-infected.

Some states in India, like Maharashtra (the western state in which India's largest city, Mumbai, is located) and Tamil Nadu (the southern Indian state whose metropolitan center is Chennai), are each larger in total population than many good-sized nations in the world. Given the great cultural diversity among India's states, they might well be thought of as separate nations. Both Maharashtra and Tamil Nadu have very high rates of HIV infection, although prevention activities in the latter state have been relatively successful, and the epidemic in Tamil Nadu may be slowing down. In the city of Mumbai, HIV prevalence among CSWs rose from less than 10 percent in the early 1990s to 50 percent in 2000 (Salunke et al., 1998), and to 70 percent in 2001. Some 2 to 3.5 percent of all women presenting themselves at antenatal clinics in Mumbai were HIV+ in late 2001, evidence that the epidemic had moved from high-risk into low-risk groups. Unless prevention programs are greatly strengthened, which seems unlikely at present, India will experience a catastrophe.

India has a relatively high rate of STDs, about 5 percent of all adults (Gaitonde, 2001). An individual with an STD is much more likely to become HIV-infected, and to have a shorter infection period before the onset of AIDS. In 2001, 4,000 Indians were becoming HIV-positive each day (Specter, 2001). In March 2002, the Indian minister of health, C.P. Thakur, announced that 2.3 HIV infections were occurring every minute. The epidemic already costs India over 5 percent of its GNP, in part because AIDS cases are concentrated in the economically vibrant western and southern states (Dube, 2000, p. 116).

The AIDS Epidemic and Economic Development

India, or at least certain states in India, experienced a rapid rate of economic development after 1991 when the nation changed over from state socialism to an economic policy of welcoming foreign investment. Several consequences of this rapid development, such as truck transportation, industrialization, and urbanization, have contributed to the AIDS epidemic. This huge country has a network of national highways and an extensive system of truck transportation. For instance, some 200,000 trucks arrive in Mumbai every evening (trucks are banned from the roads in many Indian cities during the day). There are a mind-boggling 3.5 million truck drivers in India, and they are a key means of HIV transmission. Truck drivers come mainly from Punjab and other northern Indian states, and are absent from their families for lengthy periods. Commercial sex workers are found at every truck stop in India. Often, providing female commercial sex workers is as regular a service offered by the truck stop as providing food, drink, gas, oil, and truck repairs.

Another result of India's rapid economic development in recent years is the inflow of foreign capital and a proliferation of manufacturing plants, many owned by multinational companies. These plants are located not only in India's major metropolitan centers, but also in rural market towns, especially in the economically booming states of Kerala, Karnataka, Andhra Pradesh, Maharashtra, and Tamil Nadu. It is no accident that the latter two states have particularly high HIV infection rates. Wage employment at construction sites and factories serves as a magnet, attracting millions of able-bodied men who migrate from distant villages. These migrant workers leave their wives and families behind, returning home once or twice per year. Commercial sex workers, following the demand for their services from the factory workers, often set up business in temporary tents near the factories. In 2002, an estimated 200 million migrant workers and military servicemen in India represented a prime target for commercial sex work.

Beginnings of the AIDS Epidemic in India

The first AIDS patient in India was diagnosed by Dr. Suniti Solomon, a microbiology professor at the Madras Medical College in Chennai in 1986. At that time the Chennai police were sending their assigned quota of 100 commercial sex workers per month to the city's prison. Solomon collaborated with one of her medical students in taking blood samples from one month's batch of 100 CSWs. Six were HIV-positive! Their blood samples were tested with Enzyme Linked Immunosorbent Assay (ELISA) at the Christian Medical College in Vellore, and rechecked with the Western Blot analysis in the United States. Indeed, all six cases proved to be HIV-positive. Clearly, the epidemic had reached India. Shortly, Dr. Solomon found herself giving a report about the six HIV-positive people to the Indian Parliament in Delhi. She had asked the six commercial sex workers if they had had non-Indian customers, but they reported that they had not. That meant that HIV was already circulating within India.

The epidemic was relatively late in coming to India, compared to many other countries (it was five years since the first AIDS cases had been identified in Los Angeles). The 1986 discovery of HIV/AIDS in Chennai should have served as a wake-up call for immediately launching an effective prevention campaign in India. The subcontinent could have learned valuable lessons from the earlier experiences of other countries in combating the epidemic. Thanks to a World Bank loan of $84 million in 1994 and to plentiful funding from other international agencies, adequate money was available to defeat the epidemic before it could make inroads into the population. But Indian government officials smugly and moralistically proclaimed that AIDS was a foreign disease, and that the epidemic could never spread in a family-centered society like India's. They were decidedly wrong. In 1999, 1,400 Indian citizens were being infected each day (Dube, 2000); by 2002 this figure had jumped to 5,000.

Indian government officials went through a period of denial from 1986 to the mid-1990s. The epidemic remained in a relatively minor place on the national agenda. Many Indian officials felt that the issue of AIDS was being over-hyped. Eventually, however, the Indian government was forced by international pressures, particularly from the World Bank, to face the important social problem represented by AIDS.

Studies in India show that HIV infection spreads by sexual contact in 74 percent of cases, by injection drug use in 7 percent of cases (in the poverty-stricken north-eastern state of Manipur,[5] 86 percent of drug users are HIV-positive), 7 percent are infected by blood transfusions, and 12 percent by other means (including mother-to-child transmission). From 1986 to 1991, however, many HIV prevention activities in India (representing an estimated 60 percent of the funds spent) were devoted to cleaning up the blood supply. Siddharth Dube (2000), author of a popular book, *Sex, lies, and AIDS*, an attempted national wake-up call, argued that this misallocation of AIDS control resources occurred because "everybody" is threatened by transmission via the blood supply. "Everybody" in this case includes middle-class and upper-middle-class Indians, not just the "worthless" lower-class people in high-risk groups, like commercial sex workers, truck drivers, and migrant workers. Despite extensive efforts, the blood supply in India was still unsafe in 2001, as a result of the presence of many clandestine, unregistered blood banks and "professional donors" who contributed one-third of the blood supply.

Initial Government Initiatives

India's top politicians could have thrown their weight behind the nation's AIDS control activities, and helped diminish the stigma of HIV/AIDS. Dube (2000, p. 93) states: "But in India, so far, there has been a saddening lack of top-level political commitment to HIV/ AIDS prevention." All that a prime minister of India or a chief minister (equivalent to a state governor in the United States) needs to do to boost the AIDS issue up the agenda is to give a speech about it. Only a handful of statements were made about the threat posed by the epidemic. In December 1998, Prime Minister Atal Behari Vajpayee declared that HIV and AIDS were India's most serious public health problem. However, Vajpayee's government, preoccupied with maintaining its fragile coalition government in New Delhi, has failed to sustain its anti-AIDS rhetoric, undermining the political action needed to combat the epidemic headlong.

The National AIDS Control Organization (NACO) was established in 1992 within the Ministry of Health. J.V.R. Prasada Rao, a career Indian Administrative Service (IAS, the elite government cadre) employee, was appointed as director of NACO. Thanks to a World Bank loan of $84 million from 1994 through 1999, followed by a second World Bank loan of $107 million for the 1999 to 2004 period, India has had plenty of funding for HIV/AIDS prevention.

The Department for International Development (DFID, which replaced the former British Overseas Development Council), awarded $123 million for HIV/AIDS interventions in low-prevalence states (Rajasthan, Haryana, and Uttar Pradesh) in north India, beginning in 2001. The U.S. Agency for International Development (USAID) provided another $75 million. In all, about $300 million in external funding was available for combating the epidemic in India (Dube, 2000). Money poured in from these international donor agencies because the epidemic's threat in India was so great. While funding is no longer a constraint, the AIDS program in India remains disorganized, of uneven quality, and bogged down by red tape.

One measure of this disorganization is that the Indian government failed to spend the first World Bank loan (some 40 percent remained unspent a year before its term ran out in 1999). Of the funds utilized, heavy expenditures were made in expensive conferences, planning sessions and reports, and, as noted previously, in improving blood screening (Burns, 1996). Mass media campaigns, slow to get underway, were predominantly informational (as opposed to motivational), and geared to creating public awareness of the epidemic and of the means of HIV transmission. The tone of the AIDS media campaigns contributed to fear, stigmatization, and vilification of high-risk groups. For instance, a full-page newspaper advertisement showed a basket full of eggs and asked the question: "Can you recognize which one of these eggs is rotten?" The answer said: "You can't tell who is HIV-positive by just looking at the person." India has a very strong anti-AIDS stigma.

Like many other nations, India defined the epidemic as a medical problem. It is not, and biomedical interventions alone are not effective in combating HIV/AIDS. As a top Indian doctor told the present authors in December 2001, "AIDS is not a medical problem. It is a behavioral science problem."

AIDS Control in Tamil Nadu

Within this rather dismal scene in India are several bright spots, represented by certain highly successful HIV prevention programs. One success occurred in Tamil Nadu, a state in the extreme south of India, with a population of 62 million (note that this huge population is equivalent to the national population of Thailand).

Early on, the state of Tamil Nadu was as unlikely a place as any other in India to become a success in controlling the epidemic. An HIV-positive man had been lynched in Tamil Nadu; several other lynchings occurred in India during the early years of the epidemic (see Chapter 6). The state's health minister asserted publicly that there were no prostitutes in his state (AIDS control officials promptly introduced him to 2,000 CSWs from his hometown). Some female activists in the state proclaimed that all commercial sex workers should be eliminated! In 1990, the state government of Tamil Nadu forcibly tested hundreds of CSWs for HIV, and locked up 800 HIV+ women for several months (Dube, 2000, p. 27). India's draconian approach to the epidemic, represented by its AIDS Prevention Policy of 1989 (which called for the forcible testing of anyone considered at risk of infection), was finally eliminated in 1994 as a requisite for receiving the first World Bank loan. Initially, HIV was as stigmatized in the state of Tamil Nadu as elsewhere in India.

Escaping Government Bureaucracy: The government of India is generally known for its exaggerated and unmanageable bureaucracy. In 1994, an autonomous organization, the Tamil Nadu State AIDS Control Society, was created. It channeled World Bank and USAID funding to some 35 NGO partners who conducted intervention programs aimed at various target populations. The state's AIDS Control Society was kept slim and trim, with only five professional employees and a support staff of a dozen people in 2001 (personal interview, R.C. Gandhi, director, Tamil Nadu State AIDS Control Society, Chennai, 23 December 2001). Coordination of the diverse activities of these NGOs was centered in the AIDS Prevention and Control Project (APAC) of Voluntary Health Services, an NGO in Chennai, with funding from USAID. For example, 8,000 HIV peer educators, who worked for various NGOs, were trained by APAC. They were encouraged to form a labor union. Further, APAC conducted a series of annual behavior surveillance surveys to measure the overall impacts of the AIDS control program in Tamil Nadu.

Emphasis was placed on increasing condom use by commercial sex workers (perhaps borrowing a lesson from Thailand), raising this indicator from 56 percent in 1996 to 91 percent in 2000. Among truck drivers, condom use during paid sex rose from 55 percent in

1996 to 83 percent in 2000 (APAC, 2001a; Ramasundaram et al., 2001). The broader impact of the Tamil Nadu AIDS control program is suggested by changes in the percentage of HIV-positive women visiting antenatal clinics: from 1.63 percent in 1999 to 1.59 percent in 2000, and then down to 1.35 percent in 2001 (personal interview, Dr. Bimal Charles, director, APAC, Chennai, 24 December 2001).

What lessons can be learned from the successful HIV prevention programs in Tamil Nadu? As elsewhere, political commitment was important, especially early in the epidemic, before it was too late and the epidemic had escaped out of the special high-risk groups into the general population. Chief Minister Karunanidhi of Tamil Nadu held hands with two HIV+ children in a human chain for AIDS prevention at the 1996 World AIDS Day celebration, signifying political commitment to dealing with the epidemic, and to reducing its stigma.

Administrative Leadership: Effective leadership of the AIDS Control Society was provided by S. Ramasundaram, a career IAS official. Ramasundaram, who hails from Tamil Nadu, completed graduate work at the University of Southern California in the mid-1980s, and then returned to India to pioneer effective approaches in family planning (by showing that couples were willing to adopt contraceptives if the odious government annual targets for the number of adopters were dropped). The HIV prevention program in Tamil Nadu was two-pronged, with a specialized effort, mainly through one-on-one peer communication, aimed at high-risk groups like CSWs, coupled with an intensive mass media campaign aimed at the general population. Commercial sex workers were persuaded to use condoms with their customers by the specialized communication program, and their customers were urged to use condoms with sex workers by the general media campaign. Public awareness of AIDS jumped from 23 percent in 1994 to 98 percent four years later. The intensity of the media campaign about the epidemic in Tamil Nadu rivaled that of Thailand during the Mechai period of 1991–92. Advertising and public relations firms in India were hired to mount the media campaign in Tamil Nadu.

Ramasundaram's leadership ability, and that of his successors, presented a sharp contrast to the lack of leadership shown by officials in charge of HIV prevention in other Indian states in the mid-1990s. Many were senior medical professionals nearing retirement. Such over-the-hill MDs were generally ineffective in fighting the epidemic. Many of the HIV prevention programs launched in other states failed to spend their annual budgets, which Ramasundaram and his staff consequently obtained to spend in Tamil Nadu. Even then, only a part of the $84 million World Bank loan to India for AIDS control from 1994 to 1999 could be spent. In the late 1990s, after the success of the AIDS control program in Tamil Nadu had become evident, Ramasundaram was assigned to spreading the lessons learned to other state AIDS control societies. The World Bank forced these states to form non-governmental, autonomous organizations based on the Tamil Nadu model.

A final lesson learned in Tamil Nadu was the crucial importance of gathering data about program effectiveness, and bringing such data to bear on making program decisions (as discussed in Chapter 8). Behavior surveillance surveys (BSS) were conducted annually by the A.C. Nielsen Company from 1996 onwards. The BSS included 13,000 personal interviews with such population groups as commercial sex workers, truckers and their helpers, male and female factory workers, and male patients with sexually transmitted diseases (APAC, 2001b). These data showed that the public's knowledge of AIDS had increased to 98 percent, and that condom use had increased among CSWs, truck drivers, and factory workers.

Activating Agencies

It is one thing for champions and activists to put the issue of AIDS on the national agenda, but it was much more difficult to activate international agencies to join the battle against the epidemic. Initially, most international agencies resisted becoming involved. Today, no agency can afford not to be involved.

The World Health Organization (WHO) did not establish its Global Program on AIDS until 1987, six years into the epidemic. It was only in 1996 that UNAIDS, a joint program of eight United Nations agencies, was formed, more than 15 years after the first AIDS cases were diagnosed. The United Nations General Assembly held its first discussions of AIDS in June 2001. The slow international response undermined the basic strategy of attacking an epidemic as soon as possible by throwing all available resources into the battle, before the epidemic spread further into the general population. While politicians continued to talk, the epidemic broke out of the initial high-risk groups and spread into the general populations of nations.

The epidemic has changed health organizations themselves, often in very profound ways. One example is the CDC, the U.S. government agency responsible for the worldwide control of epidemics. Not only does the CDC fight the epidemic in the United States, but around the world, working on the logic that an epidemic anywhere will eventually affect the United States. The CDC is a glamorous service because of its cadre of epidemic detectives, and it is highly respected around the world.

Before 1981, CDC employed mainly medical doctors with public health training in epidemiology. The ranks of the CDC included almost no social scientists or communication experts. Today, that situation is completely changed, due to the AIDS epidemic. Anthropologists, social psychologists, and communication scholars design and evaluate global programs to prevent epidemics. Importantly, the CDC has shifted from mainly a biomedical approach to fighting epidemics to an approach that also features the behavioral sciences in efforts to change human behavior.

In the years after the end of World War II, when many nations in Latin America, Africa, and Asia were gaining their independence, development was perceived as mainly the job of government ministries. Since the 1950s, however, non-governmental organizations have risen to carry out many development programs, in many cases with funding provided by national governments or by international agencies. The AIDS epidemic of the past two decades has resulted in a tremendous proliferation of NGOs. In many nations, NGOs carry out *most* of the prevention, counseling, treatment, and care programs, with a government AIDS control agency funding and coordinating these efforts. Non-governmental organizations are more flexible, and their employees are often more highly motivated because many are volunteers. The NGO worker may have a close family member who is HIV+ or who has died from the epidemic. In many cases, individual staff members of an NGO are HIV-positive.

AIDS advocacy and fund-raising are not just the responsibility of international agencies and government departments. Private citizens, citizen groups, and celebrities can play a role. South Africa's leading satirist and cabaretier, Pieter-Dirk Uys, who became internationally famous by highlighting the absurdities of the Apartheid system, uses his wit to highlight the South African AIDS crisis. "The battlefield has moved from politics to sex," and unless urgent, concerted action is taken, Uys notes, "AIDS will succeed where Apartheid failed" (quoted in Bergman, 2002, p. 41). Uys's 2002 show, *Foreign AIDS*, played to packed houses in the United Kingdom and the Netherlands, raising over $50,000 (U.S.) for Wola Nani (Let's Embrace in the Xhosa language), a Cape Town-based NGO that supports PWAs and AIDS orphans.

Kofi Annan: Crusader for AIDS

While the political leadership in most developing countries is denying the problem of HIV/AIDS, or at best is apathetic to it, the world is fortunate to have an international leader who has helped put AIDS on the global agenda: Nobel Laureate Kofi Annan, secretary general of the United Nations. Born in Ghana, Annan is one of the most respected Africans globally, perhaps second only to Nelson Mandela.

Annan made the fight against HIV/AIDS his personal priority, mobilizing world leaders to join hands to address the global pandemic. Under Annan's leadership, the UN Security Council prioritized HIV/AIDS as a global security issue, and in June 2001, Annan called a special UN General Assembly session on HIV/AIDS, the first such session ever devoted solely to a health issue. The UN special session brought delegates from 180 countries, 350 NGOs, and 24 heads of state to New York, culminating in a global Declaration of Commitment to HIV/AIDS. Annan called on the world community to raise $7–10 billion (U.S.) each year for 10 years toward a Global Fund for HIV/AIDS. Annan also created the Joint UN Program on HIV/AIDS (UNAIDS), a partnership among eight UN agencies, to integrate intervention efforts under a unified budget and work plan (Piot, 2001).

Annan's colleague, Dr. Peter Piot, a Belgian medical doctor who heads UNAIDS, also deserves credit for global advocacy on HIV/AIDS (Gupte, 2001). Piot impressed upon world leaders the difference that political will, backed with adequate resources, could make in combating HIV/AIDS. Under the leadership of Annan and Piot, the UN system is now speaking about AIDS openly, and with one voice.

Conclusions

In this chapter, we analyzed the agenda-setting process for the AIDS issue in South Africa, Thailand, Cambodia, and India. We touched on this policy process in Brazil, which is a unique case involving the provision of free anti-retrovirals to people living with HIV/AIDS (see Chapter 3). We described the process through which the issue of AIDS is pushed up the national agenda by visionaries, champions, and activists. This advocacy process involves communication at every step, as people favoring action influence their governments to act.

First, the issue of HIV/AIDS has to get on the national agenda. A tragic figure or event can serve as a trigger to set the media agenda. Seldom do real-world indicators alone play this role. Once the media begin giving heavy news coverage to an issue, it soon begins to climb the public agenda, measured by opinion polls in which members of the public are asked to identify the most important problems facing their nation. Once the public supports an issue, policy-makers begin to give increasing attention to the issue. In the case of the AIDS epidemic, the policy agenda leads to the establishment of a national AIDS control program, and, perhaps, to a national commitment to fighting the spread of HIV infection. The strength of the policy agenda is determined by the degree to which a nation displays political will to control AIDS.

Throughout the present chapter, we have seen evidence of the importance of political will in a nation in mounting an appropriate and timely response to the epidemic. Table 2.1 shows the degree of political commitment of our five main nations of study, measured by four indicators.

Table 2.1

Degree of Political Commitment to AIDS
Control for Five Countries

	Top National Leader Chairs AIDS Control Program?	Top National Leader Supports AIDS Control?	Funding for AIDS Control Program from Domestic Sources?	Free Anti-retroviral Drugs?	Successful National AIDS Control Program?
1. South Africa	No	No	Yes	No	No
2. Kenya	No	Yes, after earlier denial	No	No	No
3. Brazil	No	Yes	No	Yes	Yes
4. Thailand	Yes	Yes	Yes	No	Yes
5. India	No	Yes, belatedly	No	No	No

Notes

1. This color videotape, *"Time Out: The Truth about HIV, AIDS, and You,"* produced by Paramount Studios, features Magic Johnson, Arsenio Hall, and other celebrities.
2. HIV-1 subtype B (generally common in the Americas, Europe, and Japan) was most widely found in Bangkok in the early years of the epidemic, while HIV-1 subtype E was most common among the commercial sex workers in Chiang Mai. Subtype E eventually became dominant in Thailand.
3. In retrospect, such an information overload may have had some negative consequences. Further, some of the prevention ads used fear appeals, which can backfire unless the ad also tells how to take action, such as by providing a telephone hotline number to call, or the locations for obtaining an AIDS blood test.
4. Cambodia had twin prime ministers, as a means of achieving political stability after 20 years of disastrous warfare, until a coup in mid-1987.
5. HIV was first detected in Manipur in 1989; within six months, 50 percent of all drug injectors were infected. Soon, 40 percent of the wives of injecting drug users were HIV-positive. Finally, in 2001, a needle exchange program was initiated in Manipur. It was 12 years too late.

3

AIDS Drugs

■

*My idea of a better-ordered world is one in which
medical discoveries would be free of patents and there
would be no profiteering from life or death.*

The late Prime Minister Indira Gandhi of
India, in a statement to the WHO, 1981.

Proper nutrition is the best frontline drug for AIDS.

Dr. Prisca Nemapare, a nutrition expert and
director of the Zienzele Foundation in Harare,
Zimbabwe, in a statement at an HIV/AIDS
conference in Athens, Ohio, April 2002.

When 32-year-old Earvin "Magic" Johnson of the Los Angeles
Lakers announced that he was HIV-positive at a press conference
in Los Angeles on 7 November 1991, he was one of most famous
professional athletes in the world. His unexpected retirement from
basketball was a major news event (we presented data about the
effects of his announcement on the number of telephone calls to the
National AIDS Hotline in Chapter 2). On 7 November 1991, when
his blood test came back seropositive, Magic did not know the
difference between HIV and AIDS. He soon did, however, and he
helped educate the American public about this crucial distinction.
Magic Johnson became a spokesperson for condom use and other

safer sex practices. He disclosed that when he "traveled around the NBA [National Basketball Association] cities, [he] was never at a loss for female companionship." Johnson told *Sports Illustrated*, "I did my best to accommodate as many women as I could." Most of the U.S. public thought at the time that the epidemic spread among homosexuals, so Magic's disclosure of his heterosexual promiscuity publicized another means of transmission.

Although he was in robust health in 1991, it was expected that Magic's physical abilities would soon decline, and that his wife Cookie and his child should prepare for his eventual death. But thanks to his taking AZT and other anti-retroviral drugs, Magic Johnson reduced his viral load to the point at which it was not detectable. He played on the U.S. Olympic championship team. Magic remains a picture of beaming good health today, a decade after his announcement, appearing plumper (at 260 pounds, and wearing a size XXXL shirt) than in his playing days. To a multimillionaire like Magic Johnson, the annual cost of the triple cocktail is no problem. Unfortunately, most people living with HIV in developing countries do not have the resources of a Magic Johnson, who owns a nationwide chain of restaurants and movie theaters in the United States.

In the very early years of the AIDS epidemic, diagnosis of an individual with HIV was a certain death sentence. The only question was how soon an HIV-positive individual would develop AIDS, and die from an opportunistic infection. These opportunistic infections could be treated, of course, but an individual with AIDS would soon be sick with another opportunistic infection, and then another. An individual with AIDS lived in pain, dying a slow and painful death. Anti-retroviral drugs have dramatically enhanced the quality of life of AIDS patients.

What are Anti-retrovirals?

In 1986, AZT (also known as Azidothymidine, Zidovudine, or Retrovir), a drug that delayed the degenerative effects of the virus, was developed. The Food and Drug Administration (FDA) approved AZT as the first anti-retroviral therapy for HIV in March 1987. A clinical trial of AZT versus a placebo in patients with advanced HIV was terminated early, based on evidence of the experimental drug's beneficial effects on the patients' health. However, single drug therapy with AZT proved to be of limited effectiveness over time. The virus eventually reproduced a version of itself that was resistant to treatment with AZT. This familiar story had transpired with other drugs like DDT and penicillin. Resistance to AZT occurred rather quickly due to the phenomenal rate of mutation of the virus. About 80 percent of a large sample of PWAs in Canada and the United States in 1999 were carrying mutated versions of the virus that were resistant to at least one of the drugs in the triple cocktail (Sussman, 2002).

In late 1991, ddI (Didanasine) was approved by the FDA, and the world was en route to the so-called "triple cocktail." When a nucleoside analogue reverse-transcriptase inhibitor and a non-nucleoside reverse-transcriptase inhibitor were added to the cocktail, they acted to thwart HIV genes before they could integrate into the helper T lymphocyte cell to reprogram the white cell into a virus-producing "factory." By adding the third component of the triple cocktail, a protease inhibitor, a component of HIV called protease enzymes was blocked, so that HIV made copies of itself that could not infect new cells. The triple anti-retroviral therapy attacks the virus in three ways, hence the name, triple cocktail.

The anti-retroviral drugs are neither a prophylactic nor a cure for AIDS. They simply disrupt the various stages in the life cycle of the virus, as it invades the T lymphocyte white cells in the human body and converts them into factories producing further generations of HIV. The anti-retrovirals are a kind of chemical miracle, in that they reduce an individual's viral load *tenfold* within eight weeks. In six months, an individual's viral load is so low that it cannot be detected. Thus the onset of AIDS, and the opportunistic infections that come with it, are delayed indefinitely, if a person living with HIV/AIDS takes the triple cocktail of drugs for the rest of his or her life.

However, taking the anti-retrovirals involves a grueling, long-term regimen of treatments. Very unpleasant side-effects come with the triple cocktail. Nausea, headaches, and insomnia may result from AZT. A protease inhibitor in the triple cocktail like indinavir (Crixivan) should be taken with lots of water on an empty stomach to avoid dehydration. Another protease inhibitor, ritonavir (Norvir) has side-effects like vomiting, weakness, and diarrhea, and should be taken with a full, high-protein, high-fat meal (which many individuals find difficult to consume for breakfast; many others do not have such foods, due to poverty). The toxic effects of the triple cocktail are so strong that 20 to 30 percent of HIV+ individuals cannot take the anti-retroviral therapy. Certainly no one would choose to take the anti-retrovirals if they had any option. But the drugs maintain life, at least for those who can afford them and who can cope with the toxic side-effects. Of course, almost all drugs have side-effects, and some therapies are quite toxic. Many PWAs (about 70 to 80 percent) learn to manage the side-effects of the triple cocktail.

The cost of the anti-retrovirals made them completely unaffordable for almost everyone in the developing countries of Latin America, Africa, and Asia. That is, until 2001, when Cipla, an Indian drug company, announced an astounding price of only $350 per year, one-fortieth of the $15,000 previously charged for the drugs in nations like the United States! Later, we explain how this price breakthrough by Cipla occurred (Figure 3.1). A revolutionary turning point in combating the epidemic had occurred in Brazil in the mid-1990s when that nation showed that it could provide universal access to the triple cocktail. Then, in 2001, Cipla completed the revolution with its remarkable price-drop.

Brazil: A Ray of Hope

AIDS professionals often measure the passage of time in the 20-year epidemic by the alternate-year international conferences held at various locations around the world, such as Montreal, Bangkok, Vancouver, Geneva, Durban, Barcelona. These international AIDS conferences, for the first 15 years of the epidemic, were mostly filled with bad news about the mounting number of deaths. Then, at the 11th International AIDS Conference in Vancouver in 1996, the results of clinical trials of the triple cocktail were announced, receiving much acclaim. Finally, a means of holding back the debilitating effects of HIV on the human body had been found. The 2000 Durban International Conference on AIDS, enthused by the news from Brazil, declared that HIV/AIDS was a *treatable* disease. The growing armamentarium of drugs to help the human body fight HIV represented hope for the 40 million people living with HIV around the world.

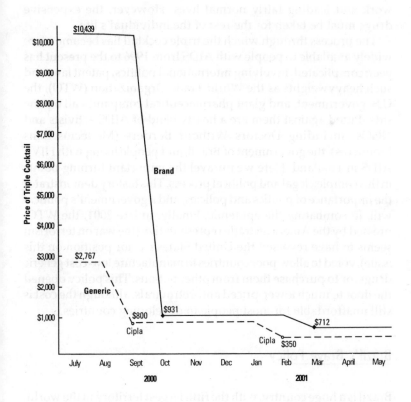

Figure 3.1 The Bottom Dropped Out of the Price of the Triple Cocktail in Developing Countries in 2000 and 2001

The effect of generic drug competition during 2000 and 2001 was to drive down the price of brand drugs for the triple cocktail, consisting of Stavudine, Lamivudine, and Nevirapine.

Source: Based on von Schoen Angerer et al. (2001).

The anti-retrovirals are not a *cure* for AIDS, the goal of a huge medical research program for the past two decades. But the triple cocktail postpones death in most cases, and can return individuals who are very sick to a healthy state. Thus, AIDS became a chronic, rather than an imminently fatal disease. In Brazil, we met people living with AIDS who had been hospitalized for months. Several weeks after beginning anti-retroviral therapy, they were back at work and leading fairly normal lives. However, the expensive drugs must be taken for the rest of the individual's life.

The process through which the triple cocktail has become more widely available to people with AIDS from 1996 to the present has been complicated, involving international politics, patent law, and such heavyweights as the World Trade Organization (WTO), the U.S. government, and giant pharmaceutical companies all on one side. Pitted against them are a hearty band of AIDS activists and NGOs, including Doctors Without Borders (Médecins Sans Frontières), the government of Brazil, and people living with HIV/AIDS in Thailand. Here we unravel the important turning points in this complex legal and political process. This history demonstrates the importance of politics and policies, and a government's political will, in combating the epidemic. Finally, in late 2001, the WTO, pressed by the American trade representative (the war on terrorism seems to have reversed the United States's prior position on this issue), voted to allow poor countries to manufacture low-cost generic drugs, or to purchase them from other nations. This policy opened the door to much lower-priced anti-retrovirals, although the cost is still unaffordable for most people in developing countries.

Brazil's Brave Policy

Brazil is a huge country, with the fifth largest territory in the world. It borders 10 other countries, and many Brazilians speak proudly of "the world of Brazil" (O mondo do Brasil). From 1964 until 1985, this Latin American nation was ruled by a right-wing military dictatorship that largely ignored the threat represented by the AIDS epidemic. Jose Sarney, the first civilian president, called the AIDS epidemic to national attention in the 1990s. Activists for a civil society (that is, for replacing the dictatorship with an elected government) then became lobbyists for government action to control the epidemic.

The first cases of AIDS in Brazil were diagnosed in late 1981 among educated and well-to-do gay men in the cities of São Paulo and Rio de Janeiro. This early pattern of transmission among gay men, similar to that in the United States, was followed by a wave of AIDS cases among injecting drug users in the port cities of Santos, Rio de Janeiro, Salvador, Recife, and Fortaleza, locations from which Brazilian cocaine is exported. Port cities, with their abundance of sailors, commercial sex workers, and injection drug users, are hotspots for AIDS transmission worldwide. The first woman was diagnosed with AIDS in Brazil in 1983. By 1985, the men-to-women ratio of AIDS cases was about 15:1 (Ministerio da Saude, 2000). In 2002, this ratio was about 2:1, indicating the rapid heterosexual transmission of AIDS in Brazil since the late 1980s.

The first AIDS program in Brazil was launched in 1983 in the state of São Paulo by Dr. Paulo Texeira, who, since the late 1990s, has served as the coordinator (or director) of the Brazilian National AIDS Program (NAP). The NAP was launched in 1986, soon after the military dictatorship ended, and public activists, including gays, women's groups, and commercial sex workers, took to the streets, demanding that the government honor their civil, health, and human rights. Several of these citizen activists became members of the National AIDS Committee (established in 1988), the National Committee on Vaccines (established in 1992), the NGO Liaison Sector (established in 1993), and the National Network for Human Rights in HIV/AIDS (established in 1996). Raldo Bonifacio, the present deputy coordinator of NAP, for instance, was a co-founder of ABIA (with Betinho), and a champion of human rights in Brazil. The National Business Council in Brazil is also composed of noted public activists, who helped pass legislation ensuring that employers cannot test employees forcibly, and that PWAs cannot be fired. Brazilian citizen-activists (such as Betinho, Bonifacio, and others) and civil society institutions (such as educational, medical, and business organizations) instigated a political response to HIV/AIDS. Nothing like this has been seen in any other country.

This Catholic nation took action against HIV/AIDS in multiple ways. The Brazilian Ministry of Health launched several daring national television campaigns promoting condoms, conversations between parents and children, and compassion for those living with HIV/AIDS. One campaign showed a conversation between a father and a son, and a mother and a daughter, about sexuality, with a voice-over that said: "You are observing the most effective HIV/AIDS counseling program in the world" (Plate 3.1). Another campaign included four entertaining spots featuring a man talking with his penis, nicknamed "Braulio," about using condoms to prevent HIV infection. This humorous ad campaign stirred considerable controversy, including angry protests from men named

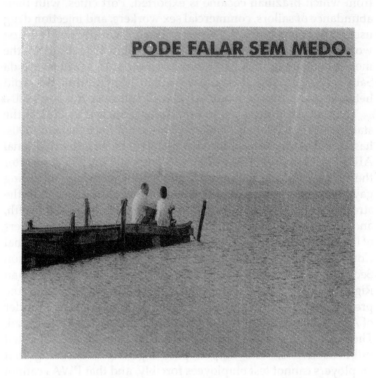

Plate 3.1 A Frame from a Television Spot in which a Brazilian Father Talks to his Son about Sexual Responsibility and HIV Prevention

The Brazilian National AIDS Program launches several daring television campaigns a year, especially during the Carnival in February, when sexual activity among strangers peaks. In this particular television campaign, parents are shown talking to their children about sexuality and AIDS, while the voice-over says: "You are observing the most effective HIV/AIDS counseling program in the world." Formative research indicated that there had been little communication between Brazilian parents and their children about sexuality. Children overwhelmingly said they would like to hear more about sexuality from their parents.

Source: Brazilian Ministry of Health.

Braulio. The National AIDS Program knew that controversy represented one means of breaking silences.

The Brazilian government also removed the 75 percent tax on condoms (called *camisinhas,* or "little shirts," by Brazilians). Some 28 million free condoms were distributed during the carefree Carnival in 2000. Condom use during first sexual encounter rose steeply among Brazilian youth, from 4 percent in 1986 to 48 percent in 1999. "Condom banks" were established by Doctors Without Borders in Rio's *favelas;* each individual received 10, 20, or 30 condoms per month, depending on their degree of sexual activity. Young Brazilians complained that they were not given an adequate number of condoms for their needs.

Despite its efforts to combat the epidemic, Brazil has the highest number of HIV/AIDS cases in Latin America. While the rate of HIV infection was only 0.6 percent in Brazil, compared to over 22 percent in South Africa, the total number of people infected was a product of Brazil's huge population of 167 million.

A personal friend of President Sarney's, a medical doctor, participated in the 1996 International AIDS Conference. When the doctor-friend returned from Vancouver, he told the president about the triple cocktail, and urged him to take action. Meanwhile, PWAs sued the Brazilian government for not upholding people's constitutional rights to live (personal interview, Jorge Biloqui, Atibaia, 18 March 2001). The Brazilian government passed a law providing free anti-retroviral drugs to every individual who tested positive for HIV. Since December 1996, free triple cocktails have been distributed to HIV-positive individuals throughout Brazil. Given that Brazil has 580,000 HIV-positive people, the cost of the drugs at world prices is staggering (actually, only about 100,000 HIV+ Brazilians have been tested and are currently receiving free anti-retrovirals). Brazilian pharmaceutical companies were ordered by the national government to begin manufacturing the drugs as "generics" (that is, lower-cost, non-brand drugs). Within a few years, eight of the dozen anti-retrovirals were being made domestically. World Bank loans of $100 million from 1993 to 1998, and of $135 million from 1999 to 2002, helped the government by defraying the cost of providing the drugs, which had dropped to around $3,000 annually per person by 2000. It dropped even further in 2001.

In the late 1990s, the death rate from AIDS in Brazil dropped by half. Valeria Saraceni, manager of the AIDS program for the state of Rio de Janeiro, recalled for us what the triple cocktail therapy had done to enhance patient care: "AIDS patients, who were close to dying, for whom we had no hope, for whom we had done whatever we could with AZT and ddI, turned around in a few weeks. They were transformed into normal beings" (personal interview, 15 March 2001). In São Paulo, the Brazilian city most affected by the epidemic, the death rate dropped by 54 percent. Brazil is the only nation in the developing world providing free anti-retroviral drugs to all citizens. Despite the considerable cost of this national policy (estimated at $444 million in 2000), the Brazilian government was saving at least as much in preventing the hospitalization of AIDS patients with opportunistic infections (Rosenberg, 2001). Further, the free AIDS drugs in Brazil cut down the transmission rates of HIV. So the treatment strategy has also had a strong prevention effect. The availability of the free triple cocktail encouraged testing by individuals to determine their HIV status. If the results were positive, anti-retroviral medicines were provided. Unfortunately, 80 percent of Brazilians who were seropositive in 2002 did not know that they were infected.

The Controversy over Patent Rights

During our meeting with AIDS activist Jorge Biloqui, a mathematics professor at the University of São Paulo who has been HIV+ since the late 1980s, in Atibaia, Brazil, he took out a pill box and popped a half-dozen drugs into his mouth. Biloqui smiled, and said, "These are my little 'lifesavers'." The following day, Biloqui purchased a cake and celebrated his 10th anti-retroviral birthday.

Who could oppose the distribution of free anti-retrovirals to save lives? For one, the international pharmaceutical companies who hold the patent rights to the drugs. They appealed to the World Trade Organization and to the United States government (several of the world's largest drug houses are headquartered in the United States) to put pressure on Brazil regarding their intellectual property rights on the drugs. Actually, the policy decision by Brazil in 1996 was legal; a loophole in the WTO agreement allows a nation to copy a patented item in case of a national emergency. Then a national government can manufacture the product, or import it as a generic from another country. In either case, intellectual property rights are conferred by what is called a compulsory license. Brazil has a compulsory license to manufacture the anti-retroviral drugs because its government declared that the HIV/AIDS epidemic represented a national emergency.

A decisive step toward a worldwide free-trade economy had been taken in 1994 when the member states of the World Trade Organization signed the World Trade Agreements. One of these agreements, Trade-Related Aspects of Intellectual Property Rights (TRIPS), called for 20-year patent protection for pharmaceuticals. Production of a patented drug by companies other than the patent-holder (this is compulsory licensing) would be allowed in the case of a national emergency. However, the U.S. government regards TRIPS as a minimum standard, and often demands additional patent protection for its drug companies, with the threat of trade sanctions. So Brazil was squeezed by the U.S., but to no avail.

Dr. Eloan Pinheiro is director of Far-Manguinhos, a government phamaceutical research laboratory and manufacturing plant in Rio de Janeiro. Back in 1996, the Brazilian minister of health had asked Pinheiro to analyze and copy the AIDS drugs contained in the triple cocktail. "From the drug companies' point of view, the assembly lines below Pinheiro's second-floor office are humming with the violation of intellectual property rights, 40,000 times an hour" (Rosenberg, 2001). Pinheiro's plant is also transforming the cost of these drugs, not only of the Brazilian-made generics, but also of their counterparts sold by the Pfizers, Glaxo-Wellcomes, and Bristol-Myers Squibbs of the world. The price of AIDS drugs with no generic equivalents decreased by 9 percent from 1996 to 2000; prices of the drugs for which there were equivalents in Brazil dropped 79 percent. For example, Bristol's d4t, whose brand name is Zerit, sells for $4.50 for 40 milligrams in the United States; Pinheiro sells a generic equivalent for only 30 cents (Rosenberg, 2001). This differential suggests that the international pharmaceutical companies are making a large profit on their drug sales.

Drug Company Investment in R&D

The drug companies argue that they must make a very heavy investment in creating each new drug, which justifies the profit margin on the drugs that they sell. The total cost of developing a new drug may total $500 million, although much of the laboratory research may be funded by the National Institutes of Health (NIH), by a private foundation, or by another source. The lengthy process of creating a new drug begins with an R&D investment. This research may be conducted in-house by a corporation, or the company may purchase the patent rights from university biomedical scientists, whose research may have been supported by the National Institutes of Health or by another funding agency (for instance, the patent for Didanosine, resulting from research by NIH, was then granted to Bristol-Myers Squibb). Sometimes the patent rights to a promising drug are acquired from another drug company. The technology licensing fee may amount to several million dollars per year. When a drug company comes into the process late in the day, it cannot legitimately claim the cost of R&D as a reason for its high drug prices. In any event, once a pharmaceutical company gains the rights to a new drug, the next phase in a decade-long process begins: clinical trials, first with animals, and then with human patients, to establish that the new drug is safe from unwanted side-effects and that it is efficacious in achieving its intended effects. Typically, the new drug is compared to the best existing treatment, in order to determine the new drug's value-added in fighting the virus.

One of the world's first medical guinea pigs may have been an 8-year-old boy who was injected with cowpox by Dr. Edward Jenner in 1796, in the hope of finding a vaccine to prevent smallpox (then an important killer). Indeed, a few weeks after Jenner injected the boy with smallpox, he was found to be immune. Today, thousands of volunteers in various nations are participating in clinical trials for new anti-retrovirals or for a potential AIDS vaccine. Why do individuals volunteer? One person in Trinidad said: "I want to take part in the trial because HIV, in a way, has devastated my life. I had a very close friend who had AIDS and the pain that I experienced dealing with it was tremendous. If the vaccine trial is the way that I can contribute to stopping this scourge, then that is what I want to do." Another Trinidadian volunteer said: "HIV is not my problem. It is our problem, and as a region with one of the highest levels of HIV, we need to find a cure for this disease" (Bartholemew, 2002b). The drug trial in Trinidad is a Phase II investigation with 40 volunteers (a Phase I trial is a safety study). The third and final step in this lengthy process is a "big league" trial (Bartholemew, 2002c).

Finally, after the results of drug trials are available, and Food and Drug Administration approval is obtained, a new drug can go on the market, and is sold for a price with a substantial mark-up so that the company is repaid for its considerable investment in the drug development process. Naturally, many new drug candidates do not gain their hoped-for effects, or are not approved by the FDA, so the corporation must earn enough from its successes to cover these losses. The company has a 20-year monopoly to sell the new drug, but often half of this period has already passed by, by the time marketing begins. In any event, pharmaceutical sales in developing countries account for a minimal portion of international drug companies' profits.

One can understand why international drug companies sought to bring the wrath of the WTO and the U.S. government to bear on Brazil. Mainly, the pharmaceutical houses worry that other nations, like South Africa, for instance, will follow in Brazil's footsteps. Doctors Without Borders is indeed encouraging other nations to replicate the Brazilian approach. Brazil has offered to transfer its drug manufacturing technologies, and to train other countries' health personnel in treating patients with anti-retrovirals.

A Complicated Regimen

Taking the triple cocktail correctly is a complex task. The complexity lies in periodicity (when to take the drugs), combination (which drugs need to be combined and which ones cannot be mixed), and food interactions (whether to take the drugs with food or not). A typical HIV patient in Brazil takes 25 to 35 pills a day. Exactly which drugs are taken depends on the patient's age, sex, and viral load. Some anti-retrovirals must be taken when the individual wakes up in the morning, others must be taken on a full stomach; some of the drugs can not be taken at the same time, or else there will be diarrhea, vomiting, and other unpleasant consequences (Plate 3.2). Health providers in Brazil paint little suns and moons on the drug bottles for each patient, and rehearse with the individual the time of day when each drug is to be taken. Despite these efforts, many problems occur. However, years of formal education are not related to the correct use of the anti-retrovirals. Individuals with at least four years of education (meaning they are literate) seem able to understand the complicated drug regimen.

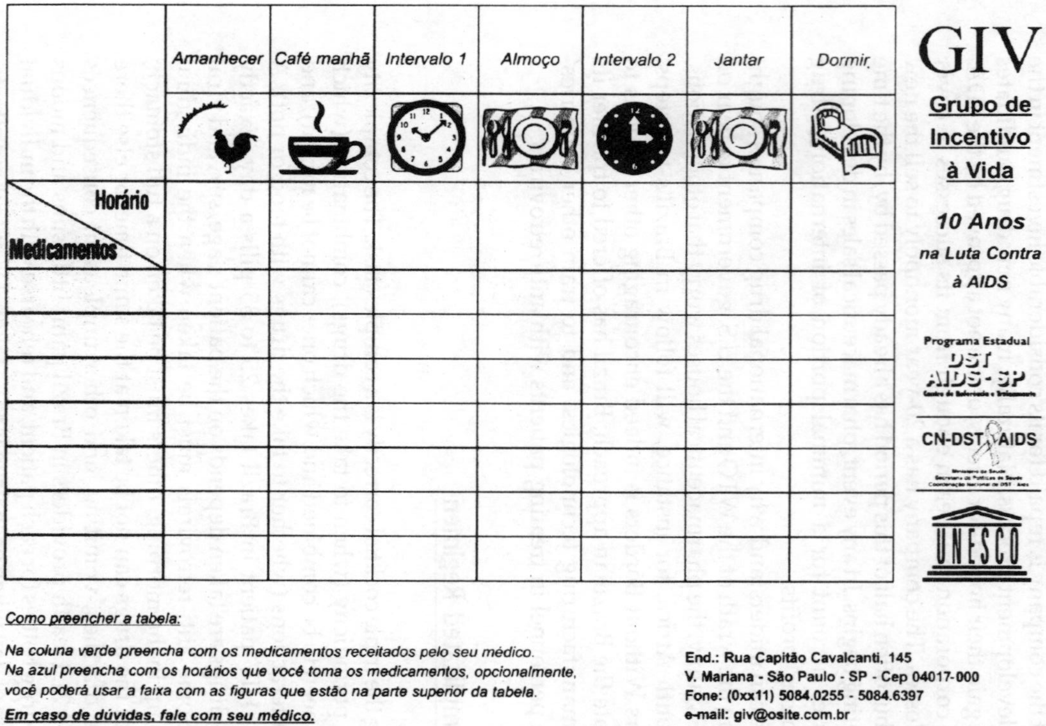

Horário / Medicamentos	Amanhecer	Café manhã	Intervalo 1	Almoço	Intervalo 2	Jantar	Dormir

GIV
Grupo de Incentivo à Vida
10 Anos na Luta Contra à AIDS
Programa Estadual DST AIDS - SP
CN-DST AIDS
UNESCO

Como preencher a tabela:

Na coluna verde preencha com os medicamentos receitados pelo seu médico.
Na azul preencha com os horários que você toma os medicamentos, opcionalmente, você poderá usar a faixa com as figuras que estão na parte superior da tabela.

Em caso de dúvidas, fale com seu médico.

End.: Rua Capitão Cavalcanti, 145
V. Mariana - São Paulo - SP - Cep 04017-000
Fone: (0xx11) 5084.0255 - 5084.6397
e-mail: giv@osite.com.br

Plate 3.2 This Matrix is Given to HIV+ People in São Paulo to Help them Understand the Complicated Regimen of Anti-retroviral Drugs they are Taking

Source: São Paulo, Brazil, Grupo de Incentivo a Vida.

The drugs in Brazil come in white plastic bottles, labeled in different colors and with chemical names. Unfortunately, the colors indicate the manufacturer, not the drug, so that the same drug may come in two or more different-colored bottles, which is confusing to people living with AIDS, particularly those who are illiterate or have poor reading skills. This confusion is unnecessary and could easily be eliminated by the Brazilian government, but it has not been, despite pleas from health practitioners. Another complication rises from the fact that an individual's particular regimen of drugs changes over time as the patient's viral load drops or rises. Further, certain of the AIDS drugs must be refrigerated. How is an AIDS patient living in a São Paulo *favela* going to refrigerate his/her supply of the drugs?

Given these multiple complications, one wonders if any person living with HIV in Brazil actually takes his or her regimen correctly. Perhaps most do. Jorge Biloqui of Grupo de Incentivo a Vida (GIV) noted how PWA group meetings helped in fostering drug regimen compliance: "In GIV's group sessions, those who have been taking anti-retroviral drugs for several years share their knowledge with those who have just begun. They answer questions, reinforce the importance of avoiding food interactions, and serve as model peers" (personal interview, 10 March 2001). Medical doctors on the staff of AIDS clinics in Brazil told us that patients frequently visited health providers with complications resulting from incorrectly taken dosages of the triple cocktail. Incorrectly taken regimens of the anti-retroviral drugs have very serious consequences, not just for the individual but also for society. When the drugs are not taken correctly, resistance to the drugs is more likely to result from HIV mutation. The mutant forms of the virus may then spread to other individuals.

Here we see the communication problems created for patients and providers by the free anti-retrovirals policy in Brazil. Some of these information problems are being solved, and eventually most will be. Why did these problems at the provider/patient interface occur? Because little attention was paid to communication factors. The colors of the pill bottles could easily have been standardized to indicate the different drugs they contained. These problems are, unfortunately, a familiar story in the worldwide battle against AIDS.

The free anti-retrovirals are not a panacea in Brazil, where the health system is strained by the drugs' cost, and by the demands of delivering complicated regimens to over a hundred thousand patients. What is the future of the triple cocktail in Brazil? Will the World Bank loan continue funding the considerable cost of the drugs? If not, will the Brazilian government assume this cost? Will widespread resistance to the drugs develop? In this sense, Brazil might be considered one huge experiment on the effects of the free anti-retroviral drugs.

In any event, Brazil serves as an exemplar for blunting the momentum of the epidemic. It is a sign of hope in the developing world.

President Mbeki's Opposition to the Anti-retrovirals

A stark contrast to Brazil, with its policy of providing free anti-retroviral drugs, is presented by South Africa, which is also a better-off developing country (see Table 1.1). Like Brazil, South Africa has a strong pharmaceutical industry and one of the highest per capita incomes of any country in Latin America, Africa, or Asia (except for the oil-rich Middle Eastern nations). Unlike Brazil, South Africa's top leadership does not want to provide the triple cocktail to its people.

In 1994, Nelson Mandela became South Africa's first indigenous president, ending decades of Apartheid rule under which only whites were allowed to vote. At the time, some 8 percent of South African adults were HIV+. The epidemic had begun in the 1980s among white gay men who had probably contracted the virus in the United States or in Europe. In the 1990s, the epidemic exploded among the African population, who make up 78 percent of South Africa's population. But President Mandela largely ignored the galloping epidemic then spreading among his followers, the South Africans who had elected him to power (Plate 3.3). Thabo Mbeki, Mandela's long-time friend in the African National Congress, was elected to succeed him as president in 1998, at the end of his term. By 2001, more than 22 percent of South Africa's adult population was HIV+.

Duesberg's Dissent

A few years ago, while surfing the Internet, President Mbeki encountered the dissident ideas of Dr. Peter Duesberg, professor of

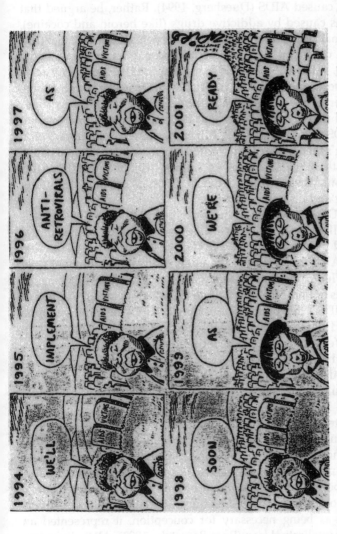

Plate 3.3 A Newspaper Cartoon Criticizing the Delays in Implementing Anti-retroviral Drug Therapy in South Africa

The Mandela and Mbeki governments of the post-Apartheid era are criticized here for their reluctance to launch a large-scale anti-retroviral program.

Source: *The Sowetan,* 16 May 2001.

biochemistry and molecular biology at the University of California at Berkeley. In 1987, Duesberg had published an article in the journal *Cancer Research*, claiming that there was no sound evidence that HIV caused AIDS (Duesberg, 1994). Rather, he argued that AIDS was caused by addictive drugs (like heroin and cocaine), recreational drugs (like nitrites), and pharmaceutical drugs (like AZT and ddI). Duesberg's dissent, championed by some media reporters, led to a 1988 article in the respected journal *Science*, in which Duesberg debated his position with Dr. Robert Gallo, the co-discoverer of the HIV-1 strain (Kinsella, 1989). Duesberg is so certain of this unusual belief that he tells people who are living with AIDS not to take AZT. Mbeki became so enamored with Duesberg's theory that he appointed him to an international panel, along with other scientists, to advise him on the HIV–AIDS connection. Mbeki wrote a letter to all heads of state, defending Duesberg and his perspective.

While Duesberg remains the most radical dissenter to the HIV-causes-AIDS theory, a more moderate form of dissension is expressed by those who believe that HIV is not always the sole cause of AIDS, even though there is a strong correlation between the two. These moderate dissenters argue that various other agents (infectious or non-infectious) serve as co-factors in the progress of HIV to AIDS. They point to cases in which HIV-negative gay men developed pneumocystic pneumonia or Karposi's Sarcoma, two key manifestations of AIDS (Root-Bernstein, 1993). The dissenters contend that AIDS researchers overlooked the role of non-HIV immunosuppressive agents (such as malnutrition, or the presence of tuberculosis and malaria which suppress the body's immune response) in explaining AIDS.

Dissenters draw an analogy with 18th century theories of how conception occurred to point to the problems with the present-day theory of how AIDS occurs. Until the 18th century, semen deposited in a woman's womb was assumed to be sufficient to produce a baby. Facts supported this archaic notion: no man, no baby; no intercourse, no baby; no semen, no baby. Subsequently, when a woman's egg was identified as being necessary for conception, it represented an important intellectual leap (Root-Bernstein, 1993). AIDS dissenters argue that while HIV and AIDS are strongly correlated, much like the presence of semen and the production of babies, the "egg" co-factor is still missing in the HIV-causes-AIDS equation.

President Mbeki has been severely criticized for his strange stance on the triple cocktail. At the 2000 International AIDS Conference in Durban, South Africa, 5,000 eminent scientists signed the Durban Declaration, which stated that HIV caused AIDS (Durban Declaration, 2000). Nevertheless, Mbeki continues to support Duesberg and his theory, comparing him to Galileo and other scientists who were once criticized for their radical ideas.

In 1997, the South African government, under Mandela's leadership, had passed the Medicines Control Amendment Act, to enable provision of affordable drugs to the South African people. The act was immediately attacked by a legal challenge from 41 global pharmaceutical companies. Later, the Mbeki government staunchly defended the act at home, and played a leading role in international trade negotiations to seek affordable drugs. Eventually, in April 2001, the pharmaceutical companies dropped the case, as world public opinion criticized drug companies for engaging in "medical apartheid." Despite these victories, Mbeki's government has still not begun to provide anti-retrovirals to its people, except for pilot-testing the use of Nevirapine at 18 sites to reduce mother-to-child transmission of HIV.

During our visit to South Africa in 2001, most observers described the AIDS policies of the Mbeki government as "confused" and "lacking in direction." On the one hand, Mbeki's government launched Partnership Against AIDS, a multi-sectoral mobilization program to confront AIDS, and increased its budgets for HIV prevention programs, including widespread condom distribution. On the other hand, it has blocked the Treatment Action Campaign's, and other activists', efforts to demand a policy change to provide affordable drugs. President Mbeki refuses to declare a national emergency, so that South Africa may resort to compulsory licensing.

Mbeki's government fought and lost three court cases over its refusal to make Nevirapine universally available to pregnant mothers in South Africa. In April 2002, after dragging its feet for four years, the government acknowledged the usefulness of anti-retroviral drugs, and agreed to provide universal access to Nevirapine to pregnant mothers and their newborn children. The government also agreed to provide free anti-retroviral drugs to rape victims who tested HIV-positive. However, these policies will only go into effect in December 2002, eight months later, during which time several thousand more children will be born HIV-positive.

While South Africa makes some progress in fighting HIV/AIDS (Mbeki recently appointed his deputy president Jacob Zuma to head the Presidential Taskforce on AIDS), Mbeki's "confused" stance on the epidemic holds lessons for policy-makers worldwide about what *not* to do as a government leader. Mbeki did too little, too late. Instead of building consensus and coalitions to tackle the raging epidemic head on, his stance fostered dissent and alienation. Unfortunately, the delays and dissent have already cost tens of thousands of lives.

Zachie Achmat, AIDS Activist

Achmat is a 39-year-old openly gay man of Malaysian descent who is an advocate for providing anti-retrovirals in South Africa. He was raised in Cape Town by his aunt and his mother, who were labor union activists in the garment industry. He joined the African National Congress and participated in student protests against Apartheid. By the time he was 18, Achmat had been jailed several times, and he believes he contracted HIV while in prison. Achmat refuses to take anti-retrovirals until they are available to all South Africans. He states: "I don't want to live in a world where people die every day simply because they are poor."

In 1998, Achmat fell ill with a systemic thrush, an opportunistic infection that attacks people with weakened immune systems. He was treated with Diflucan, a patented Pfizer medicine, but he refused to take anti-retrovirals, which cost (at that time) $6,000 per year in South Africa. Diflucan could be obtained in Thailand for one-tenth the cost of the drug in South Africa. In October 2000, Achmat flew to Bangkok and purchased 5,000 pills of Bizole, an anti-fungal drug. These medicines in Thailand cost only one-sixtieth of their price in South Africa! On his return to Johannesburg, Achmat turned the drugs over to the government for distribution to poor people, daring the authorities to arrest him for illegally importing Bizole.

Achmat founded the Treatment Action Campaign (TAC) in 1998 in order to attack the South African government's policy of not making anti-retroviral drugs available to the poor. Approximately 28 million of the world's 40 million people infected with HIV live in Africa, but only about 25,000 of these people receive the anti-retrovirals, only 0.001 percent of all Africans with HIV. One TAC poster states: "Minister [of Health] Manto Tshabalala-Msimang. Issue compulsory licenses. Produce anti-retrovirals." If a nation considers a drug to be too costly, it can declare a national emergency, and then license local manufacturers to produce generic drugs, or it can buy generic drugs from another country. Another popular poster in South Africa shows the photograph of a drug company president, and states: "AIDS Profiteer. John Kearney, CEO, GlaxoSmithKline. Deadlier than the Virus."

Mother-to-Child HIV Infection

One of the most compelling needs for AIDS drugs in South Africa is for Nevirapine (an anti-retroviral that is an alternative to AZT), which could cut the yearly total of mother-to-child HIV infections down from 70,000 babies to 35,000. In comparison, in the United States about 300 babies are HIV-infected annually. Mother-to-child transmission among HIV+ mothers may occur in utero, at the time of delivery, or through breast-feeding. This type of infection ranges from 25 to 50 percent (Guay et al., 1999), with about half of this HIV transmission due to breast-feeding. In Kenya, breast milk substitutes (like powdered milk) reduced HIV transmission to the child in 44 percent of the cases (Nduati et al., 2000). Experts recommend that mothers feed their babies with milk formula, rather than breast-feeding them, so that infection does not occur through the mother's milk. However, breast-feeding has other health benefits for the child, like reducing infectious diarrhea due to the lack of clean water for bottle-feeding (Marseille et al., 1999).

One of the primary aims of activist groups like Zachie Achmat's Treatment Action Campaign is to convince the South African government to provide Nevirapine to pregnant women. Distributing drugs to prevent mother-to-child HIV infection is one of the most compelling drug policies for a nation to adopt. Who wants to create more AIDS orphans who are themselves HIV-positive? Some experts recommend that, given the low cost of Nevirapine, it should be given to all women who are delivering babies, whether or not they have been tested for HIV.

President Mbeki maintains that AZT is too toxic for pregnant women, claiming that anti-retrovirals are "as dangerous as the disease they are meant to treat" (quoted in Baleta, 2001). The toxicity of AIDS drugs can often be managed well, much like the side-effects of chemotherapy drugs for cancer treatment. Further, the benefits of drug adoption (and the accompanying toxicity) outweigh the costs of inaction. Boehringer Ingelheim, a drug company that manu-factures Nevirapine, a drug similar to AZT in preventing mother-to-child transmission of HIV, offered to supply the medicine free of charge for five years to developing countries on request. Just one tablet of Nevirapine, taken during labor, along with a single dose for the newborn child, reduces the risk of mother-to-child trans-mission by half (Swarms, 2001). The South African government finally decided to provide the drug to the next 90,000 women to deliver at 18 sites throughout the nation. This pilot project is a step in the right direction, but it is only a drop in the bucket, as one million births occur in South Africa per year. HIV-positive mothers will eventually die from AIDS unless they receive anti-retroviral therapy, creating more AIDS orphans in South Africa. As noted previously, Nevirapine will not be available throughout South Africa until the clinical trial is completed at the end of 2002.

Doctors Without Borders

Médecins Sans Frontières (Doctors Without Borders) received the Nobel Peace Prize in 1999 for its humanitarian assistance in war-torn and impoverished areas of the world. Doctors Without Borders, often referred to by its French initials, MSF, was established in 1971 by French medical doctors who had worked for the Red Cross during the Biafran War in Nigeria, and by French journalists. The MSF is an NGO specializing in emergency medical assistance and in advocacy for certain health issues. While MSF currently has offices in only 18 countries, it has activities in over 80 nations. Much of the program activity of MSF is carried out by more than 2,500 volunteers, who are mostly young doctors.

In recent years, Doctors Without Borders mounted an Access to Essential Medicines Campaign to gain worldwide access to life-saving drugs like the anti-retrovirals. Several MSF projects deal with preventing mother-to-child transmission by making AZT or Nevirapine available near the time of birth. In many countries like Brazil, South Africa, and Thailand, Doctors Without Borders has not only served as a technical champion, but has also sought to influence national policies for making low-priced anti-retrovirals available. For instance, in 2001, MSF joined with people living with HIV/AIDS and other NGOs to put pressure on the Thai Ministry of Public Health to provide generic anti-retrovirals to many more of the one million Thais who were HIV-positive. In South Africa's Western Cape Province, Doctors Without Borders is conducting an important trial for providing the triple cocktail to very poor people.

Doctors Without Borders's global effectiveness as a champion for the cause of underprivileged people suffering from HIV/AIDS results from various factors. The MSF's interventions are usually piloted and evaluated before being scaled up. Interventions are designed to engender local participation in order to ensure sustainability. For instance, the "condom bank" interventions in Rio's *favelas* (discussed previously) were established through a network of local community leaders. The MSF also established 10-by-5-foot "information walls" at strategic *favela* locations, feeding them with posters, banners, and newspaper articles to stimulate community debate.

PWA Pressures for Drugs in Thailand

When we met with Senator Jon Ungpakorn at Parliament House in Bangkok on 2 August 2001, he had just come from a meeting with the Government Pharmaceutical Organization (GPO) of Thailand. The senator is the vice-chairman of the Senate's Health Committee, as well as the president of the AIDS Access Foundation, which represents people living with HIV and AIDS. Ungpakorn was seeking to influence the GPO to lower its prices for generic anti-retrovirals and to increase its production (Williams et al., 1999). Since the GPO had begun producing Zidovudine in 1993, the price per patient had dropped from $324 per month to $87 (in 1995). By mid-2001, about 3,000 HIV-positive Thais were on anti-retroviral drugs, many of them getting these drugs as part of a large-scale "experiment" (without a control or placebo group, so hardly an experiment in the usual sense). The goal of Ungpakorn, and of other HIV/AIDS activists in Thailand, was to raise this number from 3,000 to as many as possible of Thailand's one million HIV+ people.

Jon Ungpakorn studied engineering as an undergraduate, and then taught physics at a university in Bangkok. He found the classroom dull, at least compared to policy advocacy. He resigned from his teaching position and established the AIDS Access Foundation. When the new Thai constitution came into effect, creating a 200-member parliament in 1996, he was elected to the national legislature. Thus, he became an activist for people living with HIV/AIDS, one who also had an influential role in the elite circle of national policy-makers.

One of the populist platform planks that helped elect Prime Minister Thaksin Shinawatra to office was the 30-baht (U.S. 70¢) Health Care Plan. This scheme allows any Thai citizen to receive consultation, treatment, and medicine by paying only 30-baht when visiting a local hospital. The new health care plan went into effect nationwide in October 2001. Unfortunately, however, the health scheme did not cover the cost of anti-retroviral drugs, because the Thai Ministry of Public Health claimed that it had an insufficient budget for this huge expense.

Thanks to pressure on the GPO by Senator Ungpakorn and other activists, the price of the triple cocktail dropped from $8,100 per year in late 1999 to only $660 by December 2001. On World AIDS Day, 1 December 2001, the minister of public health agreed to include the anti-retrovirals in the 30-baht health scheme, at least as far as the Ministry's budget would allow. Immediately, 7,000 people would be included, with preference given to the 70,000 individuals with AIDS (that is, who were already showing the symptoms of opportunistic infections). This important decision by the minister came about due to pressure from 1,300 PWAs and their friends, who gathered at Parliament House to demand action. Senator Ungpakorn was one of the speakers arguing that the cost of supplying the anti-retrovirals was a wise investment, in terms of the potential economic consequences for the workforce. Then, in March 2002, the GPO reduced the cost of the triple cocktail to only $360 per year. Within a year, the GPO will be producing six million tablets of the triple cocktail each month.

Yusuf Hamied's Price Revolution

The present authors visited Cipla's headquarters in Bombay Central on 20 December 2001 in order to meet Dr. Yusuf K. Hamied, the company's president (Plate 3.4). At the time, most Americans knew of Cipla as the manufacturer of the antibiotic Cipro, short for Ciprofloxacin, which vaulted into news headlines in fall 2001

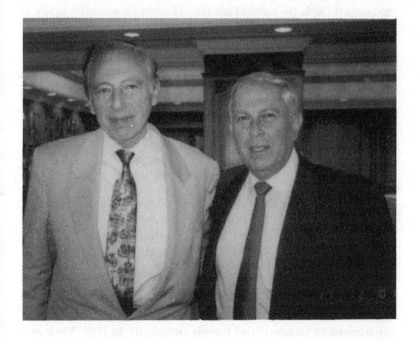

Plate 3.4   Dr. Yusuf Hamied, President of Cipla (right) with Dr. Robert Gallo, Discoverer of HIV-1, in a 2001 Event in Mumbai.

Dr. Hamied led the shocking drop in worldwide prices for anti-retroviral AIDS drugs in 2001. Two decades previously, Dr. Rolovit Gallo had led the charge to isolate the human immunodeficiency virus that causes AIDS.

Source: Cipla.

during the anthrax scare in the United States following the 11 September 2001 terrorist attacks. Cipro cost $5 per tablet in the United States, but Cipla sold generic versions of the antibiotic for only 10 cents per tablet. Among those involved in combating the AIDS epidemic worldwide, Cipla became famous for having caused the bottom to drop out of anti-retroviral prices during 2001.

The journey that brought us to Dr. Hamied involved some complicated network connections. They began with an Indian doctoral student at the University of New Mexico, Avinash Thombre, who had worked as a journalist specializing in reporting on the epidemic in Pune, a city near Mumbai. Rogers asked Thombre how to contact Cipla president Hamied. Thombre e-mailed a medical doctor friend of his in Pune, who in turn knew Dr. Jaideep Gogtay, a medical doctor who worked as an advisor to Dr. Hamied. A few e-mails later, our visit with Dr. Hamied had been arranged. It was scheduled early in the workday by Dr. Gogtay, because he knew that Yusuf Hamied, called "Doctor" by his staff at Cipla, would become extremely preoccupied with his work later in the day. That did in fact happen, with long-distance calls from London and with the visit of another drug company president.

We met in the company's boardroom at Cipla, under a photograph that showed Mahatma Gandhi, on the occasion of his visit to Cipla, with Dr. Hamied's father, also a chemist, who started Cipla in 1935 with profits earned by importing a sexual tonic from Germany (Specter, 2001). While studying chemistry in Germany in 1925, Hamied's father, an Indian Muslim, met his mother, a Lithuanian Jewess. According to Judaism, this ancestry makes Yusuf Hamied a Jew (he must be one of very few Indian Jews in this nation of one billion people).

Yusuf Hamied earned his Ph.D. in chemistry at Cambridge at age 23. Today, he maintains a home in Mauritius, as well as an apartment in London, and travels frequently to New York and Hong Kong. But he is a resident of Mumbai, an Indian citizen, and a very wealthy one. We found Dr. Hamied to be straightforward, informal, outspoken. We wanted to know how he could sell the anti-retrovirals for $350 per person per year, the extraordinarily low price that Cipla had announced earlier in 2001. We asked: "Are you such a bad businessman that you sell below the cost of production, or is the low price for the triple cocktail due to your altruism?" The answer, it seems, is a good deal of altruism for the poor people of the world, combined with rather good business sense. In the first place, Cipla manufactures 400 products, of which the AIDS drugs constitute just 12 (Specter, 2001). They represent a small portion of Cipla's annual sales of $290 million. Cipla is the second largest of 20,000 pharmaceutical companies in India, with 5,500 employees. Its plants for manufacturing the anti-retrovirals are located in Mumbai, Pune, and Bangalore, with other drugs manufactured in Mumbai, Goa, and elsewhere in India. Cipla began producing cancer drugs in the 1960s, and has an important presence in most other aspects of the drug industry.

Cipla manufactures the anti-retrovirals as generics, and thus avoids paying a technology licensing fee to the overseas pharmaceutical companies that own the patents. This unique advantage is due to the India Patents Act of 1970, which only protects the patents for a manufacturing process, but not the product patent on the drug itself. This act allows "me-too" drugs to be produced by manipulating the molecular structure of a patented drug. The purpose of the 1970 act was to lower drug prices in India, and that it has done. India has the lowest drug prices in the world today, about one-tenth of current world prices. So Cipla can legally "reverse engineer" a patented foreign drug, and then manufacture it without paying for the expensive R&D in which the overseas pharmaceutical companies invested. One can imagine why the companies holding the intellectual property rights to new drugs view Cipla as "one of the great pirate enterprises of the corporate world" (Specter, 2001, p. 74).

In Cipla's defense, Dr. Hamied points out that two of the three main drugs in the triple cocktail were developed with public funding. Didanosine (ddI) was developed with NIH funding, and Stavudine (d4t) was developed by researchers at Yale University. Both drugs are marketed internationally by Bristol-Myers Squibb.

Price Slashing by Cipla

The story of how Dr. Hamied and Cipla came to announce the shockingly low price for the anti-retrovirals involves a complicated combination of good intentions, rejection, and accident. The narrative begins with Dr. Hamied being invited to address the European Commission in Brussels in September 2000. In Hamied's brief speech, about three minutes in length, he challenged the world to sell AIDS drugs for prices that the poor could afford. He stated: "We are ready to offer this combination [Cipla's triple cocktail of Lamivudine, Stavudine, and Nevirapine] internationally at around U.S.$800 per patient per year." Dr. Hamied left the Brussels meeting expecting a bombshell of rapid reaction. Several ministers of health and heads of state of African nations were present at the Brussels meeting. But to Dr. Hamied's surprise, nothing happened.

Several months later, Dr. Hamied offered free supplies of Nevirapine, which is effective in preventing mother-to-child transmission of the virus, to the Indian government. He repeated the offer, this time personally to India's prime minister. No response.

Then, in January 2001, the nearby state of Gujarat was hit by a devastating earthquake, killing 30,000 people. Cipla responded by sending free medicines. Hamied says that the disaster woke him to a recognition of the even greater disaster of the AIDS epidemic looming in his country. He reflected on why his country was moving mountains to cope with the recent natural disaster, but was apathetic to the monumental disaster of AIDS that was unfolding. On 6 February 2001, Hamied faxed an offer to Doctors Without Borders, to sell them the triple cocktail for $350 per year, if they would distribute the drugs free to HIV+ people in developing countries. The next morning, at 2.00 A.M. Mumbai time, Dr. Hamied received a telephone call from Donald McNeil of *The New York Times*, who wanted to know if the offer was legitimate (McNeil, 2001a). Hamied confirmed the astounding price, adding that he would sell at that price to anyone who would undertake the free distribution of the anti-retrovirals. The following morning, the news was on the front page of *The New York Times*. Suddenly, Dr. Hamied and Cipla were known throughout the world. The general reaction was amazement at the ridiculously low price. How could Cipla sell the triple cocktail for a dollar a day per HIV-positive person?

The price revolution that Cipla launched caused worldwide repercussions. Shortly afterwards, Merck announced that it would reduce its price for some anti-retrovirals by 90 percent in certain African countries. The international pharmaceutical houses realized that clinging to patent laws might be bad for business in the face of the international plague. Not to be outdone by its domestic competitor, Hetero Drugs of Hyderabad announced a price of $347 per year, followed by Ranbaxy's price of $295 per year. "The impact of Cipla's decision has been extraordinary" (Specter, 2001, p. 76).

The Arbitrary Price of Drugs

What explains Cipla's rock-bottom price? The company formed a unique, affordable triple cocktail, called Triomune, that did not include protease inhibitors, which are relatively expensive. The idea of creating this affordable triple cocktail occurred to Dr. Hamied while he was listening to Judge Edwin Cameron at the 2000 International AIDS Conference in Durban, when Cameron discussed his own drug regimen of anti-retrovirals. Cipla's triple cocktail combines three drugs into a single pill, to be taken twice daily. Thus Cipla has greatly simplified the complexities encountered with the 35 pills that must be taken per day by an HIV+ person in Brazil. But Triomune can be sold only in India, because a different pharmaceutical company patents each of the three drugs. Cipla also sells a second-line triple cocktail that includes AZT, and a third-line combination, at a still higher price, that includes the relatively more expensive protease inhibitors. But it is the $350 per year Triomune that commands world attention.

Dr. Hamied points to the rather arbitrary pricing policies for most drugs. Many are pegged at 500 to 1000 percent above the actual cost of production. In short, the cost of a drug is often what the seller thinks a buyer can afford to pay. Dr. Hamied beckoned toward the suits and ties worn by his visitors on 20 December 2001 and asked, "What will drug companies charge you for their drugs? What will they charge an Indian villager for the same drugs?"

Certain costs incurred by Cipla are extremely low. For instance, Cipla's headquarters in Mumbai Central is located on prime real estate, which would rent for several million dollars per year. But the buildings were built years ago, and are depreciated to zero today. Most of Cipla's manufacturing plants are at least a decade old. The salary paid to a highly educated professional in India is approximately one-tenth that earned by a counterpart in the United States (Singhal & Rogers, 2001a). The actual costs to Cipla of producing the triple cocktail are accordingly much lower than in Euro-America.

As we were leaving after the interview with Dr. Hamied, he asked Dr. Gogtay to give us each a sample of Nevirapine oral suspension, a 25-milliliter bottle sufficient for one HIV-positive mother and her newborn baby. The instructions accompanying the medicine indicate that two 10-milliliter cups (a small plastic cup is included in the package) are to be taken by the mother, and a single dose is to be given the newborn with a small plastic syringe (also enclosed). The bottle does not have to be refrigerated, thus making it ideal for conditions in developing countries. Cipla offered this liquid form of Nevirapine free to UNICEF and to the government of India, and it is now being pilot-tested in 11 Indian hospitals.

We left Cipla with the small bottles of Nevirapine in our pockets. It seemed unbelievable, and somewhat reassuring as to the state of the world, to know that one held a drug that could save a life. It also made one feel very guilty, knowing that this simple solution to HIV infection was still not available to most pregnant women in Latin America, Africa, and Asia.

Search for an AIDS Vaccine

"Vaccination" comes from the Latin word for cow, *vacca*, because the first experiment with developing a vaccine for smallpox was undertaken by Dr. Edward Jenner, an English country doctor, who injected a boy with cowpox, a disease similar to smallpox, to develop immunity to the latter disease.

Despite the massive R&D efforts of biomedical scientists over the past 20 years, a vaccine for AIDS has not been developed and there are no good prospects of success in sight. Development of an affordable, appropriate, and effective HIV/AIDS vaccine is seven to 10 years off (Makgoba et al., 2002). Why is it so difficult to create an AIDS vaccine? One problem is the paradox of vaccinating the human immune system against a virus that attacks the human immune system itself. Another difficulty is the lack of an experimental animal on which to test vaccine candidates. Only humans get HIV (even chimpanzees, from whom HIV-1 may have evolved, only get SIV, simian immunodeficiency virus).

A further problem is that most efforts to develop a vaccine are directed toward HIV-1 subtype B, which is most common in the Americas and Europe, rather than toward subtype C, which is responsible for more than 55 percent of all HIV-1 infections globally, and which is dominant in Africa and India. Thus it is possible that an eventual vaccine will least benefit the nations hardest hit by the epidemic. Finally, most drug companies are hesitant to invest large amounts in R&D for an AIDS vaccine because of its low profit potential.

Some commercial sex workers in Nairobi's Pumwari red-light district have remained HIV-negative for up to 20 years, despite continued high-risk exposure. Similar long-time sex workers have been studied in Gambia. Such resistance to HIV infection is presumably due to the CSW's ability to mount a protective immune response to HIV (Kaul et al., 2000). These CSWs have a very high level of killer T cells. Strangely, when these CSWs retire from working in the sex industry, they often become HIV-infected! Dr. Bette Korber, an AIDS researcher at the Los Alamos National Laboratory (personal interview, 21 February 2002), suggests that the CSWs may have a low-level HIV infection (from their HIV-positive customers) that stimulates their bodies to produce killer T cells, and which prevents them from becoming HIV-positive. When they quit the sex industry, their level of T lymphocytes falls off, so that when they next have sex with an infected person, they become infected. The strange case of these commercial sex workers has been studied by AIDS researchers in order to gain insights into possible strategies for developing a vaccine. The scientific question is how to stimulate the human body to produce a high level of killer T cells.

"Joyce" (not her real name) lives in the Pumwari red-light district in Nairobi. She migrated from Tanzania in 1983, and, with three children to feed, she turned to prostitution. Joyce was a respondent in a research project directed by Dr. Frank Plummer of Canada and others (Kaul et al., 2000; Schoofs, 1999). Amazingly, despite the fact that 14 years have passed since her original HIV blood test, Joyce has maintained her HIV-negative status. She serviced up to 10 customers a day for many of these 14 years. Ninety percent of the other commercial sex workers in Pumwari have become HIV+. Joyce contracted other STDs, indicating that her customers did not use condoms. So certainly Joyce was exposed to HIV. But she did not become infected.

Developing an effective AIDS vaccine has been a process of one step forward, one step back. As Lifson and Martin (2002) remark: "Sisyphus would be well suited to a career in AIDS-vaccine research." The death of Monkey 798 at Harvard Medical School in 2000 illustrates the unexpected setbacks in the vaccine battle. Dr. Dan Barouch and his colleagues immunized eight rhesus monkeys with an experimental vaccine in early 2000, testing its effects by also injecting thĕ monkeys with a lethal AIDS virus. The unvaccinated monkeys in the control group quickly contracted AIDS and died (Schoofs, 2002). Six months later, blood tests of Monkey 798 began to show changes in the monkey's immune system. In less than six weeks, the entire virus population of Monkey 798 changed to a mutant type that rendered the vaccine helpless in fighting the virus (Barouch et al., 2002). The demise of Monkey 798 showed that the path to developing an effective vaccine would not be an easy one, given the high rate of the virus's mutation (Schoofs, 2002).

Unfortunately, vaccine production is not very good business. Current profits from all vaccine sales combined (for hepatitis B, tetanus, and others) are lower than for a single patented anti-ulcer drug (Garrett, 2001). So there is little corporate interest in developing vaccines that will be utilized mainly in developing countries.

The key steps in developing a new drug are being followed in the development of an AIDS vaccine. Many candidate drugs have made it to small-scale Phase I safety testing, and many have failed at this step. However, only one large-scale Phase III drug trial is underway. It costs $35 million and includes a large sample of 16,000 injecting drug users in Thailand who are taking Aventis Pasteur's ALVAC. The attempt here is to cut the HIV infection rate more among the treatment group that is administered the candidate drug, compared to a control sample randomly selected not to receive the drug. The AIDS vaccine will probably not cure people living with HIV or AIDS. Instead, it will likely decrease the viral load of people living with HIV. Such a vaccine with perhaps two or three administrations might have important advantages over the present anti-retrovirals, which must be taken for life.

Research to find an AIDS vaccine goes on. Perhaps someday, maybe in seven to 10 years, it will be successful. Meanwhile, the world must carry on with efforts to prevent HIV.

Nutrition, the First Line of Defense

In her opening statement at an international conference on HIV/AIDS and the African Child, held at Ohio University in April 2002, Dr. Prisca Nemapare, a nutrition expert from

Zimbabwe, said: "Let no one doubt that proper nutrition is the best frontline drug for AIDS." Nemapare heads the Zienzele Foundation in Harare, which works with AIDS orphans, empowering them through education, nutrition, and vocational training. Nemapare (2002) contends that pap (or mealie meal), the maize-based staple food of poor people in Sub-Saharan African countries, is not very nutritious, and, unless supplemented with dairy, poultry, and eggs (a rarity for poor people), it limits the body's ability to fight infections. Might such nutritional deficiency, in part, contribute to the more rapid onset of AIDS among HIV-positive people in Sub-Saharan Africa?

In the countries we visited, many HIV/AIDS programs distributed "neutraceuticals" (nutritious food packages) to PWAs, in the absence of AIDS drugs. Nemapare educates Zimbabwean families to supplement their maize porridge with milk, poultry, and eggs, and if this is not possible, to incorporate termites and caterpillars in their meals, as both are a rich source of protein and minerals.

Nutrition and anti-retroviral therapy, in combination, represent the desired therapeutic response for those afflicted with HIV/AIDS. However, in the absence of anti-retroviral drug therapy, proper nutrition is indeed the first line of defense. In Brazil, we heard of several instances of HIV-positive people trading their free anti-retroviral AIDS drugs for food. After all, what good are anti-retrovirals if people do not have enough to eat?

Herbal Treatments

In every country that we visited in the process of writing this book, we encountered numerous herbal therapies widely in use by HIV-positive people. This popular use of herbal medicines should not be surprising, given the generally unaffordable cost of anti-retroviral drugs and the rapidly growing number of HIV-positive people in developing nations. As one HIV/AIDS official told us, even if the treatment for the disease were to consist of only a glass of clean, drinkable water, 75 percent of HIV-positive people would not have ready access to it.

Indigenous Knowledge Systems

Medical professionals who introduce a new drug or other cure often assume that their target audience is like a blank slate, lacking any relevant experience with which to associate the new idea. On the contrary, any set of people to whom an innovation is introduced evaluate it in terms of their prior experience with something they perceive as similar (Rogers, 1995). Individuals make sense of the new in terms of the old. Often, a familiar name is used to refer to the new. For instance, truck drivers in India referred to HIV with the Hindi word *garmi* (heat), which they had used previously for STDs like syphilis and gonorrhea.

So to be effective, an HIV prevention program needs to understand how the target audience perceives HIV, condoms, monogamy, opportunistic infections, anti-retroviral drugs, and the herbal therapies that have been used for centuries. It is an egregious error to regard traditional practitioners of herbal drugs as quacks, and their therapies as bogus.

Most developing countries are characterized by a rather thin veneer of Western-style biomedical science, provided by modern hospitals and other facilities, staffed by a cadre of university-graduate medical doctors. This modern medical system only reaches a relatively small percentage of the total population, consisting mainly of urban individuals who are of higher socioeconomic status. Cadres of traditional health practitioners, spiritualists, birth delivery attendants, and herbalists are found in every village and in poor urban neighborhoods. In India, four alternative systems of medicine exist: ayurvedic, *unani, siddha,* and homeopathic. The ayurvedic system is over 3,000 years old and includes half a million practitioners who dispense treatment throughout India. Together, ayurvedic and *unani* practitioners conduct over 75 percent of all medical consultations in India (Mane & Maitra, 1992). In India's poverty-stricken state of Bihar, 95 percent of all medical consultations are initiated with a traditional health provider. Further, an estimated two-thirds of all babies born today in developing countries are delivered at home by traditional birth attendants. These traditional health providers have a high degree of credibility and are usually the first source of help sought by individuals when they become ill. Each year, one million seropositive women deliver babies with the help of traditional midwives (Bultreys et al., 2002). How can they be involved in reducing parent-to-child transmission?

In the process of writing this book, we encountered herbal drugs for treating HIV in Brazil, South Africa, Kenya, and Thailand. Traditional health providers have an herbal medicine for every common health problem, including HIV/AIDS. These herbal therapies may be effective in curing certain of the opportunistic infections that come with AIDS. Perhaps some of the herbal therapies have certain anti-retroviral qualities. Turmeric, a naturally occurring spice (and an ingredient in curry) has shown promise. Also, *keezhanelli*, a common weed in Tamil Nadu in South India, has been used for centuries as a treatment for hepatitis A. Dr. Suniti Solomon, director of the Y.R.G. Center for AIDS Research and Education in Chennai, took a sample of *keezhanelli* to St. Michaels Hospital in London for chemical analysis (personal interview, 24 December 2001). The results showed that *keezhanelli* had some anti-retroviral properties as a reverse transcriptase (Gaitonde, 2001, p. 220). A next step is to test this herbal therapy in a double-blind experiment. Lacking such scientific evidence of their efficacy, Western-trained medical doctors generally look upon herbal treatments with disdain. They regard traditional practitioners as "quacks," and dismiss their herbal therapies as phony. Indeed, some herbal medicines have proven to be false cures for HIV/AIDS.

In the developing countries of Asia, Africa, and Latin America, traditional healers are much better positioned than are medical doctors to care for HIV/AIDS patients. They can dispense herbal medicine to reduce opportunistic infections and to boost the immune systems of those who are HIV-positive, and can serve as caring counselors. The cost of a consultation with a traditional healer, and the price of herbal drugs, is relatively low. Further, traditional healers are perceived as being more approachable, personable, and community-centered than are medical doctors. In India, a medical doctor in a government hospital spends about two to three minutes per patient. The encounter is devoid of personal greetings, eye contact, or casual conversation (Mane & Maitra, 1992). The doctor's focus is on understanding the symptoms of the sickness, not the person behind it. The doctor–patient relationship is often hierarchical, depersonalized, and governed by biomedical principles.

Pimjai and the Don Kaew Community Health Project

A personal role model for herbal medicine is Mrs. Pimjai Intamoon, who heads the Community Health Project in Don Kaew village, Mae Rim district, located a 40-minute drive south of Chiang Mai, Thailand (Plate 3.5). Some 340 HIV-positive people currently live in the village, where the total population is 700. Half of the children in the village are HIV-positive, mainly as the result of mother-to-child infection, with the mothers having been infected by their husbands, who in turn were infected by commercial sex workers. The further spread of the epidemic has been slowed down; no new case of HIV infection has occurred in the past two years. The village, and the area surrounding it, was hard hit by the epidemic. Some 350 villagers, mainly men, have died from AIDS, and during our visit to Don Kaew the smell of smoke from a nearby Buddhist cremation site hung in the air. Pimjai says she has participated in more than a thousand AIDS-related funeral ceremonies in recent years.

Pimjai was infected with HIV by her husband, who had become infected while he was working in Bangkok. Now, 14 years after she learned that she was HIV+, Pimjai appears to be in amazing health, which she ascribes to her regimen of meditation, nutrition, and exercise. She is a welder, and her expertise with an arc welder is evident at building construction sites in Don Kaew village. Pimjai has a positive attitude toward her illness. She is always smiling, even when she received the results of her HIV blood tests. She has not taken anti-retrovirals.

Pimjai was the first person in Don Kaew village to publicly disclose her HIV status. With the help of her parents, Pimjai started the Community Health Project in 1993. It was originally head-quartered in her home. The project's purpose is mainly to organize income-generating activities for the many HIV+ widows in the village who were infected by their husbands. Initially, they produced a woven flower product that was used in cremation ceremonies. Then a sewing project was organized, which currently involves 25 HIV+ women. The project's theme is self-reliance, although in the past the project received funding from the Thai-Australian Project for AIDS Control, and the Terra des Hermes Foundation of the Netherlands.

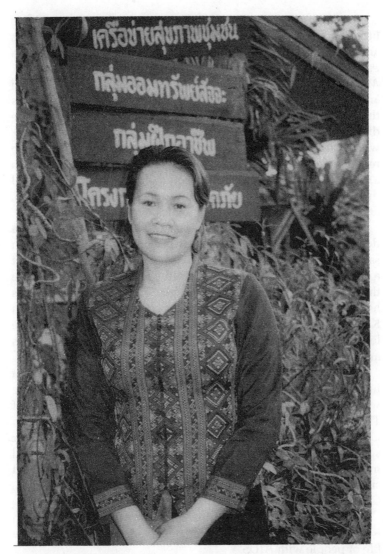

Plate 3.5   Mrs. Pimjai Intamoon Directs the Community Health Project in Don Kaew Village near Chiang Mai, Thailand

Several of the herbal plants that the project uses to make HIV therapies are growing in front of the project's building. Pimjai, who has been HIV-positive for 14 years, leads the self-reliant project in a village in which half the inhabitants are seropositive.

Source: Personal files of the authors.

The modest building owned by the project has become a veritable little factory for herbal drug production. One herb, *acanthaceae*, is an anti-diarrhea medicine that also reduces fever. Another drug, *euphorbiaceae*, is used to cure hepatitis and opportunistic infections. *Menispermaceae* is taken as a tincture to increase appetite. Pimjai and her associates gather the herbs, which they grow nearby, process them in an electric dryer, and pack them in capsules, which are distributed to HIV-positive people. Pimjai and her group of HIV+ women at the project also make an organic insecticide and a mosquito repellant from citronella grass (lemon grass); they cook the leaves in a solar boiler to produce a pungent liquid. Profits earned from herbal drug sales go to providing care for people living with HIV/AIDS, and as seed funds for further economic development.

The project started a savings society for HIV-positive women a decade ago, and today they boast of 500,000 baht ($10,000) in savings. The Thai government offered the Community Health Project a one million baht loan, but they proudly rejected the offer because they considered the interest rate too high. Seven neighboring villages have now started their own savings societies, modeled after Don Kaew's successful initiative. Pimjai serves as coordinator of the local wisdom network, through which the village savings clubs are organized.

Pimjai received various honors for her efforts in self-reliant income production and for her work with herbal medicines. She was selected for a role model award from the prime minister of Thailand. Pimjai has been on Thai national television and on CNN. She proudly showed us her day-planner, in which her speaking appearances were scheduled solidly for the next several months. The guest book at the Community Health Project contained signatures and admiring comments from visitors from India, Japan, China, Cambodia, and Vietnam.

A wooden sign hangs in front of the project building in Don Kaew village that states (in Thai): "A bit of kindness lengthens the life of people with AIDS."

Herbal Remedy in Chinese Ruins

Herbal treatments can be effective in addressing diseases that increase a person's vulnerability to HIV/AIDS. Tuberculosis,

STDs, and malaria reduce an individual's immunity and, along with HIV, serve as co-factors in speeding the progress to AIDS (Root-Bernstein, 1993).

Chinese chemists found an efficacious herbal remedy for malaria, a disease that strikes 500 million people each year (killing two million), from the sweet wormwood herb, *Herba artemisiae* (Lague, 2002). The medicinal properties of sweet wormwood for malaria treatment were unearthed during archaeologist excavations of the Mawangdui Tombs in Hunan province in the early 1970s. Based on the manuscripts they found, Chinese researchers have for the past three decades tested various extracts of this herb, isolating a crystalline compound *qinghaosu* (Artemisinin), which is poisonous to the malarial parasite, but has no side-effects for human beings. This pioneering work was conducted with inexpensive equipment in a home-style laboratory.

The discovery of Artemisinin is especially noteworthy, as widespread use of anti-malarial drugs like chloroquine led to drug-resistant strains of malaria. Doctors Without Borders (MSF) is working with various African governments to include Artemisinin derivatives as treatments for malaria.

Conclusions

Are the anti-retroviral drugs the solution to the worldwide AIDS epidemic? Hardly, due to economic factors, which make the triple cocktail unaffordable for the majority of HIV-positive people in most developing countries. When we asked Dr. Hor Bun Leng, deputy director of the AIDS control program in Cambodia, whether the triple cocktail was being distributed to HIV-positive people in his impoverished nation, he replied: "Our limited funding cannot even provide drugs to control the opportunistic infections associated with AIDS, let alone the expensive anti-retrovirals!" Even if the triple cocktail were affordable, it would still not be the solution to the worldwide AIDS epidemic. However, anti-retrovirals could be a useful part of a comprehensive program that includes effective prevention.

Further, the toxic side-effects of the triple cocktail prevent many HIV+ people from taking these drugs or from completing a full course of treatment. Then there is the worrisome problem of growing resistance to the anti-retrovirals due to the high rate of mutation of the virus. A key factor in the efficacy of the anti-retroviral drugs is improving the quality of how they are taken by people living with HIV/AIDS, so that (a) these individuals return to improved physical health, and (b) a drug-resistant virus is kept in check. For example, in India, the triple cocktail can be purchased over the counter at pharmacies (if the buyer can pay for the drugs). Many HIV+ people stop taking the anti-retrovirals after a month or two, when they have recovered their health. They mistakenly think they are cured (Dr. Suniti Solomon, personal interview, 24 December 2001). Unfortunately, the virus then returns with a vengeance, as the individual's viral load shoots up. The likelihood of infecting others also increases. Under these conditions, drug resistance is likely to develop, and the resistant strains of the virus are passed on to other individuals. As Dr. Michael Gottlieb, the UCLA medical researcher who identified the first AIDS cases in America, says: "Anti-retroviral therapy continues to evolve rapidly in response to the virus's own evolution, in a kind of biological chess game" (Gottlieb, 2001).

To date, the developing countries benefiting most from the anti-retrovirals, like Brazil, have had a well-developed domestic drug industry. But how about the smaller developing countries, like Trinidad and Tobago and other Caribbean nations, which do not have a domestic drug industry? Further, cheaper drugs are needed in developing countries for malaria, pneumonia, and other opportunistic infections. Some critics point out that free-market forces do not reward the pharmaceutical industry for R&D on these diseases of poor people in developing countries.

The role of anti-retroviral therapies, discussed in this chapter, raises questions about whether prevention versus treatment is actually a false dichotomy, at least in the case of the case of the AIDS epidemic. In Brazil, for example, widespread use of the anti-retrovirals to treat people living with HIV/AIDS has greatly decreased the rate of HIV infection. So are the drugs a treatment intervention, or are they preventive?

Nevertheless, the triple cocktail, since it became available in the mid-1990s, has demonstrated that the virus is treatable, and that means, at least for economically advantaged individuals, that HIV is not a certain death sentence. The cost of the anti-retrovirals will probably continue to drop in the future, so that more HIV-positive people in more countries will benefit. Perhaps herbal therapies will prove to be efficacious. One can continue to hope.

4

Targeting Unique Populations

■

Interventions have been developed that have the capability to reduce HIV incidence and relatively risky behaviors by up to 80 percent.

Prabhat Jha et al. (2001)

The effects of targeting interventions are illustrated by a prevention program for about 1,000 sex workers in Pumwari, a low-income area in Nairobi, Kenya. Some 80 percent of the CSWs here were HIV-positive in 1985, when the intervention program started. Free condoms were provided, and a free health clinic was established that treated STDs, gave counseling, and provided a medical check-up every six months. Outreach education was carried out through one-on-one contacts and through *barazas* (group meetings). The average CSW in Pumwari had four clients per day. This intervention prevented an estimated 6,000 to 10,000 HIV infections per year, at a cost of approximately $10 per case of HIV infection prevented (Moses et al., 1991).

If, instead of targeting CSWs, 1,000 men had been randomly chosen from Nairobi and provided similar health services, and they had achieved the same rates of condom use, only a paltry 80 infections would have been averted annually (Altman, 1997). Here we see the advantages of intervening upstream in the process of an epidemic. Note that the Pumwari program provided other health services, in addition to just condoms, that the CSWs wanted (such as the health clinic and STD treatment), which also contributed indirectly to HIV prevention (STDs are a co-factor in HIV infection). We also see how much cheaper (and more humane) HIV *prevention* can be, compared to the *treatment* of infected individuals.

This chapter analyzes lessons learned about targeting HIV/AIDS programs to such unique populations as commercial sex workers, truck drivers, injecting drug users, and others. HIV prevention programs are often targeted to these high-risk populations, especially in the initial stages of the epidemic (Chapter 1). The purpose is to prevent HIV/AIDS from breaking out into the general population. Despite the obvious wisdom of this strategy, it has seldom been effectively followed. For example, during the early years of the epidemic in India, interventions were rarely targeted to high-risk groups. In 2002, an Indian government official concluded: HIV "is no longer confined to vulnerable groups, such as sex workers and transport workers, or to urban areas" (Ramasundaram, 2002).

Targeting in San Francisco

In the early days of the epidemic in San Francisco, in 1981 and 1982, considerable disagreement existed within the gay community about how to cope with HIV/AIDS. Some outspoken individuals questioned whether sexual behavior actually spread HIV (they suspected that straight society was using the AIDS threat to close the San Francisco bathhouses, in order to limit the sexual freedom of gay men). Eventually, a certain degree of consensus was reached, and gay organizations pulled together to combat the epidemic through the STOP AIDS program. Many of the gay bathhouses were closed, not by edict of the county/city department of public health, but because the number of customers visiting them fell off sharply in the age of HIV. By 1993, only one of the dozen bathhouses in San Francisco was still in operation, and the rate of anonymous homosexual contact had decreased considerably.

The STOP AIDS Program

Soon after the epidemic got underway, gay men's organizations in San Francisco began to launch HIV prevention programs. The most noted, and effective, of these was STOP AIDS. This intervention program was founded by gay San Franciscans, and was based on social psychologist Kurt Lewin's small group communication theory and on diffusion of innovations theory (Rogers, 1995). Focus group interviews were initially conducted by STOP AIDS in order to assess how much gay men already knew about the epidemic, and what they wanted to know (Wohlfeiler, 1998). This formative research was carried out in order to design an effective intervention. Gradually, the STOP AIDS founders realized that the focus group interviews were having a strong educational effect on the participants, as group members exchanged useful information about HIV prevention. Volunteer leaders asked the group members: "What do you think about the safe sex guidelines? What makes them difficult to follow?" (Wohlfeiler, 1988, p. 233). Men were recruited on Castro and other streets in gay neighborhoods to attend the small group meetings that were held in homes and apartments. STOP AIDS employed a cadre of outreach workers to organize and lead these meetings.

STOP AIDS "relied heavily on diffusion theory, which suggests that only those early adopters, who make up a relatively small segment of the population, need to initiate a new behavior for it to spread throughout the population" (Wohlfeiler, 1998, p. 231). A well-respected individual who was HIV-positive led each small group of a dozen or so gay and bisexual men. The means of transmission of the virus were explained, and individuals were urged to use condoms and/or to seek monogamous partnerships. Questions were asked and the answers were discussed by the group. At the conclusion of the meeting, each member was asked to make a commitment to safer sex, and to volunteer to organize and lead future small group meetings of other gay men (such commitment, witnessed by other members of a group, is part of the Lewinian social psychology of individual behavior change).[1]

From 1985 to 1987, STOP AIDS reached 30,000 men through its various outreach activities, with 7,000 of these individuals participating in the small group meetings that launched the diffusion process in the gay community. A media campaign was aimed at the gay population of San Francisco to raise awareness-knowledge about HIV/AIDS. The number of new HIV infections dropped from 8,000 annually in the earliest years of the epidemic, to only 650 by the mid-1980s. Then attendance at the small group meetings fell off, and it became difficult for STOP AIDS to recruit fresh volunteers. The critical mass of early adopters of safer sex in the gay community had been reached, and the idea of safer sex would continue to spread spontaneously thereafter. STOP AIDS declared victory in 1987, and closed down its local operations. In 1990, however, STOP AIDS swung back into action in San Francisco in order to carry the safer sex message to new cohorts of younger gay men who were migrating to the city.

San Francisco was one of the first cities in the world in which prevention programs caused a major decrease in the rate of new HIV infections. Unfortunately, by the late 1980s, about half of the gay and bisexual men in San Francisco were infected and were on their way to AIDS-related deaths. Nevertheless, further infection was greatly slowed down. Why was STOP AIDS so successful in bringing about this massive sexual behavior change? This intervention (a) was highly targeted to a specific population of high-risk individuals; (b) was founded and implemented by respected leaders of the target community, rather than by "outside" professional organizers and educators; (c) depended mainly on volunteer leaders, which kept costs low; and (d) based itself on two theories of behavior change communication: Lewin's theory of small group communication and individual commitment, and Rogers's diffusion of innovations theory (1995). These theories provided a basis for the communication strategies utilized in the STOP AIDS intervention.[2]

Unfortunately, most intervention programs in the world have been designed in an ad-hoc manner, rather than conceptually. Hence, intervention programs do not benefit from behavior change communication theories.

A Proliferation of Prevention Programs

By 1993, when one of the present authors (Rogers) began investigating the relative effectiveness of HIV/AIDS prevention programs in San Francisco, there were an amazing 212 such programs (this in a city of only three-fourths of a million people). These programs had proliferated because each was highly targeted to a specific population. At this point, the epidemic had broken out of the initial high-risk population of gay and bisexual men, and had spread to other high-risk groups. For example, one of the prevention programs studied by Rogers was targeted to young Thai girls who worked in massage parlors and were also commercial sex workers. Another program was aimed at Deadheads (followers of the Grateful Dead rock musicians), who numbered only about 150 in San Francisco. Importantly, each such prevention program was typically organized and operated by members of the target audience. Thus, Filipino male commercial sex workers conducted a prevention program aimed at young Filipino men who hung out in "rice bars" in the city. Each of the 212 programs in San Francisco was an *intervention*, defined as actions with a coherent objective to bring about behavioral change in order to produce identifiable outcomes.

Funding for many of the 212 prevention programs was provided, at least in part, by the CDC, with funds channeled through the city's public health agency (Dearing et al., 1996; Rogers et al., 1995). One might wonder whether such a proliferation of prevention programs in San Francisco was an efficient use of public funds. Undoubtedly there was unnecessary duplication of efforts, and resources were wasted through competition between programs aimed at similar audiences. On the other hand, the high degree of targeting meant that the prevention programs were culturally sensitive to the target audiences.

Important problems facing highly targeted HIV prevention programs throughout the world are: (*a*) that they do not speak with one voice; and (*b*) that they waste resources by competing with each other. Usually, some sort of coordinating network or consortium is needed to integrate the diverse prevention programs.

The Targeting Strategy

Targeting is the process of customizing the design and delivery of a communication program on the basis of the characteristics of an intended audience segment (Dearing et al., 1996). The targeting strategy can emphasize cultural sensitivity, if the target audience is involved in the intervention program through formative research, as peer educators, and/or through advising the program's implementation. An example of such involvement in a program by means of formative research is provided by the Healthy Highways

Project with truck drivers in India, discussed later in this chapter. The STOP AIDS intervention in San Francisco was culturally sensitive because the prevention activities were designed and carried out *by* gay men *for* gay men, and were based on a detailed understanding of how gay men perceived the epidemic.

The ultimate targeting strategy is *tailoring,* in which a communication message is directed to an individual, who represents a very homogeneous audience indeed. Tailoring is made possible, in most cases, by the use of a computer (and perhaps the Internet) to store a large number of alternative messages on a topic like HIV prevention, and then to send one of the messages to an individual such that the message fits precisely with that individual's situation.

The high-risk groups that represent transmission hotspots may be concentrated in dense pockets, as was the case with gay men along Castro Street in San Francisco in the early 1980s, and with CSWs in Kolkata's red-light district, Sonagachi. Such spatial agglomeration enables programs to reach the members of particular populations with specialized messages, which can be a highly effective strategy for behavior change communication.

Targeting Hotspots

Ports, prisons, and peace-keeping locations represent hotspots of HIV infection, and also present opportunities for targeted interventions. Akin to commercial sex districts, seaports represent a spatial agglomeration of commercial sex activity and drug use. Ports bring together an explosive mixture of highly mobile single men: sailors, fishermen, migrant port workers, truckers, and security policemen. Alcohol and drug use are high among these high-risk groups, who routinely purchase commercial sex in the port's vicinity. In 2001, Population Services International (PSI) launched Operation Lighthouse in India, a highly targeted intervention in each of 12 Indian seaports, where a total of 200,000 migrant workers are employed (personal interview, Sanjay Chaganti, project manager, PSI, 20 December 2001).

Soldiers, whether involved in armed conflict or in peace-keeping, are at high risk for HIV infection (Fleshman, 2001).

Soldiers on duty — mostly young, single men — seek commercial sex and/or have relatively high rates of homosexual liaisons, which puts them at high risk for HIV transmission. Military culture tends to valorize toughness, aggressiveness, and risk-taking, perpetuating a sense of invincibility. Over 50 percent of Dutch soldiers on a five-month peace-keeping mission in Cambodia reported sexual contact with commercial sex workers. HIV infection rates among Nigerian soldiers who served as peace-keepers in other West African countries are double the national HIV seroprevalence rates.

Senegal has done a commendable job of keeping HIV infection rates low in its armed forces (Fleshman, 2001). The Senegalese army is the largest consumer of condoms of all armies in Africa. During peace-keeping missions, young recruits and experienced soldiers are educated about HIV, supplied with condoms, and screened for STDs. Targeted HIV prevention interventions to soldiers are critical, given their high degree of mobility, as well as vulnerability, across global borders.

Intervening Upstream

Among various target groups, *peer education programs among female sex workers have the highest impact in preventing HIV infection in developing nations* (Jha et al., 2001). The logic here is that most individuals have relatively few sexual partners, while a few individuals have many. Thus it is a wise use of limited resources to target behavior change interventions at CSWs rather than at their clients, as there are many fewer commercial sex workers. Of course, if resources permitted, *both* CSWs and their customers should be reached with HIV prevention messages, and this has been done in some settings. Commercial sex workers are a high-priority target group in almost every country, because they are "upstream" in the chain of HIV infection. Female CSWs infect men, who then infect their wives, who then infect their children when they are gestating, born, and breast-fed.

The consequences of changing the behavior of members of a high-risk group like commercial sex workers ripple out through a much larger population. For example, say that a communication intervention strategy like peer education leads one CSW in the Mumbai red-light district to begin using condoms with her customers. The average female CSW in Mumbai services about seven customers per day, so her adoption of safe sex is immediately magnified seven times through her sexual networks. Thus a given investment in targeted communication with CSWs may be leveraged many times in its ultimate effects. Peer educators (often former or present CSWs themselves, who have been given special training and supervision) operate on a one-on-one basis to reach the targeted CSW with a special message. Some of the more successful intervention programs are those targeted at commercial sex workers and their clients (Jha et al., 2001; Lamptey, 2002), as illustrated by the Pumwari program in Nairobi, Kenya (discussed at the beginning of the present chapter).

Program Effectiveness

Effectiveness is the degree to which an intervention program fulfills its objectives. If a peer outreach program with CSWs is intended to prevent HIV infection, then its effectiveness is measured as the degree to which this objective is achieved. Cost-effectiveness is calculated as the cost of each unit of behavior change achieved. For instance, the cost per HIV infection prevented is estimated at $8 to $12 for peer educator intervention programs with commercial sex workers (Jha et al., 2001).

Unfortunately, despite the fact that cost-effectiveness analyses have been conducted of interventions with various types of target groups (CSWs, truck drivers, injection drug users, etc.), the results of these analyses have often not been implemented in national AIDS control programs (Jha et al., 2001). Why not? One reason is that the most cost-effective interventions often lack advocates. Further, most countries lack adequate funding for full-scale implementation of even the most cost-effective interventions.

Homophily with Targeted Individuals

The relatively high degree of similarity of the individuals in a unique population, as compared with the much more diverse population of a nation, facilitates effective communication. Targeting communication messages at specialized audience segments is more efficient, and effective, than aiming communication messages at a general, and hence more heterogeneous, population. A communication message can be designed to be much more effective when it is targeted to a smaller, more homogeneous audience than when it is aimed at a nationwide, heterogeneous audience.

Homophily is the degree to which two or more individuals who communicate are similar. In the highly effective STOP AIDS prevention program in the early days of the epidemic in San Francisco, speakers at the small group meetings of gay men matched the characteristics of their audience. The presenters were young gay men who were respected opinion leaders in the gay community. Further, the speakers were usually HIV+, which meant they were perceived as highly credible. They knew what they were talking about concerning transmission of the virus. Their message, in part, was: "Don't do what I did. Practice safer sex."

Uniqueness is the degree to which an audience of relatively homophilous individuals differs from the larger population of which it is part (Dearing et al., 1996). High-risk groups targeted for HIV prevention interventions are examples of unique populations. Society perceives them as unique, and may stigmatize them (see Chapter 6). For example, in India, CSWs, truck drivers, and injecting drug users are all looked down upon by society. Partly as a result, the personal lives of high-risk audience segments for HIV prevention in many countries are colored by "hopelessness, despair, and bitterness" (Dearing et al., 1996). Outreach workers like peer educators are homophilous with their high-risk audience members, and do not share society's stigmatization of them. Being nonjudgmental is an essential quality of effective outreach workers.

Credibility of Peer Educators

Credibility is the degree to which a communication source is perceived as expert and trustworthy. Peer educators are selected because of their trustworthiness in the eyes of the intended audience members. Most peer educators in CSW interventions are former commercial sex workers; some continue sex work while also working as peer educators. Program experience has shown that their experience as commercial sex workers is essential to providing them with trustworthiness and credibility in the eyes of their target audience. Most sex workers are driven into their profession by poverty, and so both the peer educators and their audience members are homophilous in socioeconomic status.

When peer outreach workers begin their educational work, they are often given a brief training course about the means of HIV transmission, safer sex methods like condom use, and how to approach their intended audience members. Peer educators may distribute free condoms, or sell them at a subsidized price. The income from condom sales may constitute the peer educator's remuneration for her work. Peer educators often train CSWs in negotiating condom use with their customers.

Standard instructions for the peer outreach workers are to first develop a personal relationship with an audience individual (say, a commercial sex worker), to learn from the individual what his/her problems are, and to understand and accept the individual's situation. The peer educators must be non-judgmental, or interpersonal relationships with their clients will be ruptured. The process of getting acquainted with a commercial sex worker may take several weeks or months. Only then can the outreach worker effectively intervene with a social change communication message like practicing safer sex. Repeated contact (perhaps a dozen or more visits) with a target individual is usually necessary to change that individual's behavior.

Communication Networks

As discussed in Chapter 1, HIV spreads through interpersonal networks of transmission. The networks may involve sexual relationships among gay men, or the linking of a female commercial sex worker with her customers (Wolf et al., 2000). Examples of the network nature of HIV transmission cited previously included the CDC cluster study of 40 gay men in the United States (Klovdahl, 1985), and Jeff Kelly's study of the adoption of safe sex through the identification and training of opinion leaders in gay bars in American cities (Kelly et al., 1997).

One strategy that capitalizes on the network nature of HIV transmission is to utilize peer educators, especially if opinion leaders among the target population are selected. In a practical sense, this strategy means that outreach workers (a) must be selected from among the target audience (for example, peer educators among CSWs must themselves be former or present commercial sex workers), and (b) should be regarded as trusted sources/channels of communication about HIV prevention. The peer educators may use themselves as negative role models if they are HIV+ (that is, they tell their clients not to do what they did).

One type of network link, the bridge, is particularly important in HIV transmission networks. Bridges connect high-risk groups with the general population. Thai men who had commercial sex and then had intercourse with their wives played a bridge role in spreading HIV infection in Thailand (Morris, 1997). Another example of a bridge link is an injection drug user who conveys the virus to a member of the general population through heterosexual intercourse.

The Network Nature of HIV Transmission

One example of interpersonal networks among injection drug users is provided by Dr. Tom Valente's study of the Baltimore Needle Exchange Project. Valente, a communication network scholar, was a professor of public health at Johns Hopkins University in 1994, when he began using bar codes to identify each clean needle that was distributed free in the city's program for injection drug users. Each month, 200,000 clean needles were distributed, and almost as many were returned at various points in the city's drug-infested central core. Valente et al. (1998) found that 5,369 individuals participated in the needle exchange project from 1995 to 1997.

Valente constructed a huge network matrix, composed of the 5,369 individuals to whom the clean needles were given versus the 5,369 people who returned them (sometimes this was the same person). Opinion leaders in the network were people who distributed the clean needles to many others. Some 64 percent of all the needles were distributed by only 9 percent of the drug users, who were called "satellite exchangers." The clean needles, which were distributed at no cost, were then sold on the street for about one dollar each. Thus, entrepreneurship characterized the satellite exchangers.

About 20 clean syringes were given to an individual on each visit to the project. The average injection drug user used 149 syringes during the two years of study. But the typical satellite exchanger handled 1,046 syringes!

The network nature of needle exchange in Baltimore suggested entry points for outreach workers to promote HIV prevention through the distribution of clean needles.

Harm Reduction among Intravenous Drug users

Intravenous (IV) drug use represents the primary mode of HIV transmission in certain areas (Inciardi, 1992). For instance, in India's north-eastern states of Manipur, Mizoram, and Nagaland, which are in close geographical proximity to the drug-rich Golden Triangle Area of northern Thailand, Myanmar, and Laos, seroprevalence rates among injecting drug users (IDUs) are as high as 50 percent. HIV rates are also soaring in the former Soviet republics, driven by unchecked IV drug use and a paucity of harm reduction programs. In the Ukraine, HIV seroprevalence among IDUs was 2 percent in 1995. A year later, it had soared to an unbelievable 57 percent (Altman, 1997).

In Poland, a country with over 60,000 IV drug users, and where over half of new HIV infections occur among IV drug users, various harm reduction programs are underway. One of these intervention programs is located in a city square between Warsaw's main train station and the Holiday Inn Hotel. Disposable syringes and needles, bandages, condoms, bleach, and antiseptic are distributed to drug addicts at an appointed time every evening (Pasek, 2001). This harm reduction program employs the principle of "one for one plus one": Drug users collect used needles and exchange them one-for-one for new needles. In addition, they get one additional needle. This policy makes drug users "partners" in the needle exchange process, and reduces the incidence of needle reuse and inappropriate disposal. Jack Charmast, a supervisor of Warsaw's Streetworker Association, noted the behavior changes spurred by this harm reduction program:

"I remember times when junkies were sharpening needles on a box of matches" (quoted in Pasek, 2001, p. 18).

Amsterdam's methadone-by-bus project is a traveling harm reduction program. Buses operated by health authorities, NGOs, and private foundations visit locations around the city, dispensing methadone (a detoxification agent) to drug users, and provide clean needles, syringes, condoms, and other medical services. Bureaucratic procedures are kept to a minimum, preserving the anonymity of clients, and a comfortable, non-judgmental atmosphere is created in which intravenous drug users feel "safe" (Kapila & Pye, 1992).

The Opinion Leader Strategy

One communication strategy that takes advantage of the network nature of the epidemic's spread is to utilize *opinion leaders,* defined as individuals who are sought by others for information and advice about some topic (Rogers, 1995). Several of the early HIV/AIDS prevention programs in San Francisco, such as STOP AIDS, utilized the opinion leader strategy in their outreach efforts to control the epidemic (Chapter 1). For example, the director of one prevention program in San Francisco told us: "Well, you don't have to target everybody for a new idea [HIV prevention] like ours. Some people are just naturally going to pick it up and do it and talk about it . . ." (quoted in Dearing et al., 1996).

The effectiveness of the opinion leader approach rests on the degree to which program staff are able to select the most influential opinion leaders in a target audience. In the 1980s in San Francisco, identification of opinion leaders was not particularly difficult, as high-risk gay men lived in intact urban communities. Knowing who was especially influential in such dense, well-connected networks was fairly easy. As one program official told us: "Well, he's [an opinion leader] just such a good spokesperson for this [HIV prevention] because everybody really respects him because of what he's done for the Castro" (quoted in Dearing et al., 1996). Gay bars offered a convenient site in which to identify opinion leaders. "We watch in gay bars and approach the guys who are the most popular" (Dearing et al., 1996).

Dr. Jeffrey Kelly and his associates at the Center for AIDS Intervention Research at the Medical College of Wisconsin, in Milwaukee, utilized the opinion leadership strategy, first in a series of interventions in U.S. cities, and later in five developing nations. Bartenders were enlisted to help identify opinion leaders in gay bars in U.S. cities. These influential individuals were then trained in the means of HIV transmission, methods of practicing safe sex, and in how to communicate such preventive information to their followers. Free condoms were also made available in the gay bars. Results of these opinion leader interventions showed a measurable decrease in infection rates in the intervention cities, compared to a set of control cities (Kelly et al., 1991, 1997).

Jeff Kelly and a set of collaborators are currently testing the opinion leadership strategy in 30 poor neighborhoods in Chennai, India; large apartment buildings in St. Petersburg, Russia; 32 villages in Zimbabwe; market centers in Fujan, China; and in several cities in Peru (Chapter 8). Funding for this series of experimental evaluations of the opinion leader strategy is provided by the National Institute for Mental Health (NIMH). One of the present authors (Rogers) is a consultant to this multi-site research project that tests the opinion leadership strategy.

Commercial Sex Workers

In the course of writing this book, the authors studied numerous intervention programs for HIV prevention among CSWs, in part because such interventions are so ubiquitous. Today they are found in every city of each developing nation. In the early stages of the epidemic, in most countries, commercial sex workers and their clients are (a) the largest population at risk for HIV infection, and (b) the major disseminators of the virus to others (Ngugi et al., 1988).

Some CSW prevention programs that we studied were outstanding in their ingenuity, intensity, and effectiveness. Others were less so. The ideal intervention program should: (a) effectively select and train peer educators so that they have a high potential for influencing others; (b) provide condoms free or at a subsidized price in order to decrease susceptibility to HIV and other STDs (an important co-factor in HIV infection); and (c) make available literacy classes, health clinics, savings plans, and other services that CSWs value. Out of the variety of CSW intervention programs in diverse countries, we focus here on three programs in India, one in each of three major cities: Mumbai, Chennai, and Kolkata. These intervention programs differ widely in their effectiveness. For example, HIV prevalence among CSWs in Mumbai increased from 1 percent in 1986 to 45 percent in 1993, and to 72 percent in 1997. Meanwhile, HIV prevalence in Kolkata increased from 0 percent in 1986 to 2 percent in 1993, and then leveled off (Salunke et al., 1998). What explains these extreme differences?

Mumbai: Epicenter of the Epidemic

Half of all HIV-positive people in India live in the state of Maharashtra, and many are concentrated in its main city, Mumbai, which has a total population of 12.5 million. Mumbai is the epicenter of the AIDS epidemic in India. The biggest red-light district in the world, including 70,000 commercial sex workers, is located here. Police harassment and the fear of HIV infection in recent years led some thousands of CSWs to move out of the main red-light area in south Mumbai to two other locations in the city, Turbhe in Vashi and Hanuman Tekdi in Bhiwandi.

In the early evening, taxis filled with CSWs can be seen leaving Kamathipura, Falklands Lane, Kennedy Bridge, and other areas in Mumbai's main red-light district. They are heading for hotels and other locations throughout the city. Throngs of men begin pouring into the red-light district, starting at sunset. Different areas in the red-light district are known for their specialties: "Number 1" (vaginal sex), "Number 2" (anal sex), and "Number 3" (oral sex). The streets are differentiated by price, with the youngest and fairest-skinned CSWs charging the highest prices, up to $40 a night. The lowest price is about 50 cents per sex act.

Mumbai has more migrant workers than any other Indian city, and they form the main customer base for the sex industry. The profile of a migrant worker in Mumbai would be along the following lines: a young man in the 17 to 30 age range, doing manual work 12 to 14 hours per day, and living in a small, cramped room in a *chaal* (a dormitory-style building). The migrant worker has no access to health care, and may have only sparse or incorrect knowledge of HIV/AIDS. The migrant worker may have an STD, which increases the likelihood of his becoming HIV-infected. Once or twice a year, the migrant worker returns to his home place, where he may infect his wife.

The Process of Empowerment of CSWs: Commercial sex workers in Mumbai typically pass through a gradual process of increasing self-empowerment during their years in the red-light district. Many CSWs come to Mumbai from other states in India; therefore, they do not initially know the language spoken in Mumbai (Marathi). The present authors began a group interview with a dozen women in the red-light district by asking them where they were from: Karnataka, Nepal, Andhra Pradesh, West Bengal, Uttar Pradesh, some from Maharashtra. When they began sex work, these women were under the total control of a brothel owner. Many CSWs in Mumbai spend their workdays in zoo-like cages (they are called "cage girls").

Gradually, the typical sex worker gains a certain degree of independence, perhaps entering into a 50–50 arrangement with the brothel owner during her second year in the Mumbai red-light district. Sometimes the sex worker attracts a partner/pimp, often referred to as a "husband." The sex worker may have one or more children. By the third year or so, the typical sex worker may leave the brothel and work on her own. By this time, the sex worker is almost certainly HIV-positive. These women are often stigmatized, mistreated, or turned away from government health clinics, so they self-medicate with drugs purchased from pharmacies or on the street. Many phony doctors practice in the red-light district, dispensing expensive bogus cures. When a CSW begins to lose her health, from AIDS-related illnesses, she is likely to be thrown out of the sex business, and forced to fend for herself somehow.

The flourishing sex trade in Mumbai is operated by a brutal, powerful mafia. When Population Services International (PSI), the largest social marketing organization in the world, launched its Red-Light District Project in Mumbai in 1988, PSI officials had to meet with the mafia bosses to explain that their program sought to prevent HIV infection (which would be good for business), and that they would not urge CSWs to leave their profession. The home-grown Mumbai mafia forces brothel owners to pay them protection money, and may assist a brothel owner in squeezing a competitor out of business. Organizing commercial sex workers in Mumbai has generally been very difficult or impossible (in sharp contrast to the experience in Kolkata's red-light district).

The PSI Project: Arupa Shukla, project manager for the PSI Red-Light District Project in Mumbai, selects, trains, and supervises a cadre of peer educators (Plate 4.1). Most are former CSWs, and some are HIV+. The project headquarters is on the second floor of an old building in a poor neighborhood in the heart of the main red-light district. The peer educators are somewhat older than the average CSW, perhaps in their early 30s. They speak a variety of Indian languages, in addition to Marathi. An important factor in their effectiveness is their ability to talk with CSWs in their native tongue, so as to develop a relationship of trust.

The peer educators wear bright yellow shirts with the PSI logo, and wear identification cards around their necks (this bestows prestige, makes them look official, and enables them to deal more effectively with police harassment). Their only pay is the modest earnings from their sale of "Masti" (fun) condoms, the brand supplied by PSI. They urge CSWs to use condoms with their customers, and train sex workers in negotiation skills. Population Services International estimates that their peer educators have contacted over 30,000 CSWs in Mumbai over the past decade.

Social marketing is the use of strategies adapted from for-profit commercial marketing to the non-profit marketing of condoms, oral contraceptives, oral rehydration therapy (ORT), and other means of improving health (McKee, 1994; UNAIDS, 1998c). Population Services International was founded in 1970 by two public health students at the University of North Carolina, Dr. Tim Black and Phil Harvey. Both were experienced in developing countries, and soon PSI launched social marketing projects in Latin America, Africa, and Asia. Today, PSI is involved in HIV prevention throughout the world, mainly through social marketing programs for condoms (Harvey, 1999).

The PSI social marketing project in Mumbai operates a well-baby clinic, provides medical care for STDs and tuberculosis, and makes referrals to hospitals. Literacy classes are offered, and peer educators urge CSWs to start a savings account (some 5,000 such

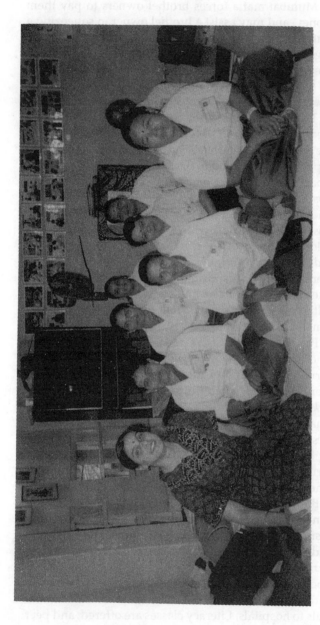

Plate 4.1 Ms. Arupa Shukla (Extreme Left) of PSI and Peer Educators of the PSI Red-Light District Project in Mumbai

The peer educators wear yellow shirts and carry identification cards as they contact commercial sex workers in one-on-one communication. These peer educators are former CSWs, and several are HIV-positive. Here the peer educators meet with Shukla in a weekly staff meeting.

Source: Personal files of the authors.

accounts have been established in the past decade of outreach programs in Mumbai). Peer educators help the CSWs buy sewing machines and develop other income-generating activities, so that they can someday leave the sex industry, hopefully before becoming HIV-positive.

Chennai: The CHES Program

Unlike Mumbai and Kolkata, there is no single, geographically concentrated red-light district in Chennai, the capital of Tamil Nadu state and an important metropolitan center in India. Instead, the sex industry is scattered throughout the city. A survey of 400 CSWs in Tamil Nadu found that 61 percent were full-time sex workers, with 12 percent also selling flowers, fruits, or vegetables. Some 11 percent of CSWs also worked as housemaids, and 6 percent were employed in the film industry (APAC, 2001a). Nineteen percent were illiterate, 27 percent had less than an elementary school education, and 43 percent had an elementary school education. An impressive 91 percent of the commercial sex workers were using condoms in 2000, up from 56 percent in 1995.

We visited Community Health Education Society (CHES), an NGO headed by Dr. P. Manorama, a pediatric gastroenterologist who was earlier pursuing a rewarding career in a government hospital in Chennai. Then, in 1993, her hospital refused to treat two HIV-positive children. So she adopted them. Then she hired some female CSWs who were HIV+ to help care for the children when she could not be at home. By 1995, she had resigned from her hospital appointment, and started CHES. Soon this NGO was offering testing, counseling, home care for people living with AIDS, an orphanage for AIDS orphans, and an HIV prevention program for men and women in the garment industry.

Its Project Thozhi (Girlfriend) employs 30 peer educators (who are themselves former CSWs) for outreach to the commercial sex workers in the area of Chennai in which CHES is responsible for HIV prevention. This area, about one square mile, has been mapped to identify the location of brothels and other sites in which sex work takes place (Plate 4.2). The map is covered with dozens of spots, squares, and other symbols, indicating various types of sex work:

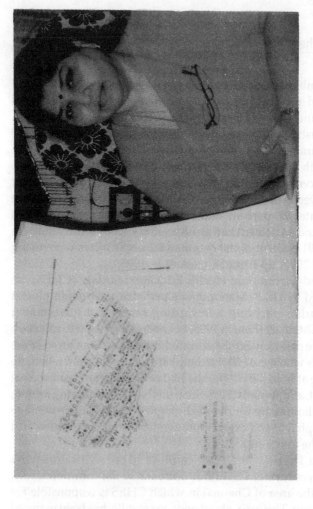

Plate 4.2   A Map of the Muthialpet-Kothwal Chavdi Area in Chennai is Held by Dr. Manorama, Director of CHES, Showing the Locations in which Commercial Sex Work Takes Place

The map depicts 28 pick-up points, 3 brothels, 4 lodges (hotels), 81 street sex workers, and 3 key informers. An initial mapping of this area facilitated the targeting of commercial sex workers in this section of Chennai by CHES peer educators.

Source: Personal files of the authors.

pick-up points, brothels, street workers, and lodges (hotels). Dr. Manorama also told us about mobile sex (in vehicles), and sex in movie theaters. The latter technique consists of the sex worker waiting near the back of a movie hall until she spots a male sitting alone. While the audience is involved in the film, the sex worker performs fellatio on her client. Sometimes sexual intercourse may take place. Then the CSW moves to another man, sits beside him, and rubs against him. With luck, the sex worker can service three or four customers during a two-hour film.

Peer educators of the CHES told the present authors that typically they needed about one month in order to persuade a commercial sex worker to use condoms with her customers. Often the relationship begins with the outreach worker offering a free condom to a female sex worker. After a dozen contacts or so, in which the peer educator becomes acquainted with the CSW's situation and her needs and aspirations, the outreach worker tries to persuade the CSW to practice safe sex. The peer educators are each equipped with a tiny 3-by-4 inch flipchart, similar to the larger flipcharts used by other types of peer educators (Plate 4.3). The 34 pages of the flipchart deal with using condoms, practicing safer sex, and avoiding unwanted pregnancy. The diminutive size of the flipchart enables CHES peer educators to use it in a clandestine manner with CSWs, often while being observed by police, customers, and others on the streets of Chennai.

The CHES peer educators are volunteers who may earn a small income from the sale of condoms. They receive family health care from CHES, help with their children's education, and a cash award for outstanding performance, such as identifying CSWs who have STDs. The fact that the peer educators are volunteers undoubtedly adds to these outreach workers' credibility in the eyes of their clients.

Commercial sex workers in Chennai have a tradition of collaborating for mutual benefit. For instance, the CSWs in a neighborhood may arrange for a *caragu* (eagle) to warn them when a policeman is approaching. The CHES peer educators encourage CSWs to band together, such as by organizing 50 or so CSWs into a *sangam* (society). This neighborhood association of sex workers may engage in income-generating activities, organize a savings system, and go together to a health clinic for monthly check-ups. The CHES peer educators may encourage CSWs in a *sangam* to teach each other

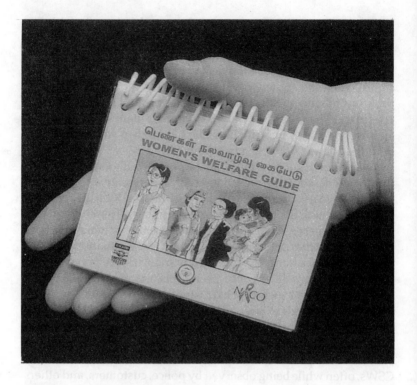

Plate 4.3   A Tiny 3-by-4-inch Flipchart is used by CHES Peer Educators
to Promote the use of Condoms, and to Educate on how to Avoid
Unwanted Pregnancy and STDs

The diminutive size of the flipchart allows the CHES peer educators to use
it in a clandestine manner with CSWs, so as not to draw the attention of the
police, customers, and others on the streets of Chennai.

Source: AIDS Prevention and Control (APAC) Project of the U.S. Agency for
International Development (USAID).

beauty tips, so that they are more attractive and can charge their
customers higher rates. The peer educators treat the CSWs like
girlfriends, which is why the prevention program is called Project
Thozhi. There is solidarity among the peer educators and between
them and the commercial sex workers. They believe that AIDS is
everybody's problem, and hence that collective action is required
(Plate 4.4).

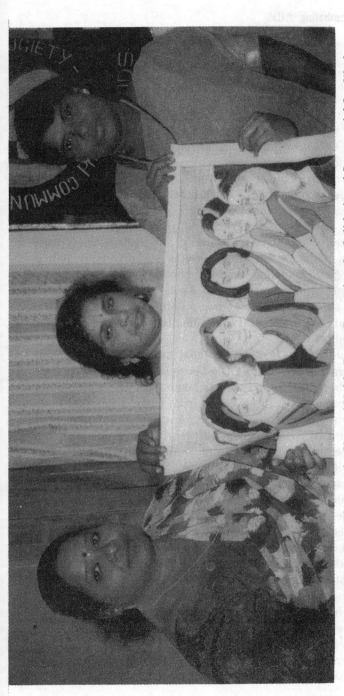

Plate 4.4 Three CHES Peer Educators in Chennai Hold a Poster Promoting the Solidarity of Commercial Sex Workers

These peer educators, former (or current) commercial sex workers, belong to a kind of informal labor union that promotes self-efficacy, which undoubtedly adds to their credibility.

Source: Personal files of the authors.

Kolkata's Empowered CSWs

The capital of West Bengal is a city with a history of powerful labor unions and a leftist (Communist) government. Some 6,000 CSWs in the Sonagachi red-light district in Kolkata (previously Calcutta) are organized in a strong labor union, the Women's Collaborative Committee, formed in 1995. This unique organization has 30,000 members, each of whom pays dues of 50 cents per year. This labor union of CSWs in Kolkata fights against police harassment, provides schools for the children of commercial sex workers, and creates savings plans for its members. The labor union is enterprising; in 2001 it smuggled Raja family planning condoms from Bangladesh, a neighboring country, into Kolkata, so that CSWs would have adequate supplies for use with their customers. The typical CSW in Kolkata keeps a small stash of condoms under her pillow.

Guided by Dr. Smarajit Jana, the slight, mustachioed epidemiologist in charge of the Sonagachi Project, the Women's Collaborative Committee has taken the lead in promoting condom use, which increased from 3 percent in 1992 to 90 percent in 1998 (Dugger, 1999). As a result, only 5 percent of Kolkata's CSWs are HIV-positive, while in Mumbai the comparable figure is 70 percent. The HIV prevention program in Kolkata employs 180 CSW opinion leaders and 100 other outreach workers, each paid about one dollar a day, and operates 12 health clinics for commercial sex workers, funded by the Indian Ministry of Health. Wearing green medical jackets over their saris, CSW opinion leaders tell brothel "madams": "If you are to enjoy the fruits of the tree, you must keep the tree healthy" (Dugger, 1999, p. A1). The total cost of the intervention program with CSWs is $210,000 per year. Through the committee, commercial sex workers in Kolkata have become leading crusaders against HIV infection.

The contrast between the Mumbai and Kolkata CSW intervention programs is instructive. The relatively effective prevention intervention in the latter city is based on creating and maintaining a feeling of female empowerment, an approach that is impossible in Mumbai as a result of the existing social structure. In Kolkata, CSWs talk openly in front of their brothel madams; in Mumbai, CSWs listen attentively or speak quietly. In Kolkata, CSWs wear "decorous saris in muted colors and look like office workers waiting impassively at a bus stop." In Mumbai, in contrast, the CSWs wear "shiny red lip gloss, midriff-baring halters, skintight velvet pants, and gaudy saris. They pose aggressively with their faces set in a sulky come-on" (Dugger, 1999, p. A1).

The CSWs in Kolkata are *organizing for social change*, the process through which a grouping of disempowered individuals gains control of their future. An individual sex worker in Kolkata has little power to change her life conditions; but, organized collectively, the female CSWs have accomplished a great deal. Hundreds of CSWs regularly *gherao* (encircle) the local police station, demanding action against pimps, hoodlums, and criminals who harass them. Sonagachi CSWs routinely intervene to rescue child prostitutes who are sold into the sex trade. In 1995, child prostitutes under the age of 19 constituted 20 percent of CSWs in Sonagachi. In 1998, with the organized intervention of CSWs, this number had dropped to 3 percent (Dugger, 1999).

Kolkata's approach in Sonagachi emphasizes the prevention of HIV infection, which negates the need for large-scale treatment programs. This approach is efficient, as prevention is much cheaper than treatment.

The Healthy Highways Project in India

In India, as in many African nations, truck drivers and their helpers are an important means through which HIV spreads geographically. The 3.5 million truck drivers in India are a high-risk group because of their numerous sexual contacts with commercial sex workers (Plate 4.5). Truckers may frequent the red-light districts of large cities like Mumbai (some 10,000 truckers arrive daily in Cotton Green, the city's huge truck terminus, the largest in India), but more often they have sex at truck stop *dhabas* (roadside stalls where one can eat, drink, and rest). Thousands of these truck stops are located along the major highways of India.

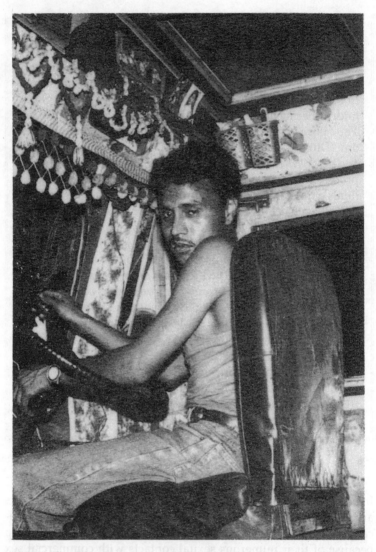

Plate 4.5   A Truck Driver on the Highway between India and Nepal

Truck drivers, like the young driver in this photo, are on the road, away from their spouses, for 25 days per month. They purchase commercial sex almost on a daily basis along the national highways. The truck's cab is decorated with pictures of family, deities, and other memorabilia, and is considered sacrosanct. Sex almost always occurs outside the truck in India.

Source: Family Health International. Photograph by Mary O'Grady.

A truck driver and his helper, often a teenage boy who aspires to become a driver someday, may get down from their vehicle after eight to 10 hours of driving, tired and hungry. While the truck is being serviced, the driver avails himself of food, alcohol, a bath, sex, and sleep. The CSW may be supplied by the owner of the *dhaba*, or she may be a freelance sex worker. Perhaps she is a housewife living nearby. The come-on may be subtle, perhaps a slight lifting of skirts or sari, a bangle left on a bench, or a ribbon tied to a tree branch, indicating a location at which sex is available. Most truck drivers consider frequent sex while on the road, away from their wives and families, a necessary part of their masculinity. Sex with a commercial sex worker never takes place in the truck cab, which is considered by truckers to be sacrosanct. It is often decorated with photographs of the trucker's wife and family, and/ or of religious symbols. Most truckers are heterosexual, but some have sex with their helpers. Trucker lingo for men having sex with men (MSM) is "reverse gear," while sex with female CSWs is "forward gear."

Learning to Think Like a Truck Driver

When the nationwide Healthy Highways Project (HHP) began in 1997, funded by DFID (the British international aid agency), one of the first surprises facing the project staff was that the truck drivers did not *want* to be helped! Some truck drivers protested against being singled out as HIV carriers. Dr. Jyoti Mehra, former technical consultant for the project, when we met with her in Delhi (personal interview, 19 December 2001), remembered that the project staff members had to first learn "to think like a truck driver." Only then could they begin to plan an effective intervention for HIV prevention with their target audience. Extensive formative research, including survey interviews and focus group interviews, was conducted. The findings were highly revealing with respect to the occupational subculture of Indian truck drivers. For instance, when truck drivers were queried as to how they could have sex in thorny bushes under a roadside tree, a typical reply was: "Bed? What bed? Her [the CSW's] body serves as the bed." When asked why they did not get their STDs (called *garmi*, literally "heat" in Hindi) treated, the truck drivers replied: "What's the point? We sit behind the truck engine for 10 hours every day. We are bound to have heat [*garmi*]." Despite the formative research results, it was not easy for the project designers to think like a truck driver.

One problem was that India's truck drivers are culturally very diverse, speaking different languages and sharing little except their common occupation. Many drivers are from northern India, especially the state of Punjab, and many are Sikhs. But many are not. So the target audience for the Healthy Highways Project was not culturally homogeneous. This diversity meant that all project materials had to be produced in several languages, and had to avoid any cultural indicators, such as clothing, facial shape, or skin color.

In the pilot phase of the Healthy Highways Project, truckers were contacted mainly at truck stop *dhabas* by outreach workers from 40 NGOs, who partnered in the HHP. These NGOs had previously been involved in family planning, reproductive health, and other such health services, and thus had experience in behavior change communication activities. However, most of the outreach workers were young men who had not been truckers, so they were not perceived as homophilous by the truckers. The truck drivers resisted these Young Turks who descended on them as soon as they parked their trucks at a *dhaba*, giving them no time to unwind after driving for up to 10 hours. The outreach workers were not viewed as *peer* educators, and their activities were perceived as an "intrusion" into the daily life of the truck drivers. At this early stage, the Healthy Highways Project had a high volume of contact with the truckers, but few were persuaded to adopt safer sex. The pilot phase of HHP yielded many lessons for refining the outreach intervention. For example, the outreach workers might have been perceived as more credible if they had worked with truckers or former truckers in outreach teams.

Refocusing through Formative Research

A health communication expert, Rosemary Romano, helped HHP create a strategy document for behavior change communication.[3] Workshops were held with project staff to sharpen the intervention. After this thorough stock-taking, consensus was reached about the next steps to be taken. Lintas advertising agency was contracted to create a set of colorful flipcharts for the project's 500 outreach workers to use with small groups of truck drivers at *dhabas*. An attractive logo in black on yellow, showing a curving highway (Plate 4.6), was designed, and used to color-brand all project materials.[4] The flipcharts, comic books, and other materials featured two stylized characters, "Ustaad" (literally "expert"), a driver wearing a scarf around his head, and "Vijay," his young helper. The flipcharts showed Ustaad pulling out a condom before sex with a CSW (Plate 4.7). The virus was depicted in the flipcharts and other message materials as a spiny round object in the body, with an evil face (Plate 4.8). Such a depiction was not medically correct, of course (for example, the virus is actually far too tiny to be seen by the naked eye), but this symbol of the virus was easily recognized by the truckers. It communicated the idea of HIV to them. When these materials were pre-tested by Pathfinder, an Indian research agency, the truck drivers appreciated the materials; as did the outreach workers (personal interview, Jyoti Mehra, 19 December 2002).

On the back of each flipchart was printed a script that the outreach worker was to follow in the presentations to small groups of three or four truck drivers. In order to overcome the linguistic problem, the material was provided in several languages, all in phonetic spelling. What if a truck driver from Tamil Nadu were in the Punjab, where the outreach worker spoke only Punjabi? Or a Punjabi truck driver found himself in Andhra Pradesh where the outreach worker spoke only Telugu? In the latter case, the outreach worker would read the script in Punjabi, written phonetically in Telugu, thus helping to overcome the linguistic divide.

The Healthy Highways Project adopted a motto that was meaningful to the truck drivers: "Sex without condoms is like driving without brakes." This line was understood by truck drivers, and made sense to them. The main persuasive appeal to the drivers was to maintain good health for the sake of their families, so as not to infect their wives and unborn children. Maturer outreach workers were hired, whom the truckers perceived as much more credible. Healthy Highways posters, featuring Ustaad and Vijay, were put up at truck stop *dhabas*, and free condoms were distributed. A colorful comic book in several languages, depicting Ustaad and Vijay, was made available to the truck drivers.

The HHP, after a year or two of getting underway, began to interface more smoothly with the truck drivers. In some Indian states, especially in Tamil Nadu, Andhra Pradesh, and Karnataka, where

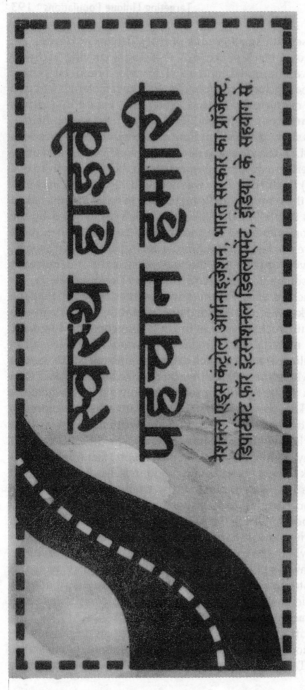

Plate 4.6 Logo of the Healthy Highways Project in India

This symbol of a curved (black) highway on a yellow background was pre-tested extensively with Indian truck drivers by project staff, and appeared on all project posters, flipcharts, and other messages. The caption in the Hindi language promotes the idea of healthy highways.

Source: Healthy Highways Project (NACO/DFID).

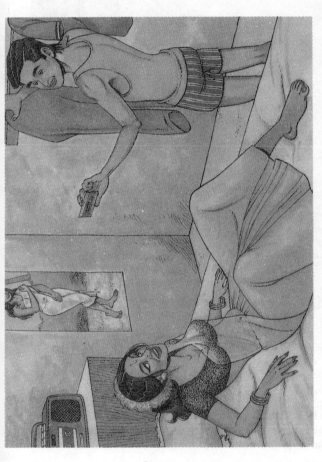

Plate 4.7 This Frame of the Healthy Highways Project's Flipchart Urges Truck Drivers to use Condoms with Commercial Sex Workers at a Truck Stop *Dhaba*

This frame was extensively pre-tested with truck drivers in India in order to determine the exact pose of the commercial sex workers, the provocative poster on the wall, and the facial appearance of the truck driver (to convey that he is an Indian, but not of an identifiable region). The striped undershorts are typical of those worn by truck drivers in India.

Source: Healthy Highways Project (NACO/DFID).

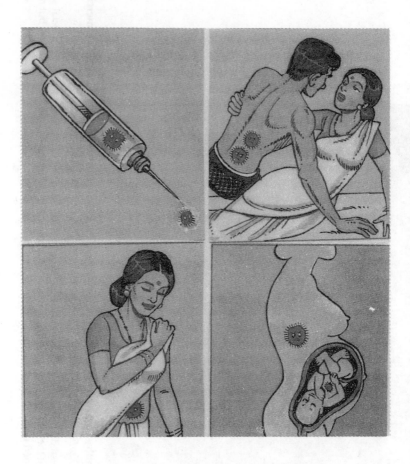

Plate 4.8   The HIV Virus is Depicted as a Large Spiny Organism in a Flipchart Frame for use with Truck Drivers by the Healthy Highways Project in India

The virus shown here is magnified greatly in order for truck drivers to understand the means of HIV transmission. Pre-testing of these messages indicated that the intended audience comprehended the virus when depicted in this form. In the flipchart, the virus symbol always appears in red, the color signifying danger.

Source: Healthy Highways Project (NACO/DFID).

NGO outreach workers were particularly well trained, the revised strategy for behavior change communication began to show the desired effects. The high rate of STD infections (around 20 percent of truckers in 1997) dropped to 10 percent in 2001 in Tamil Nadu. Condom use increased. However, in 2001, the nationwide Healthy Highways Project was decentralized by NACO, the National AIDS Control Organization of India, to each state's AIDS control society. The project lost momentum, except in states such as Tamil Nadu, and, unfortunately, trailed off to a premature death.

What lessons may be learned from the experience of the Healthy Highways Project in India? One conclusion is that the volume of individual communication contacts with target audience members is not necessarily a factor in the latter's adoption of safer sex. If the communication source is not perceived as homophilous, trustworthy, and expert, little behavior change will result. Formative research and the pre-testing of messages are important, if these messages are to make sense and to persuade their audience. High-quality and effective campaign materials do not come cheaply. The cost of the flipcharts and other campaign materials, including an audio cassette for each trucker, was high. The HHP experience also suggests that bureaucratic decisions, based on considerations other than program effectiveness, can derail a seemingly successful intervention.

Urban Slums

Kibera is one of the largest and most dismal slums in Africa. Located on the south-western side of Nairobi, this 300-acre (about half a square mile) slum is a breeding ground for all that is wrong with Kenya: its AIDS epidemic, violent ethnic animosities, and poor economic conditions (Lacey, 2001). Kibera is home to an estimated 1.5 million people. In fact, Kibera is so densely populated that for convenience people refer to various parts of the slum as "Bangladesh," "Soweto," and so forth.

More than half of Nairobi's residents live in slums like Kibera, in mud huts in the shadow of skyscrapers. The presidential palace of President Daniel Arap Moi, one of the wealthiest and most powerful of Kenya's 30 million people, overlooks Kibera.

A foreign news report described Kibera as follows: "Heaps of garbage litter the landscape. Toilets are such a rarity that most people simply use the ground. Electricity is a luxury, as is running water. Domestic violence is rampant, as are rape and incest. Diseases fester in the damp, overcrowded environment" (Lacey, 2001). Kibera is built on public land that has been overrun by squatters. As a result, people living in Kibera are not eligible for public services like garbage removal, water, or roads.

The present authors met Mrs. Anne A. Owiti, director of the Kibera Community Self-help Program (KICOSHEP), one of the largest NGOs in Kenya with 40 paid employees and 100 volunteers. This NGO is funded by Feed the Children, the Ford Foundation, and other private foundations. The CDC recently sponsored five HIV counseling and testing centers in Kibera that are operated by KICOSHEP. The NGO also provides seven centers in Kibera to care for AIDS orphans (Plate 4.9). Further, KICOSHEP distributes 30,000 condoms per month, mainly through 65 unemployed youth who charge a subsidized price (they get to keep the money from these sales). Owiti employs peer educators to promote safe sex for HIV prevention among the one hundred or so CSWs who inhabit one section of Kibera.

Owiti distributes local herbal therapies like aloe vera and ginger to HIV-positive people, along with medical drugs. During 2001, with Ford Foundation support, Owiti began providing a Chinese herbal medicine, *tabao*, which may be taken as a tea, an ointment, or in pill form. The herb seems to reduce the viral load of HIV+ individuals, and to have no side-effects (personal interview, 20 June 2001, Kibera, Nairobi). Owiti is evaluating the efficacy of *tabao* in an experiment that is currently underway in Kibera.

Using the Internet

The Internet has diffused very rapidly since 1989, first in North America and Europe, and had reached approximately 450 million people by 2002, with much recent growth in Asia (Singhal & Rogers, 2001a). The number of people living with HIV/AIDS who have Internet access must be fairly modest, given the relatively low socioeconomic status of most people living with HIV/AIDS, and the generally high status of those who have Internet access.

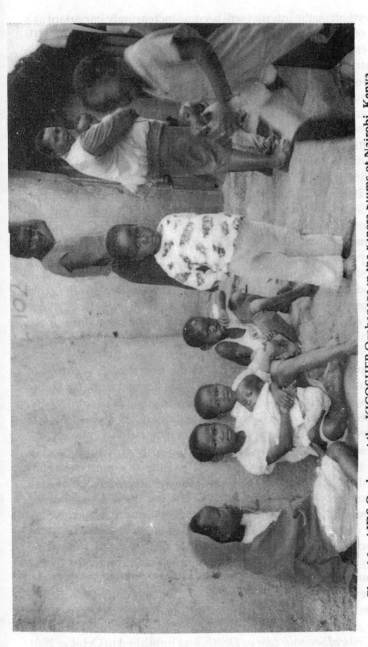

Plate 4.9 AIDS Orphans at the KICOSHEP Orphanage in the Kibera Slums of Nairobi, Kenya
Both parents of these children died from AIDS, and most of the orphans were born HIV-positive.
Source: KICOSHEP.

Nevertheless, the Internet will become increasingly important as a way of reaching certain target populations (like youth) with HIV prevention messages, at least in certain of the better-off developing countries (Reeves, 2000). Increasing numbers of young people in developing nations use the Internet at telecenters such as cybercafes and public access computer centers.

Some PWAs and their family members participate in on-line support groups. The Internet also links many NGOs in advocacy activities to combat the epidemic. Further, the Internet offers the potential of tailoring highly specialized messages to individuals, but this strategy has rarely been utilized in developing countries.

In 2001, the Romanian Society for Education on Contraception and Sexuality launched a website (www.sexdex.ro) to provide information and counseling to youth about STDs, unwanted pregnancies, and HIV/AIDS. It soon became one of Romania's most popular websites for youth, attracting over 100,000 hits during its first year (Dionisie, 2001). A medical doctor and a support staff provide confidential advice to visitors. The website also offers chat groups, a peer education forum, and links to other locally available HIV/AIDS services in Romania. The anonymous nature of the virtual interaction promotes an open discussion of taboo topics, creating a comfortable space for youth to regularly log on to.

A particularly fascinating use of the Internet has occurred in Thailand since March 2001. "Kaew" (not her real name), a young Thai woman with an M.A. degree from a prestigious Thai university, learned that she was HIV+ when she underwent a routine blood test demanded by her employer. Even before she told her family, she entered the following message on a website (www.pantip.com): "I have a little friend named HIV.... This little villainous friend has taught me a precious lesson, the value of life, the value of each passing second ...." Amazingly, she received 60 responses immediately. These e-mail messages were supportive and helpful; many came from HIV+ people.

Soon, Kaew was writing a daily diary online (www.kaewdiary.com). She told of how she was infected by her first and only boyfriend. Kaew described his growing thinness, dead eyes, and other symptoms, as he approached his death. Before he died, she forgave him for infecting her. Kaew's electronic diary drew media attention, and the interest of publishers. Her book, *The Critical Second: Life or Death*, was published in October 2001

(Plate 4.10). Within two months, the book (in Thai) was in its sixth reprinting and had sold 16,000 copies. By February 2002, Kaew's book was in its eighth edition.

Kaew continues her on-line diary on her website. On 17 December 2001, Kaew announced on her website that she was flying from Bangkok to Chiang Mai to participate in an international AIDS conference. Our Thai colleague in writing this book, Dr. Pat Chatiketu, attended a workshop session with a woman that he suspected was Kaew (she later confirmed by e-mail that it was she). Kaew reports that she is plump and in good health. She says that her viral load has remained low, although she is not taking anti-retrovirals or herbal therapy (she explains that eating cheesecake is her "drug" of choice).

Kaew wrote: "I can't fight alone. I have an overwhelming amount of support and encouragement from friends around the world . . . . Because of these friends, I have made it through the bad days."

Conclusions

Targeting is the process of customizing the design and delivery of a communication program on the basis of the characteristics of an intended audience segment. The targeting strategy has been widely utilized since the beginning of the AIDS epidemic in 1981 to reach high-risk populations. HIV prevention messages are aimed at these target audiences in order to slow or halt the spread of the virus to the general public. Because infection spreads mainly through sexual networks, using peer educators at key social locations in these networks can be an effective intervention for HIV prevention. Most HIV prevention programs concentrate on promoting condom use. Condoms can be an effective means of preventing HIV infection, but they have to be used.

While mass media communication can create awareness-knowledge of HIV/AIDS, and of the means of transmission, interpersonal communication with peers is essential to change risk behaviors. Exactly who the peer educators are, and how they are perceived by members of the target audience, determines the impact of such interventions. Evidence to date indicates that *peer educators, if carefully chosen, trained, and supervised, can be a cost-effective means of HIV prevention with commercial sex workers, and with*

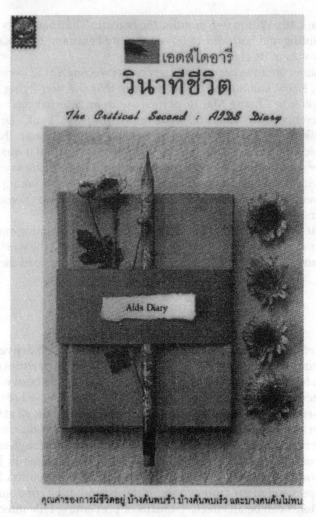

Plate 4.10   The Website for Kaew's *The Critical Second: Life or Death*

This cover page of Kaew's diary says: "Some find the value of being alive sooner, some later, and some never." The back cover of the book says: "I write a diary for remembrance because I don't know what else I could do . . . . My diary is available on-line and as a book. I hope that the diary will be helpful for others and will be something that people remember of me when I leave this world."

Source: Personal files of the authors.

other high-risk groups. Prevention is much cheaper and more humane than the treatment of infected individuals. But even in urban areas where effective peer education programs have been mounted, HIV continues to spread. This is discouraging.

Notes

1. Kurt Lewin was a German-born scholar who migrated to the United States in the 1930s in order to escape Hitler's fascism. Lewin fathered the modern field of social psychology.
2. Another behavior change theory, which was implicitly involved in the STOP AIDS program's use of opinion leaders, was Albert Bandura's (1986, 1997) social learning/social modeling/social cognitive theory. DiFrancisco et al. (1999) found that a national sample of 77 HIV prevention programs in the United States reported that Bandura's theory was the most widely used theoretical basis.
3. In addition, the Healthy Highways Project was guided by Project Officer Vidya Ganesh, and management consultant Dr. G. Balasubramaniam, in partnership with officials of NACO and DFID.
4. Yellow and black were used to mark Healthy Highways Project materials, including roadside signs close to truck stop *dhabas*, as signs using yellow and black also identify public call offices (PCOs) in India (Singhal & Rogers, 2001a). The PCOs mushroomed throughout India in the last decade, and many are visibly located along national highways where people stop to make telephone calls.

5

Cultural Strategies

■

The impact of AIDS is no less destructive than war itself, and by some measures, far worse.

United Nations Secretary General Kofi Annan (quoted in UNAIDS, 2000a, p. 39).

To prevent the spread of HIV/AIDS, you need behavioral change, and you can't have behavioral change without looking at people's cultural context.

Thoraya A. Obaid, executive director, United Nations Population Fund (quoted in Freeman, 2001, p. 13).

When the Dioro Child Survival Project[1] was begun in Mali in 1989 to reduce infant mortality and maternal deaths, formative research showed that Malian culture was both an ally and an enemy of the project's goals. The cultural ideal for a Malian husband was to be supportive of his wife during pregnancy. On the negative side, Malian Muslim culture proscribed discussion about the forthcoming birth between husband and wife. Talking about pregnancy was embarrassing for both men and women, and, as a result, women did not receive extra care from their husbands, nor added nutrition during pregnancy. This absence of spousal communication during pregnancy contributed to Mali having one of the highest infant and maternal mortality rates in the world.

Dioro Project authorities employed three traditional communication channels to overcome this cultural barrier: (*a*) a *pendelu*, a short cloth undergarment worn by married women, which, as a non-verbal and visual cue, symbolizes Malian marital roles, spousal duties, and privileges; (*b*) *griots*, who in Malian culture perform the roles of oral historians, praise-singers, social mediators, entertainers, and educators; and (*c*) folk songs, to promote improved maternal and child health, encourage communication between husband and wife, and increase pregnant women's utilization of health care services.

The communication campaign centered on creating a new visual symbol to represent pregnancy. When pregnant, Malian women were to change their traditional white *pendelu* into a green *pendelu*. Husbands could then play their idealized roles as protectors and supporters. Accordingly, the *griots'* songs encouraged Malian women to wear green *pendelus* during pregnancy, making their husbands aware of its symbolic meaning and of their accompanying spousal responsibilities.

Three months after launching the initial campaign in seven communities, spousal communication about pregnancy and maternal health rose from 3 percent of all spouses to 66 percent. About 90 percent of husbands, 80 percent of wives, and 77 percent of mothers-in-law reported knowing that the green *pendelu* represented pregnancy. When husbands were asked what they would do if their wives wore the green *pendelu*, 42 percent said they would immediately lighten their wives' workload, and 50 percent said they would ensure that their wives received good nutrition. Discussions of pregnancy were no longer taboo in the seven communities in which the green *pendelu* campaign was conducted.

The Malian case illustrates that, for health projects to be effective, the cultural values, beliefs, and practices of the targeted community need to be thoroughly understood. Only then can communication strategies accentuate the positive undercurrents of a culture, reducing (or completely overcoming) the effects of opposing forces.

This chapter analyzes the role of cultural values in HIV prevention programs to halt the spread of the epidemic. We begin by highlighting the limitations of the dominant biomedical approaches to HIV prevention, and then analyze the role of culturally based, participatory, and community-driven strategies for HIV/AIDS prevention. We review the strengths and weaknesses of each approach, calling for a more pluralistic strategy for preventing the epidemic.

Communication Challenges to HIV/AIDS

In the absence of a vaccine for therapeutic cure, communication strategies represent a key "social vaccine" against HIV/AIDS (*Population Reports*, 1989, p. 1). Communication is a necessary, but not a sufficient, condition for preventing HIV/AIDS, and for augmenting care and support programs. For communication professionals, combating HIV/AIDS presents challenges on four fronts:

1. Transmission challenges: HIV/AIDS is invisible, silent, and non-debilitating for many years, yet infectious. It can spread through multiple transmission modes, and does not discriminate on the basis of age, gender, religion, or geography. An unbelievable 90 percent of the 40 million people in the world who are HIV-positive do not know they carry the virus. The role of communication here is to help make the public knowledgeable about the existence of HIV/AIDS, the means of its transmission, and how to prevent infection.

2. Behavioral challenges: HIV/AIDS deals with human behaviors that often involve interaction between unequal parties (for example, an older paying client versus a poor young commercial sex worker); behaviors shaped by deep-rooted sociocultural traditions (for example, patriarchy and circumcision); behaviors that are private and personal (for example, sex, drug abuse); behaviors that are recurring (for example, condom use); behaviors that are highly functional in that they satisfy physio-logical, psychological, or socio-affiliative needs; beha-viors whose discussion is considered taboo by society; and behaviors that are moralized upon, stigmatized, and discriminated against by society. Here, communi-cation helps to create awareness of these inequalities, and to institute policies that may increase equality.

3. Response challenges: Efficacious responses to HIV/ AIDS involve the adoption of behaviors that depend on the compliance of more than one party (for example, condom use); behaviors that depend on the availability of products (for example, condoms) and services (for example, HIV testing); behaviors that are preventive in nature (for instance, adopting a behavior today to lower the probability of some future unwanted event); behaviors whose benefits are neither imminent nor clear-cut; behaviors whose execution is a non-event (that is, nothing happens immediately when one adopts it, so motivation for maintaining behavior change is low); and behaviors that involve foregoing or reducing pleasure and adventure. Here the role of communication is to convey the prevention message to the intended audience, and to bring about behavior change.

4. Targeting challenges: HIV/AIDS deals with populations that are often hard to reach by means of conventional media channels, such as individuals marginalized by society (for instance, gays, injecting drug users, commercial sex workers); those who are the most vulnerable and powerless (for instance, women and children); those of lower socioeconomic status (slum dwellers); those who are on the move (migrant workers, truck drivers) and are difficult to target (Svenkerud et al., 1998). Communication messages, such as from peer educators, can get through to these unique target populations.

The Biomedical Approach to Disease and Intervention

Medical school training primarily prepares doctors for private practice. About a hundred years ago, schools of public health began to be established to retrain medical doctors in sanitation, innoculation, public campaigns, disease eradication, and preventive health. Seldom can private practitioners make much profit from these public health activities. Their focus is on improving the public's health, rather than on providing private health care for profit. Today, university-based schools of public health around the world train a cadre of professionals, not only medical doctors but also many other types of health experts, including specialists in health communication. However, almost all schools of public health emphasize a biomedical approach to health interventions.

The biomedical approach focuses on the individual as the locus of a disease, and by default, of the intervention. An example of the biomedical approach to controlling an epidemic is provided by the CDC's method of attacking a health threat, such as a new disease. Epidemiologists seek to identify who is infected and to determine the means of transmission. Individuals are the units of analysis. It is assumed that the epidemic has biological causes, which can be controlled by a vaccine or some other intervention.

Epidemiologists are typically medical doctors who have completed additional training in public health (often a Master's degree in public health, or M.P.H.). Understandably, given their medical background, epidemiologists classify diseases by the human organ that is affected, such as the lungs or the stomach. They are trained to determine the biological pathways of transmission, called "vectors" by epidemiologists, such as whether a disease is waterborne or borne by insects. Epidemiologists, rather like medical detectives, search for any common exposure to a hazard that a set of individuals may have faced, such as to radiation or the anopheles mosquito. This basic approach to epidemiological analysis functioned effectively for many health problems in the past, such as malaria, the Ebola Virus, Legionnaires' Disease, and smallpox.

But there are unique factors involved in the case of HIV/AIDS. The social situation in which the infection occurs is very important. For instance, the spouse of a migrant worker can hardly say no to sex, when her husband, who may have been infected in the city, returns home after a long absence. The *context* of HIV/AIDS demands attention, along with biological vectors such as blood and semen. In recent years, UNAIDS pioneered an alternative to the biomedical approach to HIV/AIDS, as explained in a later section.

Problems with the Biomedical Approach in Zambia

A sound basis for any preventive health intervention is to conduct data-gathering on the nature of the epidemic, on how people are coping with it, and how their cultural customs affect the epidemic and its control. Unfortunately, the time and resources for such formative research are often not available in the early stages of an epidemic. But formative research should be carried out as soon as possible, and as thoroughly as time permits.

Several nations conducted surveys as a means of designing effective national AIDS control programs. A somewhat typical national survey was conducted in Zambia in 1998 with 3,695 men and women aged 15 to 49. Zambia is a relatively small African country of about 10 million people, with a very serious AIDS epidemic underway. The first AIDS case was identified in 1984; the epidemic then spread rapidly, first in urban areas and then to the rural countryside in the usual process of interiorization. National prevalence reached 20 percent of adults by 1998. About one million people in Zambia's population of 10 million are HIV-positive, and 500 new infections occur each day. About a hundred Zambians die daily from AIDS, including an average of three schoolteachers.

By the time of the 1998 survey, virtually all of the Zambian respondents had heard about AIDS, and most thought that HIV infection could be avoided. Despite this self-efficacious attitude on the part of the public, and an extensive HIV/AIDS communication campaign over several years, 25 percent of the survey respondents mistakenly thought that HIV could be transmitted by mosquitoes. Some 30 percent believed that HIV could be transmitted by witchcraft (Zambia Central Statistical Office & MEASURE Evaluation, 1999). These misconceptions, also found in other African nations, deserve attention in future prevention interventions.

Many Zambians perceived condom use, and reducing the number of their sexual partners, the two main safe sex behavior changes recommended by health/medical experts, as being of dubious value. Some 57 percent of the survey respondents said that using a condom during sex with an HIV-infected woman could not fully protect a man. Further, only 27 percent of the respondents believed that reducing their number of sexual partners would prevent HIV infection. Only 5 percent of respondents said that they had used a condom during their last sexual intercourse (this use rate was 33 percent for men having intercourse with non-marital partners, who in about half of these cases were commercial sex workers). As in Thailand, condom use was most common during sexual intercourse with strangers (like CSWs), and condoms were least often used with a regular partner or a spouse (Steinfatt, 2002).

Most Zambians who visited a health facility with a sexually transmitted disease received incorrect treatment (80 percent) and did not receive drugs, because of supply shortages. Perhaps as a result, 30 percent of the survey respondents had gone to traditional healers, and 25 percent bought drugs from pharmacies or street vendors. Four "mystery" clients (that is, individuals trained to act like typical patients) visited each of 77 pharmacies and chemists. These mystery clients had no trouble buying antibiotics and other drugs without prescriptions (often, these were inappropriate drugs for their mystery illnesses). In short, judged by almost any standard, health and medical services in Zambia for HIV-positive individuals were wretched. The average annual income in Zambia is $370, and the government can afford to spend only $14 per capita for health. The nation has only 200 medical doctors (Panos Institute, 2000).

HIV/AIDS prevention programs routinely advise women to negotiate sexual behavior with husbands/partners who are seropositive. Zambians thought that protection from being infected by a husband/partner could be achieved (a) by refusing sex, (b) by insisting on condom use, or (c) by taking medications. However, 74 percent of men and 70 percent of women felt that nothing could be done along these lines because of male dominance over women. Thus, for about three-fourths of all Zambians, sexual negotiation was not really an alternative to the risk of infection by one's husband/partner.

Certain cultural beliefs in Zambia encouraged the epidemic. For instance, when a married man dies, his widow must cleanse herself of his spirit by having sexual intercourse with one of her late husband's brothers or other male relatives. This traditional belief about purification, while slowly dying out, is particularly dangerous in spreading HIV infection. If the husband died from AIDS and his widow is HIV-positive, she may infect his brother or other male relative, who may in turn infect his wife and future children. A similar cultural belief among the Luo in Kenya is thought to be one reason for the extremely high rates of HIV/AIDS among this ethnic group, who live along the banks of Lake Victoria.

The survey in Zambia showed that people expressed a high degree of stigma toward HIV-positive individuals. Only 6 percent of the respondents said that they had had an HIV test and knew their serological status. Given the lack of drugs and other treatment measures in Zambia, perhaps many felt that it would be futile to know their HIV status. The strength of the stigma attached to AIDS inhibited people from taking HIV tests or from providing information about their seropositive status to the survey interviewers.

Some 70 percent of the survey respondents in Zambia knew someone who had died from AIDS. Such close personal contact with the epidemic's consequences exerts a powerful "educational" effect in Zambia, serving to convince sexually active individuals that they might be at risk for AIDS. Unfortunately, many Zambians, especially women, who perceived that they were at risk, felt they were helpless to prevent infection. Three-fourths of women did not believe they could negotiate with their husbands/partners. Almost 60 percent of men believed that using a condom was futile, and 73 percent felt that reducing their number of sexual partners was ineffective in preventing HIV. In any event, 30 percent of adult Zambians thought that HIV was transmitted by witchcraft.

How would you like the job of serving as director of the AIDS control program in Zambia?

Behavior Change Models

Behavior change models for HIV/AIDS communication programming (such as the health belief model, Prochaska's stages-of-change model, the theory of reasoned action, and McGuire's hierarchy-of-effects model) begin with ascertaining the knowledge, attitudes, behavioral intentions, and behavioral practices of individuals regarding HIV prevention, care, and support. Gaps in knowledge, attitudes, and behaviors among a target audience can be identified, and communication interventions are then targeted to addressing these deficiencies at the individual level. However, the results of behavior change communication strategies for HIV prevention that have targeted individuals have been mixed at best, and generally dismal (Airhihenbuwa, 1999). Why?

Behavior change communication strategies, by focusing solely on individual-level changes, subscribe implicitly to at least four mistaken assumptions:

1. Behavior change communication strategies assume that all individuals are capable of controlling their context.

However, whether or not an individual can get an HIV
test, use condoms, be monogamous, and/or use clean
needles is affected by cultural, economic, social, and
political factors over which the individual may exercise
little control.

2. Behavior change communication strategies assume that
all persons are on an "even playing field." However,
women and those of lower socioeconomic status are
more vulnerable to HIV/AIDS. When we visited South
Africa in June 2001, Thuli Shongwe, a health communication researcher based in Johannesburg, narrated to us
the helplessness faced by young girls in preventing date
rape. Her respondents exhibited resignation: "He took
me by force. . . . What could I do?" (personal interview,
7 July 2000).

3. Behavior change communication strategies assume that
all individuals make decisions of their own free will.
However, whether or not a woman is protected from
HIV is often determined by her male partner (as
illustrated by the Zambian case described earlier).

4. Behavior change strategies assume that all individuals
make preventive health decisions rationally. Why would
one logically put one's life in danger by engaging in
unsafe behaviors? A Kenyan youth whom we met in
Nairobi in June 2001 quoted a popular Kiswahili saying
to justify this non-rational action: "*Aliyetota hajui
kutota*," which means, "The one who is wet does not
mind getting wetter."

In any event, well-informed, rational intentions to use condoms
can often fall by the wayside during a passionate sexual encounter.
Physiological urges for sexual release may overwhelm previously
conceived rational intentions about "safe sex" (Singhal, 2001a).
Also, the focus on human cognitive processes underestimates,
understates, and overlooks the role of emotions in preventive health
behaviors. For instance, witnessing the death of a close friend from
AIDS, and/or seeing the grief of his or her parents, infected widow,
and child, can serve as a powerful trigger for adopting a prevention
behavior, much more so than rationally structured media messages
promoting condom use (Airhihenbuwa, 1999).

The Social and Cultural Construction of AIDS

Behavior change communication strategies are guilty of socially constructing HIV/AIDS as a life-threatening disease that is to be feared, and that results from the promiscuous and deviant behaviors of the "others," the high-risk groups (Paiva, 1995). Hence, past communication approaches have been mostly anti-sex, anti-pleasure, and fear-inducing. While "sexuality" involves pleasure, behavior change communication strategies have rarely viewed sex as play, as adventure, as fun, as fantasy, as giving, as sharing, as spirituality, and as ritual (Bolton, 1995). Behavior change theorists, in their models and frameworks, have failed to see how the social construction of "love" — which requires risk-taking, trusting, and giving — contributes to unsafe sex.

Because they are focused on biomedical concerns, most HIV/AIDS intervention programs rarely take into account how sexuality is socially and culturally constructed in a society. Hence, HIV/AIDS intervention programs are culturally rudderless and flying blind. Here, anthropologist Richard Parker's work on the social and cultural construction of sexual acts in Brazil is illustrative (Daniel & Parker, 1993; Parker, 1991). Parker argues that the "erotic experience" is often situated in acts of "sexual transgression," that is, the deliberate undermining in private of public norms. Common Brazilian expressions such as "*Entre quarto paredes, tudo pode acontecer,*" "Within four walls, everything can happen," or "*Por de baixo do pano, tudo pode acontecer,*" "Beneath the sheets, everything can happen," signify how the erotic experience lies in the freedom of such hidden moments (Daniel & Parker, 1993). This social and cultural construction of eroticism may explain why a happily married man, with a steady home life and children, visits commercial sex workers. Within four walls, a CSW may perform a range of sexual acts that a "proper" wife would shun.

Parker's (1991) work in deconstructing "sexuality" provides social and cultural explanations for why the act of anal sex is perceived as relatively more routine in Brazil than in most Asian or African country contexts. Parker explains that anal sex is widely practiced in Brazil both among men and between men and women, and that such sexual scripts are learned early. In the game of *troca-troca* (exchange-exchange), adolescent boys take turns inserting their penises in each other's anuses (Daniel & Parker, 1993). Sexual encounters between adolescent boys and girls also routinely involve anal intercourse to avoid pregnancy and the rupturing of the girl's hymen, still viewed as an important sign of a young woman's sexual "purity."

Behavior change communication interventions for HIV/AIDS rarely take into account such contextually bound cultural and social constructions of sexuality. Hence, dissatisfaction with their relative ineffectiveness is growing. Many communication scholars believe that it is time to move away from individual-level theories of preventive health behaviors to more multi-level, cultural, and contextual interventions (McKinlay & Marceau, 1999, 2000; Salmon & Kroger, 1992). Metaphorically speaking, new voices are urging communication programmers to go beyond analyzing and influencing the bobbing of individual corks on surface waters, and to focus on redirecting the stronger undercurrents that determine where the cork clusters end up along the shoreline (McMichael, 1995).

At a UNAIDS meeting in Geneva in 2000 (in which Singhal was a participant), a representative from Kenya talked about how young schoolgirls in Kenya rendered sexual favors to urban, middle-class and affluent men (commonly known as "Sugar Daddies") in exchange for the three Cs: cash, cell phones, and cars (driving in expensive cars like the Mercedes-Benz and BMWs) (Plate 5.1). Sugar Daddies initiate the seduction process by asking young girls: "Let me buy you chicken and chips," or "Let me give you a lift in my car." Such exchanges put these schoolgirls at risk for contracting HIV. In fact, rates of HIV infection among young girls in Kenya are five times higher than among young boys, with exploitation by Sugar Daddies contributing to this difference. Ethnographic research with schoolgirls in Kenya showed that they were well aware of the high risks they faced in contracting HIV, but were willing to take their chances. Why say no to such glamorous adventures, when the alternative was to struggle through school and college, find a job, and, once married, to attend to domestic chores and reproductive roles?

In Kenya, as elsewhere, strong cultural undercurrents about masculine sexuality, belief in the virility associated with bedding young girls (who represent "trophies"), and the power and prestige

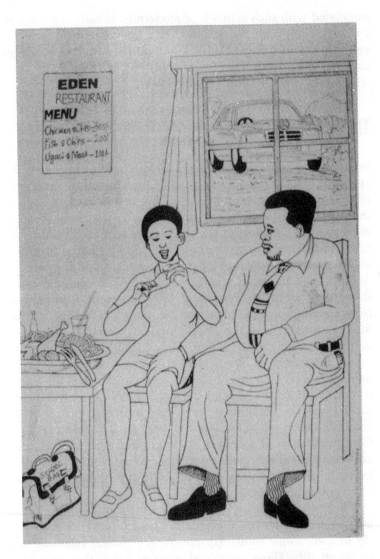

Plate 5.1 A Poster from Kenya Showing a "Sugar Daddy" with a Young Schoolgirl

Young schoolgirls often render sexual favors to older, affluent men (known as "Sugar Daddies") for cash, cell phones, and cars, putting themselves at high risk for contracting AIDS. Notice the Mercedes-Benz car visible through the window.

Source: PATH, Nairobi.

associated with such symbols of modernity as cash, cell phones, and cars, complicate the design of HIV interventions directed at young girls and at Sugar Daddies. Individually directed messages such as "Stay away from Sugar Daddies" or "Stay away from schoolgirls" will certainly be ineffective.

The UNAIDS Framework

International agencies can play a unique role in attacking the epidemic in ways that are not possible for national governments. For example, the spread of the epidemic across borders, such as through sexual tourism, migrant workers, fishermen, and the movement of commercial sex workers, is best addressed by an international body. It can also inject new thinking into strategizing about communicating for HIV prevention, care, and support.

Influenced by social scientists, the UNAIDS communication framework (UNAIDS/Penn State, 1999) represents a move away from focusing on individuals as the main target of preventive interventions. Instead, the UNAIDS model provides a multi-level, cultural, and contextual guide to designing HIV/AIDS communication interventions. The UNAIDS framework urges program managers and communication specialists to ascertain the role of communication in influencing the social and cultural environment for HIV/AIDS prevention, care, and support, including the communication action needed to create access to health services. Communication is ascribed an important role in grassroots advocacy, mobilizing political action, and in creating the context for more gender-sensitive and culturally appropriate HIV/AIDS intervention programs.

The UNAIDS framework calls for refocusing communication interventions on five key contextual domains: (a) government policy; (b) socioeconomic status; (c) culture; (d) gender relations; and (e) spirituality. These contextual domains, while they lie outside the skins of individuals, influence HIV/AIDS-related health behavior. The UNAIDS approach offers a promising contrast to the definition of HIV/AIDS in strictly biomedical terms, as adopted initially in many countries. Through this approach, UNAIDS seeks to reframe the strategies for preventing HIV/AIDS. It performed a useful function by publishing reports documenting successful AIDS control programs (several of which are cited in this book).

The five contextual domains of the UNAIDS communication framework signify that the forest is more important than the individual tree. Understanding the context allows one to appreciate the ways in which individual trees are shaped, and to discern the order that exists among these trees, including the roles, connections, and relationships that exist among them (Airhihenbuwa, 1999). Understanding the forest reveals why certain trees tower over others, which trees nurture others, and other nuances of their inter-relationships. By focusing on the five contextual domains, communication experts can create a flexible, culture-based, holistic strategy in which the interventions are located in the social patterns of relationships among individuals, as may be determined by their age, seniority, gender, socioeconomic class, and cultural and spiritual beliefs (Pasick, 1995).

Consider spirituality as an example. During the first decade of the epidemic, in the 1980s, spirituality and religion had little part in AIDS control efforts. Gradually (as we describe later in the book), religious leaders like Father Valeriano in Brazil, Phra Phongthep Dhammagaruko and other Buddhist monks in Thailand, and various spiritual organizations played an increasingly important role in AIDS control. Many NGOs conducting prevention programs and many hospices for people living with HIV/AIDS have religious affiliations.

Culture as an Ally

Communication strategists often viewed culture as static, and mistakenly looked upon people's health beliefs as cultural barriers. This is a predominantly negative view. Culture has often been singled out as the explanation for the failure of HIV interventions (Brummelhuis & Herdt, 1995; Moses et al., 1990; Parker, 1991). However, culture can also be viewed in terms of its strengths, and attributes of a culture that are helpful for HIV/AIDS prevention, care, and support programs should be identified and harnessed (Airhihenbuwa, 1995). The metaphorical coupling of culture and barriers needs to be exposed, deconstructed, and reconstructed so that new, positive cultural linkages can be forged (Airhihenbuwa & Obregon, 2000). For instance, the green *pendelu* campaign identified the cultural strength represented by the husband's supportive role during pregnancy, and harnessed the marital symbolism associated with the *pendelu* to promote improved maternal and child health in Mali. Similarly, certain smoking cessation programs among Latinos identified the cultural strength represented by the value of *familismo* (family ties), a positive Latino cultural norm, and harnessed it to reduce smoking (Airhihenbuwa, 1995, 1999; Diaz, 1997). Similarly, close family ties are an important strength of Indian society, where the definition of the family includes neighbors and colleagues (referred to as "family friends"). This strong family bond should be harnessed by HIV prevention interventions, and by care and support initiatives (Mane & Maitra, 1992).

Several sociocultural and spiritual dimensions of Senegalese society strengthened the nation's effective response to HIV/AIDS; for instance, the cultural norms with respect to the universality of marriage; the rapid remarriage of widow(er)s and divorced persons; moral condemnation of all forms of sexual cohabitation not sanctioned by religious beliefs; and extended social networks of parents, cousins, relatives, neighbors, and others, that served to control irresponsible sexuality (Lom, 2001). The fear of dishonoring one's family and the subsequent "What will they say?" syndrome exercises a strong check on individual behavior (Diop, 2000; UNAIDS, 1999b). So, cultural beliefs assist HIV prevention in Senegal.

Most HIV/AIDS communication campaigns in Latin America, Africa, and Asia undervalued traditional oral communication channels and the strength of aural comprehension. In these cultures, the oral tradition is rich in visual imagery, and is the basis on which learning is founded (Airhihenbuwa, 1999). Proverbs, adages, riddles, folklore, and storytelling are thus important communication tools. The narrative tradition offers the potential of cultural expression, particularly words of advice and encouragement that are often couched in adage, allegory, and metaphor (Airhihenbuwa, 1999).

HIV/AIDS programs fare better if scientific explanations of HIV/AIDS are couched in terms of local contexts of understanding

(Harris, 1991). Such context-based explanations are called "syncretic explanations" (Barnett & Blaikie, 1992). HIV/AIDS interventions in Africa should frame prevention messages to fit with prevailing local magico-religious myths. A diarrhea prevention campaign in northern Nigeria illustrates the importance of providing syncretic explanations. When missionaries in Nigeria became alarmed about the number of infant deaths due to diarrhea, they tried to teach mothers about water-boiling. The mothers were told that their children had died because of little animals in the water, and that these animals could be killed by boiling the water. Such talk about invisible animals in the water was met with skepticism. Babies kept on dying. Finally, a visiting anthropologist suggested a solution. There were, he said, "evil spirits in the water; boil the water and you could see them going away, bubbling out to escape the heat" (Okri, 1991, pp. 134–35). This message had the desired effect, and infant mortality due to diarrhea dropped sharply.

How can communication programs tap people's cultural domain to prevent HIV/AIDS? What are the positive and negative cultural attributes of the local community with respect to HIV/AIDS?

Tapping the Strength of the Nguni Culture

The cultural attributes of the Nguni people in southern Africa reveal points of entry for implementing HIV/AIDS behavior change communication. For instance, among the Nguni, responsibility for providing sexuality education to the young at the onset of puberty is usually delegated to an aunt or an uncle. Cultural emphasis is placed on sexual abstinence. A strong taboo exists against bringing one's family name into disrepute. Members of the extended family take turns in caring for the sick, to avoid burdening one person. There are no orphans, as extended family members take care of children without parents.

The practice of *ukusoma* (a Zulu term for non-penetrative sex), both to preserve virginity and to prevent pregnancy, is common. The woman keeps her thighs closely together while the man finds sexual release. Other groups use a bent elbow for a similar purpose. Similar non-penetrative sex practices exist among certain groups in Ethiopia (practices commonly referred to as "brushing"), the Kikuyu in Kenya, and other communities.

Culture as Enemy along Lake Victoria

One often thinks of Patpong, the well-known Bangkok red-light district, or a truck drivers' *dhaba* on an Indian highway, as an HIV transmission hotspot. In addition, there are certain key locations around the world, geographical spaces in which HIV/AIDS is particularly concentrated. One such location is Nyanza Province in Western Kenya, the Luo ethnic heartland bordering Lake Victoria. The Luo are unusually tall people, and the Nyanza area was blessed with a fertile agriculture and with a plentiful catch of fish from Lake Victoria. Nyanza was one of the most heavily populated areas in Africa, with more than 1,000 people per square kilometer.

Nyanza's fortunes began to sink in the early 1990s. Due to rapid population growth and increasingly intensive cropping, soil fertility became depleted and crop yields dropped. Worse, water hyacinths that had been planted as decorative flowers in neighboring nations washed down-river into Lake Victoria, clogging the harbors along the shores of the lake. Fishing craft were blockaded from landing. Further, a large game fish had been introduced into the lake by the British during Kenya's colonial era. It multiplied rapidly, devouring the other fish (the new fish were about the same size as an adult human).

Even more unfortunately for the Luo people, HIV entered the Nyanza area in the mid-1980s and spread rapidly. Like many other East African cultures, the Luo practice widow inheritance (also called "home guardianship"). When a man dies, one of his brothers or cousins marries his widow. This tradition guarantees that the children remain in the late husband's family, and that the widow and her children are provided for. Sexual intercourse with her late husband's relative seals the bond between the widow and her new family (Blair et al., 1997). However, this cultural practice has had disastrous consequences in the era of AIDS. Thomas McOwiti, who comes from a village near Kisumu, has almost no living male relatives. All were lost to AIDS-related deaths. Experts in Kenya say that the Nyanza area has one of the highest rates of HIV infection in the world, perhaps almost 50 percent of all adults.

Focus group discussions in Nyanza showed that the widow-cleansing practice continues as the Luo strongly wish to avoid *chira*, a curse that befalls a person who does not perform traditional rites. However, focus group discussions with community elders suggested possibilities for replacing the rite of "intercourse" with alternative rites, such as the male relative placing his leg on the widow's thigh, or hanging his coat in her home (Blair et al., 1997). Elders noted that such alternative rites were quite acceptable, as the Luo had practiced them decades ago. The Nyanza area and Luo culture deserve further study to derive lessons about the role of culture in HIV prevention that might apply locally, and in other areas.

Cultural insights from Nyanza Province suggest that HIV/AIDS program managers should go beyond the identification of harmful cultural practices (such as "wife-cleansing"), in order to create and implement culturally acceptable alternative rites. The Program for Alternative Technology in Health (PATH) in Nairobi created an alternative ceremony for young girls in Kenya, called "Circumcision with Words." To date, some 3,000 girls have participated in these ceremonies, thus avoiding the risk of HIV infection during circumcision ceremonies.

Individualistic Versus Collectivistic Cultures

As noted previously, behavior change communication interventions have focused on influencing individual decision-making with respect to HIV prevention, assuming that the individual is autonomous. Messages utilizing this approach appeal to an individual's sense of sexual responsibility. However, the cultural attributes of a society, such as its emphasis on individualism as opposed to collectivism, beliefs in efficacy as opposed to fatalism, and its focus on guilt as opposed to shame, strongly mediate in how HIV prevention messages are processed by individuals (Yep, 1997). Behavior change communication directed at individuals, which fails to account for the influence of cultural undercurrents, is likely to be ineffective in collectivistic cultures.

People in collectivistic cultures (such as Thais or Chinese) are not comfortable talking about personal issues, especially those related to individual sexuality. *Collectivistic cultures* are those in which the collectivity's goals are valued over those of the individual (Rogers & Steinfatt, 1999, p. 86). In many Asian societies, discussions of illness and death are taboo. Fatalism means that births and deaths represent "God's will." Individuals in collectivistic societies, given their cultural orientation to groups, families, and extended kinship structures, are "shame-driven" (a collectivistic emotion). Discussing one's HIV status is taboo, as it brings long-lasting shame to the entire family

People in individualistic societies, such as in the United States and Western Europe, are more comfortable talking about personal issues, including open discussion of sexual preferences. *Individualistic cultures* are those in which the individual's goals are valued over those of the collectivity (Rogers & Steinfatt, 1999, p.86). In individualistic societies, *self-efficacy*, the belief that an individual can control his/her circumstances, is normative, and individual actions are driven more by "guilt" (an individualistic emotion).

Maldonado (1990) analyzes the influence of Latino culture on sexuality, gender roles, and condom use, and the implications for HIV prevention campaigns directed to Latino men. In traditional Latino culture, men are socialized to be informed about sexuality, to initiate sex in a relationship, and to have sexual contacts outside of marriage. Women, in contrast, are not expected to be knowledgeable about sexuality, are expected to be sexually submissive, and are expected never to raise the topic of condom use. Further, condoms are viewed as a means of birth control, which goes against the teachings of the Catholic Church. Given the "machismo" element of Latino culture, prevention campaigns could consider supporting aspects of machismo that "focus on a male's responsibility for protecting his family" (Machlica, 1997, p. 259). Messages that emphasize HIV/AIDS as a threat to the family, and that promote condom use as a means of protecting the family, will then be more effective.

Use of Cultural Artifacts

HIV/AIDS communication should integrate "modern" and "traditional" entertainment, and "big" and "little" media technologies.

Communication interventions should go beyond the mass media of television, radio, film, video, and print, to include crafts, art, textiles, murals, toys, and other culturally situated expressions. For instance, in South Africa, "positive pottery" and colorful AIDS ribbons etched with traditional African motifs are created by HIV-positive individuals. In East Africa, *khangas*, the traditional fabric wraps worn by women, now carry HIV prevention messages.

In Peru, *grafichangas* and video plazas are used to stimulate discussion on HIV and reproductive health issues in public places. *Grafichangas*, a term combining graffiti and *pachanga* (fiesta), are short stories written by individuals in public places, open for others to comment upon, criticize, and debate. Video plazas present short, impromptu theatrical performances in crowded public plazas, followed by open discussion and debate. *Grafichangas* and video plazas are helping to break the silence on HIV/AIDS.

In San Francisco, AIDS outreach workers use fortune cookies and Chinese red envelopes to carry messages to high-risk Asian Americans. Fortune cookies, eaten after a Chinese meal, may include messages about safe sex and the toll-free number of an AIDS helpline. Chinese red envelopes, traditionally used to give money gifts on the Chinese New Year, have been adapted to give the "gift of life" (condoms, the address of HIV testing facilities, etc.). Such cultural artifacts, distributed in face-to-face outreach encounters, are non-threatening, face-preserving, and culturally appropriate for the targeted audiences (Yep, 1994).

The Role of Spirituality

Some HIV/AIDS communication programs tap the spiritual domain. HIV/AIDS deals with issues of life and death, care and compassion, and hope and support, which are core spiritual values. Spirituality is a broader concept than religion, although the two terms have often been used interchangeably.

Spirituality includes values and beliefs about love, tolerance, compassion, sacrifice, hope, courage, patience, and faith; reflections on what is right and wrong, fair and unfair, true and untrue; ponderings on the meaning and purpose of life, the inevitability of mortality, and the relationship among mind, body, and soul (Relv,

1997). Spirituality as a conceptual tool is very powerful, as it cuts across age, gender, class, language, religion, culture, geography, and occupation.

How might communication programs tap people's spiritual domain in preventing HIV/AIDS? How much influence is wielded by local religious and spiritual leaders (including traditional healers, voodoo priests, and others)? Which spiritual and religious organizations (such as the Islamic *madrasa* schools in Uganda) may engage in HIV prevention?

A Spiritual *Jihad* on AIDS in Uganda*

Since 1992, the Islamic Medical Association of Uganda (IMAU) has trained over 8,000 Islamic religious leaders and their volunteer teams in 11 districts of Uganda to launch a spiritually motivated grassroots movement to change HIV/AIDS-related behaviors in Muslim communities. About 20 percent of Uganda's 20 million population is Muslim. This spiritual movement taps into the existing nationwide network of Islamic leaders, including the Mufti, who heads the Uganda Muslim Supreme Council. In 1989, the Mufti declared *jihad* (a holy war) on AIDS. The Mufti supervises 33 district religious leaders (*khadis*), who supervise six county religious leaders (sheikhs), who in turn supervise about 40 imams, each of whom heads a local mosque, serving as a spiritual leader to some 75 to 100 families.

In the Muslin community, imams are highly respected and trusted local spiritual teachers (Plate 5.2). They are role models for appropriate social behavior. The imams teach about AIDS during congregational prayers, home visits, and at intimate family ceremonies such as marriage, birth, and burials. As Imam Ali noted: "Everyday I visit two homes. I use the teachings of the *Qur'an* to educate people about AIDS—especially the dangers of promiscuity. My visits are not new. The people here expect me because this is my duty as imam. People feel free to talk to me" (quoted in UNAIDS, 1998b, p. 17).

The imams incorporate accurate information about HIV/AIDS in Islamic teachings, promoting messages of mutual

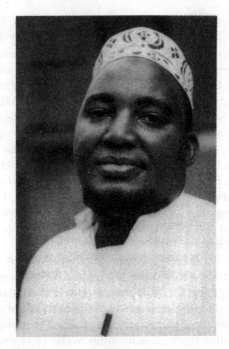

Plate 5.2 Imams, Highly Respected Religious Leaders in Uganda, Joined the Battle against HIV/AIDS by Declaring a Spiritual *Jihad* on the Epidemic

The Islamic Medical Association of Uganda (IMAU) trained thousands of religious leaders and volunteers to change the behavior of Uganda's Muslim population.

Source: United Nations.

fidelity and moral responsibility. They also educate community members about the risks of contracting HIV through traditional Muslim practices such as male circumcision (when an unsterilized razor is used for several infants), and ablution of the dead (when body orifices are cleaned without wearing protective gloves). The preventive aspects of using sterilized razors and protective gloves are especially promoted.

The imam's work on HIV/AIDS prevention, care, and support is aided locally by respected male and female assistants, who are strongly committed to HIV prevention and are respected by the community. In addition, five male and female community members are chosen by the local mosque to serve as family AIDS workers. They are respected by their peers and are perceived as being easily approachable.

Inspired by the Mufti's call to wage a *jihad* on AIDS, Islamic leaders are highly committed to their HIV/AIDS mission. As Sheikh Mohammed Bukenya noted: "People must be educated about AIDS. Many think it is caused by witchcraft. We have to tell people the truth about how the virus is transmitted. I include AIDS teachings when I conduct prayers, *khutba* [the Friday sermon], and when I speak to families at birth, wedding, and funeral ceremonies. In fact, I will not perform a marriage ceremony until both people have gone for an AIDS test. Couples usually thank me for this" (quoted in UNAIDS, 1998b, p. 19).

In Uganda, IMAU reaches Muslim children through another initiative called the Madrasa AIDS Education and Prevention Project (MAEP). Imams and their assistants teach children about AIDS through a special curriculum designed for *madrasas*, the informal schools attached to mosques. The AIDS education curriculum includes 36 short lessons, tailored to be age-appropriate. In over 350 *madrasa* schools in Uganda, students learn about HIV/AIDS. They learn about caring for AIDS patients and support community initiatives to improve their quality of life.

The experience of IMAU in Uganda suggests the importance of using existing religious institutional networks, and the power of spiritual discourse, to fight the epidemic.

* This case draws upon UNAIDS (1998b).

Coping with AIDS Spiritually[2]

In northern Thailand's Mae Chan district, bordering Myanmar and Laos (often referred to as the "Golden Triangle" area), several hundred monks regularly incorporate HIV prevention messages in their sermons, pay home visits to PWAs, provide counseling, and produce and distribute herbal medicines. Spiritual care is also an integral part of the Sanpatong Home-Based Care Project in Thailand, where Buddhist principles of kindness, compassion, altruistic joy, and equanimity help the afflicted cope with AIDS. Buddhist monks teach meditation to people living with HIV/AIDS to help them find tranquility and to boost their mental strength to continue with life. Spiritual guidance is provided on how to protect oneself from suffering and how to see the natural hand in the human cycle of life and death. Discourse covers how to come to terms with one's mortality or that of a loved one. Individuals suffering from HIV/AIDS often participate in week-long retreats at Buddhist *wats* (temples), where they meditate, re-examine their spiritual beliefs, and benefit from a regimen of diet and exercise.

People in six of the 10 countries in the Association of Southeast Asian Nations (ASEAN) subscribe to Buddhist principles. Buddhist principles forbid the taking of life (for instance, by exposing others to HIV infection) or the consumption of substances to alter the natural body state (for instance, alcohol or injection drugs), providing an effective spiritual platform to address high-risk behavior. So, from Myanmar to Vietnam, Buddhism offers a means of HIV prevention.

Several thousand miles away, David Malquez, a clinical social worker in the Milagros AIDS Project in East Los Angeles, uses culturally specific spiritual healing strategies in his intervention with several hundred HIV-infected gay Latino men, mostly recent immigrants from Mexico and Central America. Over 90 percent of Malquez's clients believe that AIDS is their "punishment" from God for their "deviant" behavior (Arguelles & Rivero, 1997). Malquez uses a combination of Mexican and Chicano healing practices and conventional psychological clinical techniques. These spiritual practices include *conocimiento* (literally, becoming acquainted with), a technique to reconnect clients with their ancestral roots, and *limpias* (implying cleansing of body, mind, and spirit). Many of Malquez's clients, with the assistance of *sobadores* (traditional masseuses), *yerberos* (herbalists), and acupuncturists, now feel empowered to cope with their HIV status (Arguelles & Rivero, 1997).

Spiritual leaders and institutions can play a key role in stemming the tide of HIV/AIDS in the African American community in the United States. However, to date, little of this potential has been realized. Since the 1990s, African Americans have accounted for a large proportion of new cases of HIV/AIDS in the United States. In

1997, African Americans were diagnosed with AIDS at a rate six times higher than were whites, suggesting an "epidemic of color" (Stolberg, 1998). Most African Americans have strong ties with neighborhood churches. Some 75,000 black churches exist in the U.S., with a membership of 25 million (Lincoln & Mamiya, 1991). Black churches have a strong tradition of leading and caring for their constituents, especially in times of suffering. For instance, the civil rights movements of the 1950s and 1960s, under the leadership of Dr. Martin Luther King, Jr., were born and sustained through direct church action in the South. However, black churches and leaders have been "reticent" on the issue of HIV/AIDS. Denial of the problem is common, and black ministers engage in "pulpit euphemisms," i.e., downplaying the problem (Swain, 2000). The promotion of sterile, rational, abstinence-only messages have helped HIV make quick inroads into the African American community.

Spirituality as an Enemy

Like culture, spirituality can cut both ways; that is, it can act as an asset or as an obstacle to HIV prevention. In a survey of 26 churches in the island nation of Trinidad & Tobago in the Caribbean, all pastors said that AIDS was a result of "sin." Each pastor promoted abstinence as the best protection against HIV/AIDS. The position of the Hindu temples in this island country was no different. Pundit Gyandeo Persad, president of SWAHA, an alliance of Hindu temples, said: "Cancer, or diabetes, is not caused by promiscuity, unfaithfulness, or drug abuse. HIV/AIDS has its genesis in acts that are condemned by scriptures" (quoted in Newton-Small, 2001, p. 8). Accordingly, the Ministry of Education in Trinidad banned the discussion of condoms in the island's schools, as promoting promiscuous behavior. Youth groups in Trinidad, hard-hit by HIV and AIDS, characterize these abstinence-only messages as "genocide," especially given the norm on sex among the island's youth. They wonder how the church and the government can feign such blindness, when coffins are being sold next to coconuts in many local marketplaces.

In the Catholic countries of Latin America, much as in the Caribbean, church leaders promote abstinence and fidelity as "God's way" of staying away from "sin" and from the "punishment" of HIV/AIDS. However, Latin American church groups are increasingly involved in care and support of PWAs, which, over the long term, may help reduce AIDS-related stigma.

Community Approaches to HIV/AIDS Prevention

The Local Responses Initiative of UNAIDS is a community-based, people-driven HIV/AIDS response. It believes that people need to "own" this health problem, and be involved as partners in socially acceptable actions for HIV/AIDS prevention, care, and support in the places where they live. This initiative hopes to create AIDS-competent societies by strengthening the local capacity of people to accept the reality of AIDS, to assess its effects on their daily lives, prevent it so as to live with it positively, and learn from their actions. Getting a target audience involved in perceiving the epidemic as *their* problem, rather than as a topic that their national government preaches about, is fundamental.

Local UNAIDS initiatives are currently underway in Uganda, Tanzania, Burkina Faso, Thailand, the Philippines, and several other countries. In Uganda, for instance, people living with AIDS actively participate in local decision-making by their village, parish, and sub-county councils. In Magu, Tanzania, thanks to community directives, traditional healers must follow a strict one-patient one-blade regimen to make incisions, or risk being fined a cow. Female guardians at schools involve teachers and students to curb unwanted pregnancies, rapes, and sexual exploitation (Phillips, 2001). Residents have outlawed the harvest rite *chagulaga* (choose), in which young men chase unmarried women into the bush, coupling for the night. In Gaoua, Burkina Faso, the struggle against AIDS has become "everybody's business": Members of the local community, government sectors (such as education, agriculture, the military, and prisons), and the voluntary sector (such as churches and women, youth, and farmers' cooperatives) have collaboratively designed a plan to combat HIV/AIDS.

These local initiatives depend on both internal and external facilitation. The purpose of such facilitation is to create an enabling environment so that local actors can take responsibility for finding solutions to their AIDS problem in a manner that is suitable for them. The premise of local initiatives is consistent with the contextual focus of the UNAIDS communication framework, which argues that "people are the subject of the response to AIDS, not the objects of our interventions." People's involvement is fundamental (Gumucio Dagron, 2001).

CEFRAN: The Community Cares

In São Paulo, Centro Franciscano de Luta Contra AIDS (CEFRAN) runs an innovative, holistic, community-centered program to restore the physical, emotional, mental, and spiritual well-being of people living with HIV and AIDS. At any given time, 400 PWAs and their families are enrolled in CEFRAN's program. All PWAs are welcome, irrespective of their skin color, gender, sexual orientation, or religious denomination. Founded in 1994 by a Franciscan priest, CEFRAN fosters compassion among community members toward PWAs, and, in turn, empowers PWAs to become valuable community citizens.

Among all the HIV programs we visited in our five-country study, CEFRAN was the most creative in its use of "food" to anchor its community-based intervention program. The PWAs enrolled in CEFRAN's program receive 250 packets of non-perishable food items (including rice, pasta, beans, oil, sugar, salt, etc.), over a four-month period. At CEFRAN, it is known that free anti-retroviral drugs and nutritious food are both essential to restore the health of PWAs. To receive these food packets, PWAs need to attend CEFRAN's weekly physical, psychosocial, and spiritual therapy sessions. Attendance is close to 100 percent. When we visited Miguel Sanchez, a PWA and assistant to the director of CEFRAN, he noted: "Food provides an incentive to attend but that is only a small part of the motivation. Through our program HIV-positive people feel that they are not alone and that the community cares" (personal interview, Miguel Sanchez, 11 March 2001).

A PWA attends 17 weekly group sessions at CEFRAN's facilities, of which the last four are devoted to enhancing occupational skills. Yoga, massage, meditation, and non-judgmental spiritual counseling are provided. Further,

CEFRAN trains PWAs in painting, arts, and crafts, and works closely with community-based employment agencies and vocational training institutions to place PWAs as electricians, plumbers, carpenters, data-entry clerks, and office secretaries. Community institutions, groups, and individuals are viewed as full "partners" in addressing AIDS, promoting compassion, and reducing stigma.

Thus far, CEFRAN has worked with over 2,000 PWAs and their families in São Paulo. But this holistic, community-centered approach has affected many more lives. Over 1,000 people, mostly community members who volunteer in CEFRAN's programs, attended CEFRAN's 2000 Christmas celebrations. "We were the biggest party in town," noted Sanchez.

Creating Sexual Subjects through Freirean Approaches

When we visited Brazil in March 2001, we encountered several HIV/AIDS prevention programs that were inspired by the participatory approaches of the late Brazilian educator, Paulo Freire. Exiled by Brazil's military regime for over two decades, Freire returned to São Paulo in the mid-1980s to serve as secretary of education for the city of São Paulo. Freire is best known for his classic book, *Pedagogy of the oppressed* (1970), in which he argues that most political, educational, and communication interventions fail because they are designed by technocrats based on their personal views of reality. They seldom take into account the perspectives of those to whom these programs are directed. Freire's dialogic pedagogy emphasizes the role of "teacher as learner" and the "learner as teacher," with each learning from the other in a mutually transformative process. The role of the outside facilitator is viewed as working *with*, and not *for*, the oppressed, to organize them in their incessant struggle to regain their humanity (Singhal, 2001b). True participation, according to Freire, does not involve a subject–object relationship. There is only a subject–subject relationship.

In Freirean pedagogy, there is no room for teaching "two plus two equals four." Such a pedagogy, according to Freire, is dehumanizing, because it views learners as empty receptacles to be "filled" by expert knowledge. Freire criticizes this "banking" mode of education: "Deposits" are made by experts. The scope of action allowed to students (or intended beneficiaries) "extends only as far as receiving, filing, and storing the deposits" (Freire, 1970, p. 58). Instead, Freire advocates problem-posing as a means of representing to people what they know and think, not as a lecture, but as an involving problem. So a lesson on "two plus two" might proceed in the following dialogic manner (Singhal, 2001b):

> Teacher: How many chickens do you have?
> Poor farmer: Two.
> Teacher: How many chickens does your neighbor have?
> Poor farmer: Two.
> Teacher: How many chickens does the landlord have?
> Poor farmer: Oh, hundreds!
> Teacher: *Why* does he have hundreds, and you have only two?

So goes the dialogic conversation that over time stimulates a process of critical reflection and awareness ("conscientization") on the part of the poor farmer, creating possibilities of reflective action that did not exist before. Freire emphasizes that the themes underlying dialogic pedagogy should resonate with people's experiences and issues of salience to them, as opposed to well-meaning but alienating rhetoric. Once the oppressed, both individually and collectively, begin to critically reflect on their social situation, possibilities arise for them to break the "culture of silence" through the articulation of discontent and action.

A Pedagogy of HIV Prevention

In 1990, Vera Paiva, a psychologist at the University of São Paulo and an expert on HIV/AIDS and gender issues, used Paulo Freire's participatory approach and Pichon Riviere's (1988) group process methodology to involve students and teachers in the low-income schools of São Paulo city in HIV/AIDS prevention. Based on a deep understanding of the sociocultural dimension of risk, the goal of the intervention was to create a generation of "sexual subjects" who could regulate their sexual lives as opposed to being objects of desire and the sexual scripts of others (Paiva, 2000). A sexual subject is one who engages consciously in a negotiated sexual relationship based on cultural norms for gender relations; who is capable of articulating and practicing safe sexual practices with pleasure, in a consensual way; and who is capable of saying "no" to sex.

In collaboration with students, teachers, and community members, Paiva developed a pedagogy of HIV prevention that sought to stimulate collective action and response from those directly affected by HIV and living in a vulnerable context. Face-to-face group interaction with girls and boys pointed to the importance of understanding the role of sexual subjects in various "sexual scenes," composed of the gender–power relationship between participants, their degree of affective involvement, the nature of the moment, the place, sexual norms in the culture, racial and class mores, and others (Paiva, 1995). Words such as AIDS, *camisinha* (little shirts, or condoms), and others were decoded, and participants proposed new words and codes for naming the body and gender rules, thus generating new realities.

Paiva employed a variety of creative techniques to help participants formulate a pedagogy of prevention: group discussions, role-playing, psychodrama, team work, home work, molding flour and salt paste to shape reproductive body parts and genitals, games to make condoms erotic, and art with condoms (to be comfortable in touching them with one's bare hands). To overcome inhibitions during role plays, a "pillow" was placed in the middle of the room, symbolizing a sexual "subject." For example, the pillow could represent an "in-the-closet" gay or a lesbian; a virgin schoolgirl; or a bisexual schoolboy. Participants could adopt the pillow to have internal discussions with the subject, experience themselves in the place of the other, or understand their own fantasy. The pillow provided a vehicle for them to speak out through an imaginary character, while preserving their privacy (Paiva, 1995).

Group processes showed that sexual inhibitions could be broken down in the context of *sacanagem* (sexual mischief), accompanied by "exaggerated" sexual talk and eroticization of the context (Paiva, 1995). Condoms became easily discussable when both the boy and the girl were ready to "loosen the hinges of the bed," or "turn over the car" while engaging in sex. In essence, the pedagogy of prevention was based on an "eroticization" of prevention.

Evaluation of the project was based, not on counting the number of condoms used, but on the progress made by students, teachers, and community members in becoming "sexual subjects." They were collectively empowered to make choices, and to act them out in culturally appropriate ways.

Paiva's project, based on Freirian principles, was to create an organized school community that could talk freely about the challenges of HIV/AIDS, and, much like the UNAIDS Local Responses Initiative discussed previously, create effective, participatory, and sustained behavior change.

Safe Sex as "Play"

Vera Paiva's work in Brazil, and the dissatisfaction with biomedical, individual-oriented behavioral change approaches, point to the importance of thinking boldly, radically, and culturally about HIV prevention. Greater attention must be paid to pleasure-enhancing approaches to HIV prevention, as opposed to pleasure reduction approaches. More community-based, dialogic approaches are needed, as opposed to individual-based "banking" approaches.

The biomedical metaphor of safe sex as "negotiation" needs to be replaced with the metaphor of safe sex as "play" (Adelman, 1992). Negotiating safe sex is a sterile, rational, and non-emotional strategy, devoid of sensuality and sexuality (Metts & Fitzpatrick, 1992). It denotes "time out" in a passionate sexual encounter, an abrupt pausing of a sexual script. For instance, in Latino cultures, where male sexuality is often signified by the expression "*Cuando la de abajo se calienta, la de arriba no piense,*" "When the bottom [penis] gets hot, the one on the top [brain] can't think," constructing safe sex as "negotiation" is a cultural faux pas (Diaz, 1997).

On the other hand, the metaphor of safe sex as "play" connotes improvisation, creativity, fun, affection, banter, and mischief. Play can manifest itself communicatively in the creative uses of language (such as in jokes, puns, or use of baby talk) or in interactional acts (such as jostling, mock wrestling, and/or playing with body parts and objects) (Adelman, 1992). A scene from the hit Hollywood film, *Pretty Woman*, illustrates how safe sex might be creatively constructed as "play." Just prior to sex, Julia Roberts, who plays a prostitute, turns to her wealthy customer, holds up her several colored condoms, and says: "Pick your color. [Then smiling sensually and coyly] You look like a gold man" (quoted in Adelman, 1992, p. 74). The playful allusion to "gold" status brings new meanings to prophylactic consumption.

In Greece, HIV/AIDS intervention programs directed at commercial sex workers creatively combine harm reduction techniques and "play"-based safe sex practices. Health authorities encourage commercial sex workers to register themselves, which obliges them to report for bi-weekly health checks for STDs and for an HIV test every three months (Kapila & Pye, 1992). Privacy and confidentiality concerns of CSWs are handled carefully. Further, CSWs learn various techniques to eroticize safe sex. Condoms are available in various shapes, colors, textures, and scents, and CSWs engage in playful sexual talk (including fantasies) to incorporate them in sexual acts. As a result, STD and HIV rates have decreased substantially, and condom usage is up (Kapila & Pye, 1992).

HIV prevention programs must seriously consider, where appropriate, constructing sex talk as "healthy passion" as opposed to the sterile biomedical construction of "safe sex." Intervention programs need to teach people how to have "good sex" that is "safe sex," as opposed to "genocidal" prevention messages promoting sexual abstinence, or "don't shoot drugs." Plate 5.3 depicts a poster from Kenya promoting good sex, forging a positive link between sexual enjoyment and safe sex behaviors. Similarly, in India, an HIV/AIDS prevention poster celebrated the *Kama Sutra*'s (literally, sex strategy) message of erotic sex and partner fidelity: "Many [sex] positions with one is better than one [sex] position with many." Authored by Vatsyayana in the 4th century, the *Kama Sutra* valorizes the art of seducing women, as well as the pleasurable and erotic aspects of sex. Such bold, radical, and culturally anchored prevention messages are rare, however, in the face of the worldwide AIDS epidemic.

The Power of Sports

What role can recreational games and competitive sports play in HIV prevention? All cultures value games and sports. In India, people are fanatical about cricket. In the countries of Europe, Africa, and Latin America, soccer evokes similar emotions. Sports bring

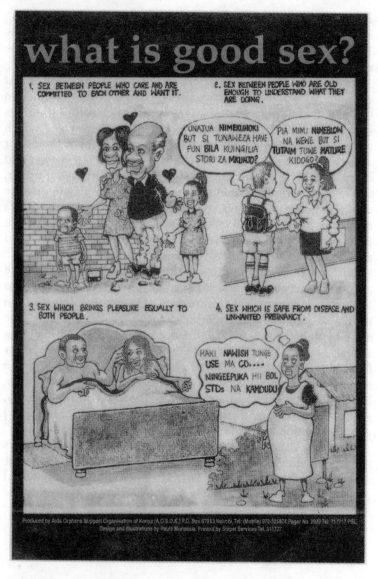

Plate 5.3 This Kenyan Poster Promotes Good Sex and Safe HIV/AIDS Behaviors

Enjoying sex can be consistent with being safe from HIV infection.

Source: Youth Exchange Network, Nairobi.

people together, serving as cultural glue that binds individuals across age, gender, religion, nationality, and ethnicity.

In 1999, Johns Hopkins University's Population Communication Services (JHU/PCS) launched the Caring Understanding Partners (CUP) Initiative in several African countries to promote HIV prevention among soccer players, and through them to target other youth (JHU/CCP, 1999). Between 1997 and 1999, some 165 national and league soccer players died of AIDS in Uganda and Kenya, pointing to the vulnerability of athletes.

Partnering with UNAIDS, DFID (the British development aid agency), the United Nations Population Fund (UNFPA), Voice of America (VOA), and other local partners, JHU/PCS launched a high-profile, male-friendly communication campaign centered around a planned regional African soccer tournament in Nairobi's National Stadium. Over 130,000 spectators, 95 percent of them male, arrived at the stadium to watch the tournament, while tens of millions watched it on television. The JHU/PCS multimedia campaign included television and radio spots on HIV prevention, endorsements by soccer celebrities, pre- and post-game events, banner displays in the soccer stadium, health stalls during championship games, and tens of thousands of posters, stickers, and calendars.

Some 168 soccer players and coaches from Uganda, Kenya, Ethiopia, Sudan, Rwanda, and Eritrea were trained in HIV prevention in order that they could counsel youth in community sports camps and high schools in their respective countries. In addition, in Cameroon, 22 national and regional soccer coaches were trained for a similar purpose (*Daily Nation*, 1999). Training the coaches meant that young boys attending soccer camps in these countries learned soccer as well as lifeskills to protect themselves from HIV. They learned about dribbling, tackling, and scoring, and, through soccer analogies, about "developing a game plan," "using their heads" (Plate 5.4), "knowing their opponent," "playing safe," "passing when in danger," and "wearing socks" (or using condoms).

The popularity of soccer in Africa, and the accompanying cultural resonance and acceptance of phrases such as "use your head," contributed to the effectiveness of the CUP Initiative. The idea of basing the CUP Initiative on soccer, and using soccer analogies, was inspired by a highly effective soccer-centered polio eradication

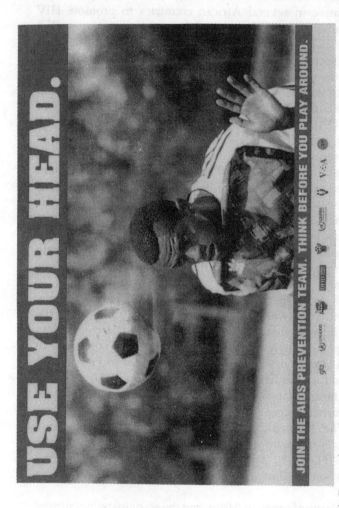

Plate 5.4 This Poster from the Caring Understanding Partners (CUP) Initiative's Multimedia Campaign in East Africa uses Soccer Lingo to Promote HIV Prevention among Male Youth

Soccer is a highly popular sport in countries of Europe, Africa, and Latin America. Soccer lingo is universally understood and accepted.

Source: Johns Hopkins University, Center for Communication Programs.

campaign in Nigeria. The campaign's catchy slogan was: "Can't be a winning team with lame legs."

While in South Africa, we learned of Y-Centers (short for Youth Centers), a project of loveLife, an organization that targets youth to reduce teenage pregnancy, HIV infections, and sexually transmitted diseases. loveLife has built over a dozen Y-Centers across South Africa, providing youth with a multipurpose recreational center equipped with basketball courts, a sexual health education center, and a counseling facility. The Y-Center represents a non-clinical, non-threatening, and friendly space, where youth can mingle, learn, and play in a safe community environment. Basketball clinics for the youth are held at these Y-Centers, and NBA-style championships with play-offs foster a competitive spirit (Lungi Morrison, personal interview, 13 June 2001). The basketball clinics go beyond teaching how to pass and shoot; they teach young boys and girls about lifeskills, about taking care of their bodies, and about sexual responsibility. loveLife also holds loveGames, a competitive nationwide mini-Olympiad in which youth compete in popular local games such as soccer, rugby, and track and field events. Through their sports and educational programs, Y-Centers train youth members to serve as peer educators in their communities. Each Y-Center comes equipped with a mobile broadcasting unit, which empowers youth to voice their opinions on the air, and helps to report on local events.

loveLife is funded mainly by the Henry J. Kaiser Family Foundation, and its advisory board is chaired by Mrs. Zanele Mbeki, South Africa's first lady. The Bill and Melinda Gates Foundation provided computers to each Y-Center for training and education purposes.

In Rio de Janeiro, Brazil, we visited Project Mangueira, located at the base of *favela* Mangueira, a hillside urban slum close to Rio's world-famous Maracana Football Stadium. Youth living in Rio's many hillside *favelas* are especially vulnerable to HIV. They are also "soccer and samba crazy," as our guide to Project Mangueira told us. The project is a community-based youth development program, combining sports and music with education, health services, and vocational training. Its Olympic Sports Complex of 35,000 square meters includes a swimming pool, a running track, an outdoor soccer field, and basketball and volleyball courts. The Astroturf for Mangueira's soccer field was funded by soccer legend

Pele during his tenure as Brazil's minister of sports. Ronaldo, the current soccer celebrity, funded the dental clinic on Mangueira's premises. Project Mangueira is built on land donated by the Federal Railroad Network Company of Brazil, and several of its youth programs are sponsored by private corporations, government ministries, and local community-based organizations. Xerox sponsors Mangueira's sports activities, and operates a state-of-the-art information technology training center.

Some 4,500 youth participate in Project Mangueira's programs, and over 35,000 have benefited since the project's inception in 1987. The school run by Project Mangueira boasts the highest school attendance of any public school in Rio, and crime in Mangueira is the lowest of any *favela* in Brazil. Sports, recreation, dance, and music represent the foundational pillars of Project Mangueira, which support a superstructure of education, health, lifeskills development, and community-building. Photo displays at Project Mangueira show that its visitors have included Bill Clinton and Nelson Mandela.

Conclusions

Culture can be a positive or a negative factor in HIV prevention. In this chapter, we encountered examples of both. Culture, context, and spirituality can play an important role in HIV/AIDS prevention. Past HIV/AIDS interventions have overemphasized individual-level strategies of behavior change communication, often ignoring the influence of cultural context and network influences on such change. Program managers must identify cultural attributes that will buttress HIV/AIDS initiatives, and harness these attributes.

Program managers must pay greater attention to pleasure-enhancing approaches to HIV prevention, as opposed to preachy, pleasure reduction approaches. Behavior change communication strategies must be reoriented to viewing sex as a playful, fun, and sharing activity. Community-based, dialogic approaches must replace individual-directed "banking" approaches. The cultural importance of recreational games and competitive sports for HIV prevention should be recognized and harnessed.

Bolton (1995) asks whether HIV prevention programs with gay communities can recruit attractive gay men to educate their partners about the joys of safer sex. Contrary to present-day prevention approaches, is it possible to liberate sexuality (as opposed to denying or repressing it), increase the sum of sexual gratification (as opposed to reducing it), and adopt healthy sexualities (as opposed to continuing with unhealthy ones)?

Notes

1. This case draws upon www.comminit.com/drum_beat_55.html.
2. This case draws upon UNAIDS (1999a, p. 71).

6

Overcoming Stigma

■

We have to face the fact that Thai people still view AIDS-afflicted people with pity and think they are bad or promiscuous.

"Kaew," a young Thai woman living with HIV/AIDS, on her website, and in her book, *The Critical Second: Life or Death*, 2001.

HIV/AIDS is like a huge rock in society. Only if everyone in society keeps breaking the rock into smaller pieces will it eventually become dust.

Sommai Punnyakamo (2001, p. 25), a Buddhist monk who counsels PWAs in Mae Chan district of northern Thailand.

On Sunday, 26 April 1998, in Chenneerkuppam, a village 25 kilometers from Chennai in the southern Indian state of Tamil Nadu, a crowd of 400 people gathered around a stranger in his mid-thirties who was dressed in a T-shirt and shorts. He had a cell phone and a pager, and carried a hypodermic syringe. He might have been a drug user. There had been rumors in the village for several days about a North Indian gang that was raping women and giving people "AIDS injections." Someone suggested that the stranger might be a member of the AIDS injection gang. The crowd demanded answers to their questions from the stranger, but he did not speak Tamil. The mood of the crowd turned ugly. They tied the man to a tree and began beating him. Someone in the crowd shouted that the man might have AIDS and that his blood could be infected. The only way to stop the man was to burn him. The stranger was dowsed with diesel fuel from a nearby truck. Then someone tossed a match. Police arrived too late to intercede (Gaitonde, 2001, p. 116).

Lynchings like this one, and others reported in India, South Africa, and in other nations, are extreme manifestations of the stigma attached to people living with HIV/AIDS. In every nation, and among the members of every culture, the stigmatization of people living with HIV and AIDS is a severe problem. Perhaps no illness in the history of humankind has generated such a strong stigma as has HIV/AIDS, with the possible exception of leprosy in Biblical times. The stigma associated with HIV/AIDS has interfered with the gathering of accurate information about the extent of infection, it is a barrier to prevention programs, it inhibits effective testing and counseling, and in many cases stigma interferes with effective treatment and care.

The purpose of this chapter is to analyze: (*a*) the nature of the stigma associated with HIV/AIDS; and (*b*) communication strategies for overcoming this stigma. We distill appropriate lessons from anti-stigma interventions around the world.

The Difficulty of Overcoming Stigma

Most nations launched communication efforts seeking to decrease the stigma of HIV and AIDS. Although useful lessons have been learned, few of these anti-stigma programs have been successful. Anti-HIV stigma remains a major problem throughout the world, and in some nations, like India, it is extremely serious. In other nations, the stigma of HIV/AIDS decreased somewhat as a result of extensive communication efforts.

Uganda, one of the handful of developing countries with a successful AIDS control program, is perhaps a kind of opposite case to India's regarding stigma. At a recent AIDS conference in Geneva, a representative from Uganda stated that stigma in his country had been completely overcome. When the first five AIDS cases were identified in Kampala, the Ugandan government immediately implemented a national AIDS control program. President Yoweri Museveni served as chair of the program. An aggressive condom use campaign was launched with commercial sex workers. Methods of HIV transmission were explained to the public through a mass media campaign, decreasing fear about being in personal contact with infected people. Urgent attention was given to the stigma associated with HIV/AIDS. Uganda's experience in fighting stigma is unusual.

AIDS Stigma in India

In India, the present authors heard many reports of AIDS patients being refused help by one hospital after another, as they sought assistance from medical doctors and nurses who refused to treat them. One top Indian medical doctor even told us that there was really no AIDS epidemic underway, because he and his medical colleagues saw very few patients with AIDS in their hospitals. He was probably correct in his observation about seeing few AIDS patients, although he was certainly wrong in concluding that the epidemic was not making inroads into his country. Until recently, it was a common practice to place a large sign saying "HIV+" on the hospital beds of HIV-positive people as a warning to hospital staff. The medical charts of HIV-positive patients were marked in red.

This odious labeling has stopped in recent years, and some public hospitals now have AIDS wards, given the rise in the numbers of AIDS patients. If medical staff attach such stigma to HIV-positive people, one can imagine that public stigma is very strong indeed. Violation of the rights of people living with HIV/AIDS to confidentiality concerning their seropositive status continued to be a serious problem in India in 2002. We heard frequent accounts of HIV-positive people committing suicide when their HIV status became known in their community through leaks of confidential medical information.

In India, most marriages are arranged by parents and others; given this practice, an individual's HIV status becomes a very important factor in his/her own marriage prospects and those of other family members. In 1998, the Indian Supreme Court ruled that the confidentiality of an HIV blood test could be broken for purposes of partner disclosure before marriage. As one might imagine, stigma prevents many people in India from coming forward for testing and counseling. As a result, no one has accurate figures about the numbers of HIV-positive people in India. The range in estimated numbers is very wide indeed. Further, individuals who are ignorant of their seropositive status delay seeking care.

The stigma is so strong in India that, unlike in most other nations, no famous movie star or other celebrity has disclosed their HIV-positive status. It is not that no famous Indians are infected, but rather that they go to extremes to hide this fact. Dr. Suniti Solomon, one of the most experienced medical doctors advising HIV/AIDS patients in India (she has seen over 6,000 such individuals since she identified the first HIV+ people in Chennai in 1986), says that she regularly treats famous people who fly from Delhi and other distant sites (personal interview, Chennai, 24 December 2001). These elites want confidential treatment and care, which Dr. Solomon's Y.R.G. CARE provides them.

Dr. Solomon told us about a particularly poignant case, the wife of a computer engineer who had infected her. She traveled 350 kilometers to Y.R.G. CARE in Chennai for testing, while nine months pregnant. An obstetrician in Chennai promised to deliver the HIV+ woman, but then the obstetrician left on vacation. The woman eventually found someone to deliver her, by not telling them she was seropositive. Fortunately, the baby was not infected with HIV. Here we see the high degree of stigma in India, and the problems that it causes in the lives of those who are HIV-positive.

Stigma is Everywhere

At an international conference on HIV/AIDS and African Children held at Ohio University in April 2002, a participant shared with the audience the plight of a fourth grade student in a Soweto school, on the outskirts of Johannesburg. The student, an AIDS orphan who lived with her grandmother, tearfully asked the teacher: "Why are my friends laughing at me? Is it because my parents died of AIDS?" Sadly, society stigmatizes those afflicted with AIDS and those affected by it, including orphaned children.

Even individuals who are neither afflicted nor affected by AIDS do not escape stigma. Dr. Smarajit Rana, who helped organize the CSWs in Sonagachi, Kolkata (discussed in Chapter 4), faced hostility and resentment from colleagues: "Sometimes, doctors are worst. They ask me: 'Why do you go in for this nonsense? Why don't you just do your proper work?'" In many countries in Sub-Saharan Africa, a woman who does not breast-feed her baby is assumed by her neighbors to be HIV-infected. They shun her, due to the stigma of HIV (Sepkowitz, 2001).

Dr. Adriana Mauro Nunes (personal interview, 16 March 2001) of Doctors Without Borders in Rio de Janeiro told us of the strong anti-HIV/AIDS stigma that exists in many *favelas* (slums). A drug lord in one *favela* demanded that a health clinic give him the names of all people living with HIV in his area. He intended to force them to leave his *favela*. In Colombia, the revolutionary guerilla group, FARC, forced all adults who lived in FARC-controlled territory to undergo HIV tests. Those found positive were forcibly evicted. In Brazil, too, we heard of PWAs who chose not to register themselves for free anti-retroviral drugs out of fear of being stigmatized. Of those who registered, many were apprehensive about carrying their plastic sacks of drugs home from a health clinic, for fear of being killed. Some *favela* dwellers left their drugs at the clinic, located outside their slum, and walked to it several times a day to take their drug therapy.

Sometimes, a stigmatized group organizes to fight the negative perceptions that society holds about it (McNeil, 2001b). The Indian Network of People Living with HIV/AIDS (INP+) struggles to fight the stigma attached to the epidemic. Some 1,000 PWAs are members, but most HIV-positive people in India do not want to identify with others of seropositive status, because of the stigma.

The Network of Zambian People Living with HIV/AIDS (NZP+) has 4,000 members, which is impressive, even though this number includes only a small percentage of the approximately one million HIV-positive people in Zambia. The self-organization of people living with HIV/AIDS to combat stigma is a promising strategy, but it is still in its infancy in most nations. The stronger the AIDS stigma, the more difficult it is for PWAs to organize to fight the stigma.

ACT UP: Fighting Stigma

The AIDS Coalition to Unleash Power (ACT UP) fights stigma in the United States boldly, radically, and creatively. ACT UP drew attention to injustices against PWAs, helped to speed up the FDA's approval of AIDS drugs (such as AZT), and lobbied for improved health care access for PWAs. ACT UP revolted against the label of "high-risk groups," emphasizing that it is *what* one does, not *who* one is, that places an individual at risk.

ACT UP popularized the slogan "Silence = Death," and staged high-profile demonstrations in places considered "safe" from AIDS, such as New York's Shea Baseball Stadium, Manhattan churches, and Wall Street, to show that AIDS was everybody's problem (Fabj & Sabnosky, 1993). ACT UP coopts existing linguistic symbols for maximum impact. At Shea Baseball Stadium, ACT UP's banners read: "No glove, no love" and "AIDS is no ball game." Its Wall Street demonstrations borrowed corporate language: "AIDS is everybody's business."

ACT UP believes in using explicit language, guerilla tactics, and shock treatment to make its point. Its activists are not shy of grabbing microphones, yanking plugs, jamming fax machines, and putting stickers on public telephones that say: "Touched by a person with AIDS." Its key message is that nobody is safe. Once, while the Sunday sermon was in progress, ACT UP activists organized a mass sit-in outside New York's St. Patrick's Church, and a mass "die-in" inside the church: Members played dead on the church floor to symbolize the consequences of the bishop's inattention to AIDS (Fabj & Sabnosky, 1993).

ACT UP's founder, Larry Kramer, a New York-based author, playwright, and AIDS activist, was inspired by Mahatma Gandhi's techniques of *satyagraha* (literally "insistence on truth" through civil disobedience), which Gandhi used to end British colonial rule in India. In 1947, Britain, the most powerful nation in the world, was shamed into withdrawing its colonial administration from India, when 350 million Indians, led by Gandhi, peacefully refused to cooperate with the oppressive structures of the colonial administration. Inspired by the writings of Leo Tolstoy, Henry David Thoreau, John Ruskin, and Ralph Waldo Emerson, and the Indian epic poem, *Bhagavad Gita*, Gandhi believed in non-violent action, wherein the dignity of the oppressed and the oppressor was equally respected. In India, Gandhi fought not only the British but also oppressive Indian social customs, such as the "untouchability" that stigmatized Indians of low birth, and fostered discrimination against them. Gandhi reduced the stigma of untouchability by welcoming these families into his ashrams, cleaning their latrines (a task typically associated with an "untouchable"), and renaming them "Harijans" (Children of God).

Gandhi's techniques of non-violent political action were suitably adapted by Dr. Martin Luther King, Jr., in the civil rights struggle in the U.S. in the early 1960s. Dr. King, in turn, inspired the generation of activists in the U.S. who launched the feminist, environmental, and anti-war movements of the 1960s and 1970s. Larry Kramer of ACT UP was one such activist. Through mass demonstrations, sit-ins, and die-ins, ACT UP made the injustices faced by PWAs more "visible," thus provoking a desired response from the U.S. government (Kramer, 1990).

The Nature of Stigma

The term "stigma" goes back to the days of Greek civilization, when it referred to a tattoo mark branded on an individual's skin for a wrong-doing (Crawford, 1996). The physical mark publicly identified the blemished individual as one to be avoided. So *stigma* is prejudice and discrimination against a set of people who are regarded by others as being "flawed, incapable, morally degenerate, or undesirable," and who are treated in a negative way. Prejudice is an attitude, while discrimination is overt behavior. The two usually go together. A stigmatized person is one who possesses "an undesired difference" from members of mainstream society, which leads society to discredit them (Goffman, 1963). A person with leprosy, AIDS, or some disability may be stigmatized. The stigma may be obvious (for example, a missing arm), or the marker may be less obvious (for example, being gay). Being identified with AIDS transforms a person from discreditable (for instance, secretly gay) to discredited (publicly gay) (Herek & Glunt, 1988).

Society officially opposes racism, sexism, ageism, ableism, and other types of prejudice, and the unequal treatment of certain individuals. For example, in the United States, civil rights legislation specifies that all of these varieties of discrimination are illegal. Outlawing discrimination, however, is seldom very successful in changing human behavior. Stigma, which is very deep-rooted, can only be modified over a period of several generations, even when laws and policies demand such change. Here we distinguish between the ideal versus the real aspects of society. Ideally, most societies want to decrease all types of stigma, and many societies outlaw discrimination. However, most people in most nations continue to be stigmatizing. That is the sad reality.

When people discriminate against others in society, coercive government policies may follow. By 1990, 104 countries had enacted HIV-related legislation, including policies ranging from compulsory detention and restriction of movement of certain groups, to regulations ensuring the confidentiality of persons with HIV (Malcolm et al., 1998). In 1991, about 40 countries required proof of HIV-negative status before allowing foreign visitors to enter (Mann et al., 1996). Foreigners have been blamed for the spread of HIV in many countries, particularly Africans, for instance, who were attending universities in India, the former U.S.S.R., and in parts of Europe (Malcolm et al., 1998). For example, in 2002, a young Kenyan man traveled to Singapore to study theology. On arrival, he was found to be HIV+ and was promptly returned to Nairobi.

In the United States, in the months after Magic Johnson retired from the Los Angeles Lakers in November 1991, he regularly came to each of the team's practice sessions, hoping to continue his relationship with his former teammates. They let him know that he was unwelcome. Magic was forced to shoot baskets by himself on another court. Finally, one young player agreed to play one-on-one with Magic at practice sessions. Some time later, when Magic announced that he was considering a return to professional basketball, various players around the National Basketball

Association publicly stated that they would refuse to play (Crawford, 1996). Karl Malone of the Utah Jazz was particularly outspoken, announcing that Magic's opponents might be at risk if he sweated on them. The educational value of this controversy was that the public gained greater knowledge about the means of HIV transmission. Eventually, the NBA adopted new rules, for instance, prescribing that in the case of injuries in which blood was involved, the game be immediately halted until the injury was bandaged. The brouhaha about Magic's return illustrated the high degree of stigma with which HIV/AIDS was regarded by professional athletes and by the U.S. public in the early 1990s.

Why is HIV/AIDS Stigmatized?

Through an accident of history, AIDS became a disease of already-stigmatized groups. In the initial era of the epidemic in most countries, HIV infection spread through sexual networks of gay men, commercial sex workers, and/or injecting drug users. These marginalized groups were already heavily stigmatized by society, and this prejudice was carried over, and strengthened, when such individuals became identified as carriers of HIV. This "double stigma" of AIDS stemmed from the identification of AIDS as a serious illness, and from the identification of AIDS with already-stigmatized groups (Herek & Glunt, 1988).

The gay community in the United States has often been blamed for starting the epidemic. Members of the Christian right and other political conservatives in the U.S. proposed a quarantine, reinstating state sodomy laws, and eliminating the civil rights of HIV-infected gays that protect them from discrimination (Herek & Capitanio, 1999). A Gallup poll conducted in the mid-1980s showed that 50 percent of Americans agreed that "most people with AIDS have only themselves to blame." Those who contract AIDS through behavior that is controllable (for example, through commercial sex work or sharing needles) are perceived as "guilty" and hence assigned more blame, receive less sympathy, and face more anger, than those who are perceived as "innocent victims" (for example, individuals infected while receiving a blood transfusion) (Wiener, 1993).

In later eras of the epidemic in each country, as pointed out previously, people living with HIV/AIDS tended to be of lower socioeconomic status. These personal characteristics associated the epidemic with people who were already perceived negatively, creating and strengthening the stigma of HIV/AIDS. AIDS-related stigma would have been far less had the epidemic first been identified, for instance, among upper-class, straight, heterosexual individuals, hemophiliacs, or children.

Previously in this book, we described how the managing editor of *The New York Times* in the early 1980s insisted that his reporters use the word "homosexual" rather than "gay." He insisted that there was nothing happy about being homosexual. Homophobia was common in the United States when the epidemic began. In a 1986 Op/Ed piece in *The New York Times*, a highly conservative political writer proposed that "everyone detected with AIDS should be tattooed in the upper forearm, to protect common-needle users, and on the buttocks, to prevent the victimization of other homosexuals" (quoted in Herek & Glunt, 1988, p. 886). Homophobia is an important reason for stigma in many nations. Under the penal code of India, intercourse between men is illegal. Nevertheless, men who have sex with men (MSM) exist in India, as in other nations, and are an important vector of HIV transmission. Most prevention programs in India do not target gay men, but the Naz Foundation in Delhi has reached 5,600 men who have sex with men. In addition, *hijras* (literally, not man, not woman) may be involved in HIV transmission in India, but this group is so taboo that little is known about their role. *Hijras* are a high-risk special grouping in the Mumbai and Chennai sex work industry.

Another important reason for the stigma attached to AIDS, based in large part on ignorance of the means of transmission, is a common fear that by associating with people living with AIDS, individuals might put themselves at risk. Such fear of infection, even among people who know and understand the actual means of transmission, may be based on an irrational reaction. The lethal nature of HIV/AIDS undoubtedly raises the level of fear.

Only providing knowledge about the means of virus transmission, as social psychologists of prejudice have found, is seldom sufficient to change such strongly held attitudes as stigma. Prejudice and discrimination are emotional matters, and are not based on facts alone. In Colombia, a 2001 national health survey revealed that 60 percent of women had positive attitudes toward PWAs. However, 85 percent strongly felt that HIV-positive people should not have sex (even with condom protection). Interventions to overcome the stigma of AIDS must attack emotionally based, strongly held attitudes and behaviors. HIV/AIDS is a disease of ignorance and intolerance. HIV-positive people are often defined by the public as "the other," and treated accordingly as an out-group. The lynching in India, described at the top of this chapter, shows how the crowd defined the stranger as the "other," as not one of "us," leading to his death.

In 1995, a center to care for HIV-positive people opened in Nonthaburi, a Bangkok suburb. The center was operated by the St. Camillus Foundation of Thailand. Community opposition to the new center was "immediate and fierce" (Steinfatt & Mielke, 1999, p. 397). Residents of Nonthaburi expressed fear about the center's water and garbage disposal, fearing that HIV infection might spread via these means (it cannot). Shots were fired into the building, followed by verbal abuse, intimidation, and bomb attacks. After nine months of operation, the center closed its doors to people living with HIV/AIDS, just as the local government ordered the center to move out of the community. In the case of this center, increased knowledge about HIV transmission might have lessened the stigma. But it was more a matter of irrational fear than of ignorance.

Measuring Stigma

Many efforts have been made to measure the degree of stigma associated with HIV/AIDS. Such measurements are needed, for instance, to determine the effectiveness of anti-stigma campaigns. A version of the Bogardus Social Distance Scale might be formulated to measure HIV/AIDS stigma. The Bogardus scale was initially used to measure an individual's social distance/closeness to various racial and ethnic groups in the United States. Five typical scale items were: I would not like to have Chinese (for example) people as neighbors, as work associates, as friends, as a date, or as a marriage partner. Then these five questions might be repeated for another racial/ethnic grouping, such as Italians or Mexicans. One of these categories might be people living with HIV/AIDS. This metric measured the relative closeness or distance of a respondent from people in other categories.

Kelly et al. (1987) developed the Prejudicial Evaluation Scale to measure AIDS stigma, consisting of items such as how deserving the person is of illness, how responsible the person is for contracting the illness, and the danger that the infected individual poses for others. Another measure is the Social Interaction Scale (Kelly et al., 1987), which includes items such as willingness to attend a party where an HIV-infected individual prepared the food, willingness to continue a friendship with an HIV-infected person, and willingness to share office space with an HIV-infected individual. Studies in the United States indicate that there is a far greater degree of stigma associated with AIDS than with other life-threatening illnesses like leukemia and breast cancer (Crawford, 1996).

One problem with creating such measures is that they are usually highly interrelated with homophobia. Such scales are obviously inappropriate when measuring stigmatizing attitudes toward heterosexual women or other categories of people with HIV/AIDS. O'Hea et al. (2001) created Attitude Toward Women with HIV/AIDS (ATWAS), a 27-item scale composed of four sub-factors: child care, myths/negative stereotypes, reproduction/contraception issues, and sympathy/transmission. Typical scale items for each of these four sub-factors are:

1. I think women who give birth to babies who are HIV+ should be prosecuted for child abuse.
2. Most women with HIV/AIDS are prostitutes or sex workers.
3. A woman owes it to her husband to have unprotected sex with him even if he has HIV/AIDS.
4. I have little sympathy for women who get HIV/AIDS from sexual promiscuity (sleeping around).

Overcoming Stigma

What role can communication strategies play in overcoming the stigma associated with HIV and AIDS? Communication strategies can help (*a*) break the silence about AIDS, and (*b*) move the discussion of HIV/AIDS from the personal-private to the public-policy sphere. Through interpersonal discussion about HIV/AIDS, individuals and communities can be moved along the continuum from a high degree of stigma toward lessened stigma.

Breaking the Silence

At a recent family reunion, one of the authors began to describe his current research on sexuality and AIDS. The discussion was abruptly terminated by an elderly relative who remarked that "such topics were not worthy of family discussion." AIDS is clearly a *taboo* topic, one that is so sensitive that it usually cannot be discussed openly. Because HIV/AIDS deals with sexual intercourse, morality, and death, many people talk about it in hushed tones. If HIV/AIDS were *completely* taboo in a society, of course, there could be no communication about this issue, no effective intervention programs, and no testing and counseling. In reality, the topic of HIV/AIDS lies somewhere on the continuum from relatively highly taboo to relatively less taboo. In most nations, HIV/AIDS is closer to the high taboo end.

The communication challenge is how to move the issue of HIV and AIDS from the high taboo end toward the less taboo end of the continuum. Only by making a topic less taboo can silence about it be broken at the individual, community, and national levels. It is only through spurring private, public, policy, and media discussion that the issue of AIDS can become increasingly non-taboo and thus be destigmatized. Therefore, communication activities are really at the heart of overcoming stigma about AIDS. The following are some promising ways of breaking the silence on AIDS.

Harnessing Symbols: One strategy for coping with a taboo topic is to represent it with a symbol, the red ribbon in the case of AIDS. To millions of people in today's world, the red ribbon *is* AIDS. Given that the virus is so small as to be invisible to the naked eye, and that most PWAs do not show outwardly evident symptoms of infection for many years, a widely recognizable symbol for AIDS is key to giving greater visibility to the epidemic.

Warren Parker, director of the Center for AIDS Development, Research and Evaluation (CADRE) in Johannesburg, played an important role in making the red ribbon a highly recognizable symbol in South Africa. When we met with Parker in June 2001, he emphasized how the red ribbon logo provides an opportunity to "brand" HIV/AIDS communication activities. Distribution of red ribbon pins and beaded ribbons, T-shirts and caps with the red ribbon, and the red ribbon logo with the toll-free AIDS helpline number on posters and pamphlets, represent symbolic ways of promoting HIV/AIDS prevention, care, and support.

Symbols such as the red ribbon "speak" despite their inanimate nature, breaking the silence on AIDS. At a recent dinner gathering in New Delhi, India, when one of the authors wore a red ribbon pin on his coat lapel, he was asked: "What does the ribbon signify?" An animated conversation about AIDS ensued. Here, the red ribbon pin helped stimulate talk about AIDS. Similarly, while riding into Manhattan in June 2001, one of the authors noticed the 50-meter-tall, lighted, ribbon-like symbol on the UN building (Plate 6.1). The taxi driver informed the author that the UN building was the site of AIDS deliberations that week, the first-ever UN special session on a health issue. The lighted ribbon symbol was a sobering sign of the global devastation caused by AIDS. The United Nations discussion, led by Secretary General Kofi Annan, resulted in the creation of a global fund for fighting the epidemic.

Symbols like the red ribbon can be further modeled through the mass media to break the silence on AIDS. The present authors were invited to an informal meeting in Johannesburg with creative writers and producers who were planning an AIDS television drama series. The discussion centered on how funerals in South Africa, typically attended by hundreds of people, were usually silent about AIDS as the cause of death. How could this silence be broken by the television series? Many ingenious suggestions flew around the room. One individual suggested that the AIDS red ribbon be displayed on the coffin of a young protagonist who dies of AIDS. Another television scriptwriter suggested that a wreath be placed on the coffin by a family elder with a large red ribbon in its center. Another person suggested that while the coffin was being lowered into the grave, a moment of great poignancy, the father of the dead person should hand out red ribbon pins to those present. The emotional poignancy of such media depiction results from the use of a symbol to break the silence.

Culturally Appropriate Humor: One strategy for overcoming the taboo surrounding HIV/AIDS is to use culturally appropriate

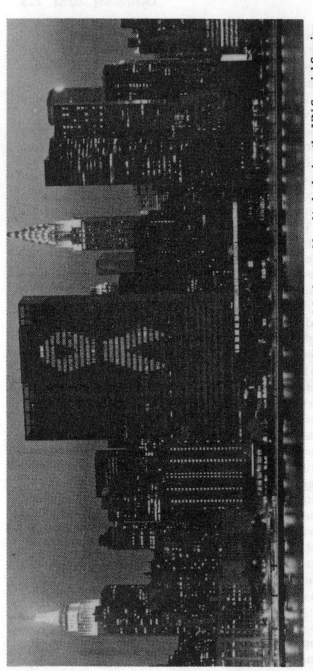

Plate 6.1   The 50-meter-tall AIDS Ribbon on the UN Building in Manhattan, New York, during the UN Special Session on HIV/AIDS in June 2001

Symbols, such as the AIDS red ribbon, "speak" loudly despite their inanimate nature. The lighted ribbon on the UN building is a sobering sign of the global devastation caused by AIDS.

Source: United Nations. Photograph by Eskinder Debebe.

humor. The "Braulio" campaign to encourage condom use in Brazil (mentioned in Chapter 3), and Mechai's efforts to popularize condoms in Thailand, are based on the use of humor. Mechai's condom-blowing contests in Patpong (the red-light district) and his famous Cabbages & Condoms Restaurant in Bangkok are examples of the utilization of humor to encourage discussions about condoms. When the authors visited this restaurant on Sukumvit Soi 12 in Bangkok, they noticed that the menu's cover caption said: "Our food is guaranteed not to make you pregnant." They ordered a condom salad as starters, and ended the meal with a condom jelly dessert. When they paid their bill, the small change came in the form of condoms. As they exited the restaurant, a large colorful sign, hanging from a tree, said: "We do not have mints, but please take a condom instead." Beneath this red and yellow sign were two boxes with condoms. One was labeled "Thai size," the other "International size." People laughed about condoms, and handled them; some even opened the packages to measure which one was larger — the Thai-sized condom or the international-sized condom. Thai people believe in *sanuk* (having fun), and Mechai's Cabbages & Condoms Restaurant exemplifies how to have fun with condoms, and, in doing so, how to break the silence on condom use.

Not much is humorous about the 40 million people in the world today who are infected with an incurable virus, of course. But jokes can be made about condoms. We were given a postcard in Rio de Janeiro in March 2001 when we visited ABIA. The card showed an erect penis with a humorous comment about using condoms. In South Africa, we saw a poster of an erect penis wrapped in the South African flag.

Comfortable Spaces: The use of barber shops to stimulate discussion about AIDS demonstrates the strategic use of space in addressing the taboos associated with AIDS. Many Indian men are too embarrassed to buy condoms at a drugstore or to talk freely about sex with health counselors or with family members. But one place in which they feel comfortable "letting their hair down" is the barber shop (Jordan, 1996). The Indian state of Tamil Nadu trained barbers to be its frontline soldiers in the fight against the AIDS epidemic. In the poorer and blue-collar areas of Chennai, Tamil Nadu's capital city, men often have their hair and beards trimmed before visiting a commercial sex worker. Now they pick up a free condom on their way out of the barber shop. Participating barber shops in Tamil Nadu provide free subsidized condoms to their clients; some barbers offer a premium "pleasure pack" at subsidized rates, from which they earn a 25 percent commission.

Mr. Mani, a local barber, cuts hair and dispenses advice on safer sex, which represents a new dimension in his 20-year-old career. He starts by talking to a client about his family and children. Slowly, he gets to women, HIV/AIDS, and condoms (Jordan, 1996). The barber program was launched in 1995 in Tamil Nadu, and within a year recruited 5,000 barbers who receive AIDS training on Tuesdays, their day off. The barbers are not paid to promote HIV/AIDS prevention, but they appear to take considerable pride in their new responsibility.

Over the centuries, India's barbers have been regarded as traditional healers, confidants, advisors, and matchmakers (Jordan, 1996). In rural areas, the barber's wife is often a *dai*, a traditional birth attendant, a low-status but highly respected role in an Indian community. "To get the king's ear, tell his barber," goes a popular saying. Reinforcing the image of barbers as healers, the local trade group is called the Tamil Nadu Medical Barber Association.

Although HIV/AIDS may be taboo in a society like India, there are special places like barber shops where this topic can be discussed openly. Women's beauty parlors and gay bars may represent other spaces where discourse about HIV/AIDS can take place comfortably.

Pink Triangle Malaysia (PTM), a non-governmental organization, operates an innovative outreach program targeted at injecting drug users (IDUs) in Chow Kit, a poor red-light community in Kuala Lumpur, the nation's capital city. This organization creatively uses space to reduce stigma and prejudice (UNAIDS, 1999a). A culturally sensitive research protocol to assess the clients' needs, prior to launching the PTM program, pointed to the importance of creating an Ikhlas ("sincere") Community Center (ICC), a "safe space" where the IDUs would feel comfortable dropping in. The Ikhlas Community Center provides meals to IDUs, medical care and treatment, referrals to hospitals and drug treatment centers, counseling and psychological support, access to condoms and other risk reduction services, and referrals to job placements. Clean bathroom and toilet facilities are also provided so that drug users can bathe, wash their clothes, and maintain their hygiene.

The IDUs participate in running these ICC activities: They cook and clean, serve as outreach workers and volunteer counselors, and carry out administrative work. This involvement helps them take ownership of the Ikhlas project, and builds their self-esteem. The IDUs of the ICC now routinely liaise with volunteer groups from hospitals, nursing schools, the corporate sector, and colleges, and thus feel more accepted by the general community. Their active involvement also makes Pink Triangle Malaysia's Ikhlas program highly cost-effective and efficacious.

The Ikhlas program represents a non-stigmatized, non-judgmental space for IDUs in Malaysia, a country where drug use, according to the local law, is punishable by death. However, the humane environment created by ICC is palpable enough for law enforcement authorities to look the other way. As such, the Ikhlas Community Center achieves harm reduction, rather than seeking to eliminate injection drug use.

The principle of harm reduction is also the basis of several Dutch initiatives that create comfortable spaces for commercial sex work, legalized in the Netherlands in 2000 (Kapila & Pye, 1992). Many local municipalities have established *gedoogzones*, streets where soliciting is allowed during predetermined hours. The city of Utrecht has an *afwerplek*, a special car park with parking bays divided by high fences, where commercial sex work is transacted. Many Dutch towns established *huiskamers* ("living rooms"), where counseling, care, and assistance are available to CSWs. Utrecht's Huiskamer Aanloop Prostitutes Foundation established a mobile, caravan-style *huiskamer*, which is parked in local *gedoogzones* during permitted hours. Commercial sex workers stop by to rest, take a shower, to buy condoms, receive counseling, and medical care (Kapila & Pye, 1992). This mobile *huiskamer* is an example of creating a mobile "comfortable space" for those at risk for HIV. The Dutch projects, much like Ikhlas in Malaysia, are respectful of people's lifestyles, non-judgmental, and create comfortable spaces where people can take refuge and responsibility for their personal decisions.

The Program for Appropriate Technology in Health (PATH) created youth-friendly drugstores in Thailand and Cambodia. Studies indicated that 40 percent of young men seeking health products viewed pharmacies as the access point for buying condoms and STD treatment. Pharmacies in Thailand averaged as many as

50 youthful clients at a drugstore per day. The strategy adopted by PATH in creating "friendly drugstores" involved training Thai pharmacists to interact with young people in a compassionate, non-judgmental manner, and to refer them, if needed, to appropriate clinical services.

Safe Virtual Spaces

Comfortable spaces can also be created virtually, for instance, through telephone helplines. AIDS helplines abound throughout the world, some directed at the general public, while others are targeted to gays, injection drug users, CSWs, and other groups. Some telephone helplines are managed by professionals such as the Italian Telefono Verde AIDS, which employs trained physicians and psychologists, while others such as AIDS-Linien in Denmark are staffed by volunteers (Kapila & Pye, 1992).

In New Delhi, India, a telephone helpline called Talking about Reproductive and Sexual Health Issues (TARSHI) provides AIDS- and sexuality-related information, counseling, and referrals, in both Hindi and English to Indian men and women of all ages, castes, and socioeconomic classes. Of the 30,000 calls received since its inception in 1996, 80 percent were from men, and about 70 percent of the callers were in the 15 to 30 age group (Chandiramani, 1998). The anonymity and confidentiality of telephonic communication, as well as the non-judgmental attitude of trained telephone counselors, make it possible for people to feel "virtually" comfortable in discussing their concerns. Callers often begin with a question on one topic, for instance, masturbation, but then move to related issues like genital size, premature ejaculation, sexual relations with multiple partners, and HIV/AIDS (Chandiramani, 1998). *These callers are moving on the continuum from less taboo toward highly taboo topics.*

Disque Saude is a telephone hotline operated by the Brazilian Ministry of Health. The director of Disque Saude, Ellen Lita Ayer, told us in 2001 that the hotline received 8,000 calls per day, about three million per year. Some 50 percent of the calls concerned HIV/AIDS, and another 20 percent dealt with STDs. The 145 telephone operators are mainly medical and dental students in Brasília, who work five hours per day. Disque Saude will double its size in 2002. A popular television show, *Laços de Família* (Family Links), which frequently deals with health problems, places the hotline's telephone number at the bottom of the television screen. When this tie-in with Disque Saude first happened, a major increase in the number of calls promptly occurred. The callers use only their first names, and the anonymity thus provided helps overcome the stigma of HIV/AIDS that may prevent individuals from seeking information from other sources.

The anonymous information gleaned by counselors at TARSHI and Disque Saude represents a goldmine of data for understanding prevailing cultural beliefs about sexuality and HIV/AIDS, including levels of ignorance and misconceptions. For instance, when talking about HIV and AIDS, male callers to TARSHI often say: "I can't understand how the virus can get *into* my body. After all semen comes *out* of my body. Nothing flows into it!" Only comfortable spaces virtually created through telephone helplines allow for such candid discussion. The most widespread misunderstandings suggest what messages are needed for HIV/AIDS prevention.

In sum, telephone helplines provide a confidential, accessible, sympathetic, non-judgmental, and non-embarrassing virtual space for discussion of HIV/AIDS issues. Telephone helplines are highly relevant for callers, as their individualized needs can be served. Further, callers take the initiative, so they are more likely to follow the advice that is provided. As a bonus, telephone helpines are an invaluable source for collecting data about the general public's perceptions of AIDS, including their feedback on specific intervention programs (Kapila & Pye, 1992).

Spiritual Leadership: A few decades ago, an anthropologist was asked to investigate why some village wells in Thailand were maintained in working order, while most soon fell into a state of disrepair. The pump mechanism broke and was not repaired, or a pool of muddy water formed around the well, resulting in pollution of the pumped water. In some villages, however, the pump was repaired if it broke, and a concrete base was built to prevent a muddy pool from forming. By accident, these village wells had been drilled on *wat* (temple) grounds, and the Buddhist monks took responsibility for their upkeep (Niehoff, 1964). This illustrates that religious leaders can be an effective force for development and social change.

In Thailand, Buddhist monks played an important role in caring for AIDS patients, educating people about HIV prevention, and thus moving a highly taboo issue on the continuum toward a lesser taboo status. Because of the high regard in which Thais hold monks, these Buddhist religious leaders are credible sources for persuasive messages about HIV/AIDS. We visited the Friends for Life Center directed by Phra Phongthep Dhammagaruko in Chiang Mai (Plate 6.2). Initially, Phra Phongthep had formed a study group for applying *dhamma* (religious teachings) to the problems of everyday life, but this effort was unsuccessful because of its abstract nature. In 1993, this monk decided to focus his work mainly on HIV/AIDS. He gave speeches in villages in Chiang Mai province, using an overhead projector, and conducting an AIDS "Quiz Show" with audience members. The prize for correct answers was an audio tape that Phra Phongthep made, with the story of an HIV-positive mother on one side, and of a male PWA on the other. Phra Phongthep preached that HIV-positive people should not spread the virus to others.

Few Buddhist monks were involved in activities to combat the epidemic in 1993, and Phra Phongthep's efforts met with severe criticism. Other monks told him that preaching religious philosophy, not AIDS, was his job. When he opened a hospice for AIDS patients on his 1-acre *wat* grounds, his neighbors complained that their drinking water might be polluted. He responded that his land was the lowest plot in the area, and that, as far as he knew, water ran downhill.

Phra Phongthep's Friends for Life Center has 10 beds. When we visited the hospice in December 2001, eight patients with AIDS were in residence, following a regimen of medication, prayer, and fresh air in the tranquil hospice. Over the past eight years, the Center has treated 800 outpatients and 400 inpatients. Some 115 died in the hospice and 56 in nearby hospitals, while others spent their final days with their family members. The monk has no funds

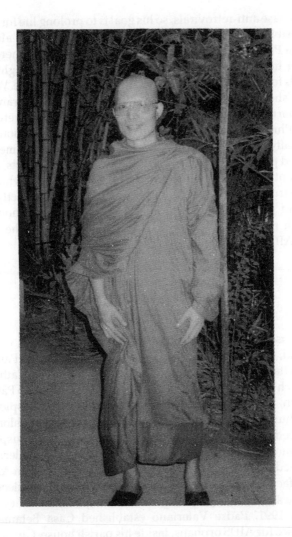

Plate 6.2 Phra Phongthep Dhammagaruko at his Friends for Life Center in Chiang Mai

In Thailand, where most people are Buddhists, a monk like Phra Phongthep is highly respected. He cares personally for people living with AIDS in his hospice. This monk works to reduce the stigma associated with HIV in Chiang Mai, an area hit very hard by the epidemic.

Source: Personal files of the authors.

to purchase anti-retrovirals, so his goal is to prolong life for as long as possible. He is non-judgmental, treating all patients alike.

Phra Phongthep recounted for us how a dying commercial sex worker had collapsed along a roadside, and was brought to the Friends for Life Center, where he provided her with care. Within a week, she died. She was an undocumented immigrant from neighboring Myanmar (Burma), and the Thai police refused to allow Phra Phongthep to prepare the body for cremation. So he personally called the chief of police in Chiang Mai, and immediately received permission to cremate the body. Buddhist priests, by dint of their otherworldly nature and the high respect with which they are regarded, can cut through lines of authority, go directly to the top, and get fast action. Spiritual leaders like Phra Phongthep, through their dedicated work, are helping to break the silence about AIDS in Thailand.

Imirim's Children

We visited another spiritual leader in another part of the world, who addressed AIDS head on. Padre Valeriano Paitoni is an Italian priest who migrated to Brazil to serve a Catholic church in Imirim, a middle-class neighborhood in São Paulo. When, in 1984, Padre Valeriano opened an AIDS hospice in his church to care for people living with AIDS, his parishioners reacted violently. Angry protesters stoned the hospice, breaking its glass windows. Three years later, Padre Valeriano opened Casa Alliance de la Vida (Alliance for Life), an AIDS care facility at a far distance from their community, a reflection of the stigma and prejudice surrounding PWAs.

In 1991, Padre Valeriano established Casa Betania, a hospice for AIDS orphans, inside his parish house. Given the central location of the hospice, and Padre Valeriano's Sunday sermons on AIDS, members of the community began to stop by Casa Betania to care for his tiny charges, holding them and feeding them (Plate 6.3). "Volunteerism is easy with children," Padre Valeriano remarked. Over the next several months, the community members gradually changed their attitudes and behavior from rejection of PWAs, to acceptance. This change

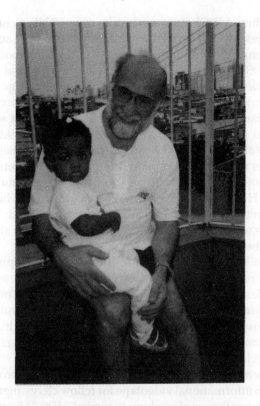

Plate 6.3 Father Valeriano and an AIDS Orphan in São Paulo

This Catholic-priest-turned-AIDS-activist used the care of AIDS orphans to reduce his community's stigma toward people living with HIV/ AIDS in São Paulo, Brazil.

Source: Personal files of the authors.

occurred through the AIDS orphans. Everyone loves children, even if they are HIV-positive. Working closely with the Imirim community, Padre Valeriano established two other hospices for AIDS orphans, Casa Siloe (in 1994) and Casa Lars Suzanne (in 1998). Community members "took ownership of these hospices. Weekly contributions tripled after we established Casa Siloe," noted Padre Valeriano (personal interview, 12 March 2001).

The three AIDS hospices in Imirim serve 50 HIV+ children, from ages 1 to 5. These HIV+ children attend local schools, sensitizing other children and school authorities about HIV and AIDS. The hospice staff works closely with local health authorities to monitor the viral load of the tiny charges, who are all on anti-retroviral drug therapy. Community members are invited to their birthday parties, which attract several hundred guests. In the past decade, only three children in Padre Valeriano's AIDS hospices passed away (these low numbers reflect the therapeutic effects of the anti-retroviral drugs, and the high quality of care, support, and nutrition that the HIV+ children receive). When we asked him how the community members reacted to their deaths, he replied: "These children were the community's children. Everybody showed up for their funeral."

Padre Valeriano's work in Imirim is greatly inspired by Paulo Freire's* philosophy of critical pedagogy and by principles of liberation theology. He talks about the need for church leaders to go beyond pulpit sermonizing to put "faith in action." His parish hosts meetings for Alcoholic Anonymous and Narcotics Anonymous, and offers adult literacy classes to the underprivileged.

A few months before we visited Valeriano, he had produced an AIDS informational videotape for fellow clergy members, emphasizing the use of condoms to combat AIDS. "My primary duty is to defend life," he told us (personal interview, 12 March 2001). Archbishop Claudio Humes of São Paulo published a statement in the leading local newspaper condemning the use of condoms and reprimanding Padre Valeriano. Valeriano politely retorted that condoms were not about religion, but about public health. The Brazilian Ministry of Health supported Padre Valeriano's position and released a condom advertisement showing an angel and a devil during the pre-Carnival celebration in 2001. The caption read: "No matter what side you are on, wear a condom" (Plate 6.4).

Brazil, the country with the world's largest Roman Catholic population, is the only country in the world where the Catholic Church has its own AIDS commission. Despite the Pope's denunciation of condoms, and Archbishop Hume's support of the Pope's position, several Catholic groups, such as Padre

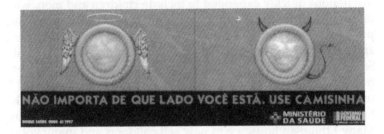

Plate 6.4   A Daring Multimedia Campaign by the Brazilian Ministry of Health during Carnival Time in 2001 Showed Condoms as Angels and Devils

The caption reads: "No matter what side you are on, wear a condom." This campaign was designed to address the Catholic Church's opposition to condoms, emphasizing that wearing condoms was good public health.

Source: Brazilian Ministry of Health.

Valeriano's church in Imirim, promote condom use and provide care and support to PWAs in order to reduce stigma.

* Paulo Freire served as secretary of education in the early 1990s in the city of São Paulo, where Padre Valeriano's parish is located.

Capitalizing on Social Rituals:[1] In Ethiopia, coffee ceremonies are a social ritual. Friends and family members get together in neighborhoods to socialize over a cup of coffee. Some innovative HIV/AIDS programs in Ethiopia piggybacked on the cultural popularity of these coffee ceremonies to initiate discussion about HIV/AIDS among housewives. Unlike youth, who may have access to AIDS prevention information in their schools, and adult men, who may learn about AIDS in the workplace, housewives are more difficult to reach through conventional channels.

In one innovative program in Ethiopia, a group of peer educators was recruited from among housewives and trained to launch informal discussions about HIV/AIDS with their friends and neighbors during coffee ceremonies. These housewife-centered discussions quickly expanded to include children and men, who informally joined the groups. Such family-based HIV discussions, previously taboo, increased dialogue between husbands and wives, and between parents and children, about how to reduce HIV risk. Some women now pack condoms for their husbands when they are traveling, saying it should be available "for use in an emergency." In some neighborhoods, the coffee conversations catalyzed the formation of local AIDS action teams and anti-AIDS youth clubs. Many Ethiopian housewives now sell condoms and many youth serve as peer educators.

Coping with Death through Memory Boxes: The idea of creating memory boxes was first initiated by a psychologist in Uganda in the mid-1990s, as a way of employing oral narrative therapy to proactively prepare individuals for their imminent death from AIDS. HIV-positive people create cardboard boxes (about the size of a small suitcase), which are usually opened at the time of their public funerals by relatives and friends (Plate 6.5). They decorate their memory boxes on the outside with favorite pictures of themselves with friends and family, and put such personal effects as jewelry, clothing, letters, and diaries inside, to help others remember them.

Most memory boxes include personal narratives by the afflicted persons, describing their life stories, including how they became HIV-positive, and perhaps the discrimination and stigma they faced from family, friends, and community members. These narratives are often read publicly at their funerals, providing a poignant setting for grieving relatives to collectively reflect on how they deal with AIDS on a day-to-day basis.

We visited the AIDS Counseling Care Training (ACCT) Center at the Chris Hani Baragwanath Hospital in Soweto, on the outskirts of Johannesburg. A special room is filled with memory boxes made by PWAs. Glen Mabuza, who directs ACCT with the help of 22 outreach workers (all PWAs), showed us the memory box made by Judith Makie Lufhugu, who died of AIDS-related complications in May 2000. Raped at age 13 by her step-uncle, Lufhugu learned of her HIV status when she was in her early twenties, and became a volunteer counselor at ACCT. During Lufhugu's funeral ceremony, her memory box was opened and her self-penned autobiography

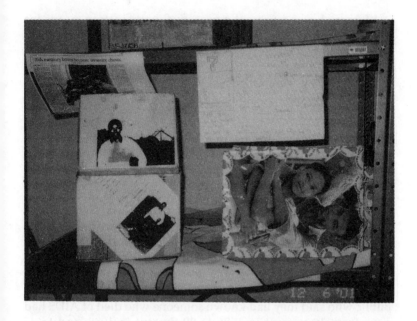

Plate 6.5   Memory Boxes at the AIDS Counseling Care Training Center in the Chris Hani Baragwanath Hospital, Soweto, South Africa

These memory boxes, prepared by individuals living with HIV/AIDS in Soweto Township, contain photographs, letters, poems, clothes, and other memorabilia. The photograph in the memory box at lower right is outlined with condom stickers that say "Condoms Keep Lovers Safe."

Source: Personal files of the authors.

was read to her family members. She talked about the trauma of rape and the overt discrimination she faced from her family members. Those present at the funeral ceremony wept openly, and apologized for their actions. Often, when an ACCT client passes away, a chartered bus takes other ACCT clients and outreach workers to the funeral, in a display of solidarity. The ACCT workers sing and chant before the funeral service. One recent funeral drew 700 individuals from the community for the service. The opening of the memory boxes during these services is a poignant and educational experience.

Memory boxes represent a proactive, participatory means for PWAs to cope with their own deaths. In countries like South Africa, where the idea of memory boxes is catching on through the efforts of several NGOs, the creation of these boxes goes hand in hand with counseling. Honoring the dead is a highly cherished social norm in every country, and memory boxes use the time and space dimensions of this event to influence the family and community discourse surrounding HIV and AIDS.

An important HIV prevention strategy is knowing of someone who has died of AIDS. As the epidemic spreads in a nation, and as more and more individuals die from AIDS, the motivation of the living to adopt preventive actions should become stronger and stronger. This, however, occurs only if relatives and friends know that AIDS was the cause of death. In the early years of the epidemic in the United States, newspaper obituaries indicated the cause of death for individuals who had died of AIDS as "causes unknown." As HIV/AIDS stigma gradually decreased during the 1980s, this situation changed. Surveys found that the percentage of the U.S. public who said they had known someone who died of AIDS had risen from 10 percent in 1986 to 20 percent in 1988, and to 45 percent in 1990. Thus, the AIDS-related deaths of half a million Americans have been a strong influence on HIV prevention.

An investigation of Uganda, Kenya, and Zambia (Macintyre et al., 2001) found that knowing someone who had died from AIDS was a strong predictor of adopting three HIV prevention practices: (a) using condoms; (b) reducing the number of sexual partners; and (c) restricting sexual relations to one partner. The correlation between knowing someone who had died of AIDS and prevention behavior was especially strong in Uganda, perhaps because HIV/AIDS was discussed relatively openly, compared to neighboring Kenya and Zambia. In fact, all of the Uganda survey respondents who had adopted all three of the preventive actions knew someone who had died of AIDS. Some 92 percent of the 1,733 Ugandan male respondents knew someone who had died of AIDS, while this figure was around 74 percent in Kenya and Zambia, where stigma was stronger. In all three nations, knowledge of AIDS and of the means of its transmission was very high.

So reducing stigma to the point at which individuals talk about people who died from AIDS can have a strong HIV prevention effect. The study in the three African nations suggests that "it's not what you know, but who you know" that matters in HIV prevention (Macintyre et al., 2001, p. 160).

Home-based Care Programs:[2] A common observation is that where HIV/AIDS is widespread and health workers have considerable contact with PWAs, discrimination is less and stigma is reduced. For instance, a study of 878 general practitioners in Australia showed that their direct contact with people living with HIV/AIDS significantly reduced their fear and prejudice (Bermingham & Kippax, 1998).

Similarly, home-based care programs for AIDS patients make HIV/AIDS more visible in the community, and, over a period of time, reduce stigma and discrimination, as the experience of Tateni Home Care Services in Mamelodi, South Africa, shows. Tateni Home Care Services was started by a group of retired nurses in Mamelodi, a black township of 1.5 million people on the western fringes of Pretoria, the capital of South Africa. In response to the growing need for care and support of local AIDS patients, Tateni developed a home-based care policy and training materials in cooperation with local health authorities. Tateni's credo is based on the values of empathy, acceptance, and the removal of discrimination against those infected with HIV/AIDS.

Tateni's program complements existing health care services, rather than duplicating or competing with them. Family members of AIDS patients are trained to enlarge the base of primary caregivers, thereby boosting the community's internal capacity to handle HIV/AIDS. Tateni was careful not to copy home-based care models from industrialized countries, where clients usually receive formal, home-based health care, mostly in senior citizen homes or in nursing home facilities. African traditions emphasize complex family and community relationships of support, obligation, and consensus. Cost-effective, family-based home care is provided by Tateni in a way that is respectful of cultural norms and traditions. Tateni mainly provides enabling palliative care, but HIV/AIDS prevention, education, and surveillance are also an integral part of its work. Tateni's outreach workers teach home care using life-sized dolls made of foam rubber and cast-off clothes. They show caregivers how to look after patients while guarding themselves against HIV infection (for instance, by wearing protective gloves).

Sesame Street, the popular children's television program produced by Children's Television Workshop (CTW) in the United States, and co-produced by CTW in many other nations, will now combat the stigma of HIV/AIDS. In 2003, one of the muppets in the South African co-production of *Sesame Street* will be HIV-positive! Cer-tainly, starting with children aged 2 to 5 (the intended audience for *Sesame Street*) is a sound strategy for fighting the stigma of HIV/AIDS.

The strategies just discussed, ranging from using symbols, to humor, to using appropriate spaces, are means of getting people to talk about the topic of HIV/AIDS, and thus of breaking the silence about the epidemic.

From the Personal-Private to the Public-Policy

In addition to breaking the silence, discourse about HIV/AIDS needs to move from the personal sphere to the family, community, public, and policy spheres. Some illustrations of how this movement occurs now follow.

Humanizing HIV/AIDS through Disclosure: As more and more people disclose their HIV-positive status, the taboo surrounding the infection lessens. When former Zambian president Dr. Kenneth Kaunda, a highly respected African statesman, disclosed that his son had died of AIDS, it humanized the AIDS epidemic in Zambia. Often, however, the first individuals in a nation to disclose that they are HIV+ are punished severely. Previously, we mentioned the sad case of Gugu Dlamini, a young woman living in a Durban township in South Africa. After she declared her HIV status in a radio broadcast on World AIDS Day in 1998, Gugu was stoned and stabbed to death (see Chapter 2).

It is important to humanize stigmatized individuals who are, or become, well-known public figures: Nkosi Johnson, Ryan White, Magic Johnson, Betinho, and so forth. These courageous figures help set the media agenda for the issue of AIDS, but they do much more. They show that individuals living with HIV/AIDS are people just like everyone else. They are children, women, and men; gay and straight; wealthy and poor; famous athletes, movie stars, and ordinary people. In their public appearances, these "poster people" for the epidemic stress that they want to be treated the same as everyone else. They want to pursue their education, earn a living, maintain their health, and help others. These spokespeople for overcoming AIDS stigma alone are not enough, however, because an organized campaign approach is necessary. Repeated, targeted messages are needed.

"Little Sheila," a 4-year-old HIV+ girl in São Paulo, was an important champion for the destigmatization of HIV in Brazil in 1991. An AIDS orphan, Sheila Cortopassi de Oliveira was adopted by a wealthy couple after the death of her mother. Her adoptive parents tried to enroll Little Sheila in the Colegio San Luis, an elite Jesuit school in São Paulo, but she was rejected for admission. Her parents sued the school in a widely publicized lawsuit, and won. The dispute attracted considerable news coverage in Brazil, and helped construct HIV/AIDS as a human rights issue. In Little Sheila's memory, an annual award is given to Brazilians who champion the human rights of HIV-positive people. The 1999 winners of the award were Father Valeriano Paitoni (discussed earlier), and AIDS activist Jorge Beloqui.

Grieving Publicly: The AIDS Quilt: As discussed in Chapter 1, when the AIDS Memorial Quilt was first displayed on the Mall in Washington, D.C., in 1987, it had 1,920 panels, each panel representing an individual who had died of AIDS. By 1996, it had grown to 40,000 panels, large enough to cover 26 football fields; and by 2001, the number had grown to 45,000, representing one-tenth of the total number of AIDS deaths in the United States since the disease was first identified in 1981 (Holland, 2001). The quilt does not discriminate: It honors the memory of different individuals irrespective of color, sexual orientation, socioeconomic status, age group, or gender (Hawkins, 1993). Collectively, the quilt is an enormous canvas representing those who have died of AIDS. It poignantly depicts the growth of the epidemic.

When Cleve Jones started the quilt in 1986 to honor his friend Marvin Feldman who had died of AIDS, it was a symbol of personal grieving (Plate 6.6). As the idea of honoring the dead spread among other grieving individuals in other locations, the panels began to be sewn together into vast quilts, representing a move toward public grieving. For several years, the quilts were displayed on football fields at multiple U.S. locations. In 1996, all the quilts were sown together and displayed on the Washington Mall by AIDS activists and grieving relatives.

Symbolically, the ever-growing quilt moved the issue of AIDS from the space of personal grieving to that of public grieving, reducing the stigma associated with AIDS deaths. The quilt helped break down the "social distance" between the dead and the living: Those watching the quilt said they felt "similar" to the PWAs, and

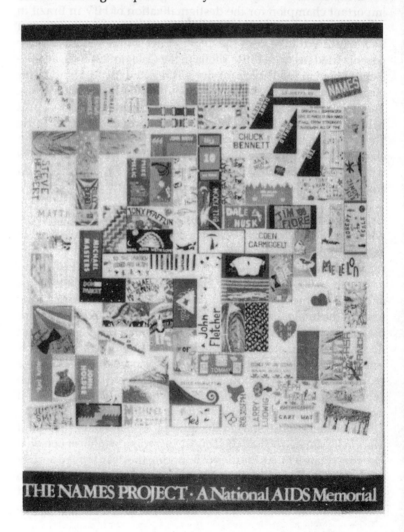

THE NAMES PROJECT · A National AIDS Memorial

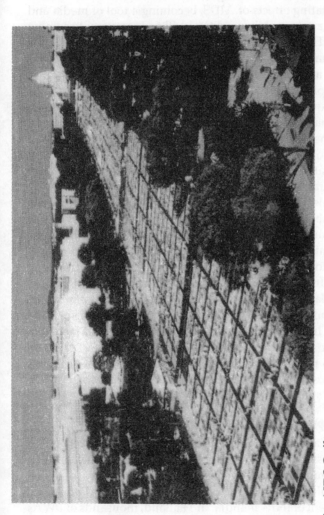

Plate 6.6 The AIDS Quilt

At this early stage (1986) in the HIV/AIDS epidemic in the United States (see plate on previous page), the AIDS quilt only represented a few dozen individuals who had died. In 1996, when the quilt was displayed on the Mall in Washington, D.C. (above), it covered 26 football fields. By 2001, the quilt had grown to 45,000 panels.

Source: The AIDS Names Project, San Francisco. Personal files of the authors.

that "AIDS is their problem" (Knaus & Austin, 1998). Through the AIDS quilt, relatives and friends did not grieve alone. A sense of collective efficacy was built among grievers to cope with their loss.

The quilt also served as a highly visual and permanent symbol of the devastating effects of AIDS, becoming a tool of media and public advocacy to mobilize political will and resources to combat the disease. The quilt is a memorial for the dead, much like the Vietnam Memorial. However, unlike other memorials, the quilt is (*a*) moveable, and (*b*) a meta-memorial (i.e., a memorial of memorials). It can be displayed at many locations in smaller sizes.

The AIDS quilt, which can now be accessed through the Internet, is also a virtual memorial. Relatives and friends post the pictures, voices, and memorabilia of their loved ones, which can be accessed by anyone from anywhere in the world. Through such electronic postings, relatives and friends grieve and lend support to each other in virtual space.

Wall murals (Plate 6.7), candlelight vigils (Plate 6.8), and traveling exhibitions about AIDS also represent public sphere activities to break a community's silence on AIDS, and to spur public discourse on the epidemic. During the 2000 Durban AIDS Conference, loveLife, an organization devoted to enhancing sexual responsibility among the South African youth (discussed in Chapter 5) launched its loveTrain (Plate 6.9). The loveTrain, the world's largest movable HIV/AIDS billboard, provides clinical services, counseling, and HIV testing. In 2000, as the colorful train made its journey from Cape Town to Durban, it stopped in various towns to host celebrity concerts and provide HIV tests and counseling. The loveTrain's journey across South Africa received extensive coverage in the mass media, spurring talk about HIV/AIDS.

Organizing PWAs: People living with HIV/AIDS often organize into support and action groups, so that when networked into a nationwide association, they can influence national policies. Many PWA organizations mount effective campaigns to decrease stigma.

An example is the poster (Plate 6.10) featuring the late Ashok Pillai, president of INP+ in India. In Thailand, thousands of PWAs are organized into hundreds of local groups. These HIV-positive people demonstrate their numbers every Valentine's Day. In Chapter 3, we told of how these PWAs staged a demonstration at Parliament House in Bangkok on World AIDS Day, 2001, in order

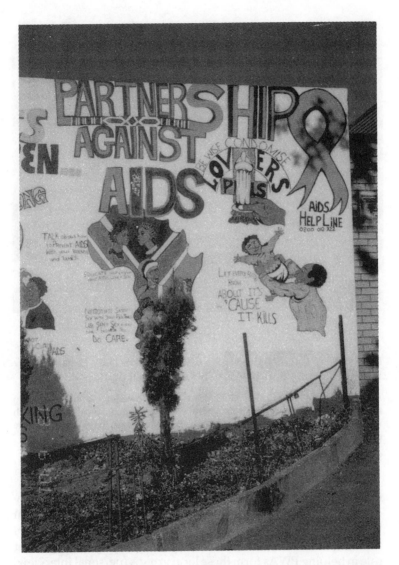

Plate 6.7   A 20-by-30-foot Wall Mural on the Community Center in Alexandra Township, Outside of Johannesburg, South Africa

This mural, painted by the residents of Alexandra Township, is a permanent, visible symbol of the degree to which the community faces the HIV/AIDS epidemic.

Source: Personal files of the authors.

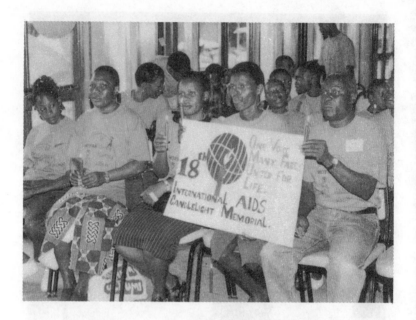

Plate 6.8   A Candlelight Vigil on World AIDS Day, Organized by Women Fighting against AIDS in Kenya (WOFAK)

A candlelight vigil for the AIDS dead was followed by a march of two thousand people through Nairobi's main street, ending at a local church. Such vigils, well reported by the press, spur dialogue about the epidemic in the public and policy spheres in Kenya.

Source: WOFAK.

to lobby for free anti-retrovirals. Thailand has a more highly organized population of PWAs than other nations. Senator Jon Ungpakorn, the chairman of the AIDS ACCESS Foundation, says that hospital staff and other health providers play an important role in helping PWAs form these local groups (personal interview, Bangkok, 1 August 2001). However, hospital social workers often then try to control these PWA groups, channeling them toward a social support function and away from lobbying activities.

People living with some disease, and their family members, can form powerful organizations to lobby for benefits, such as

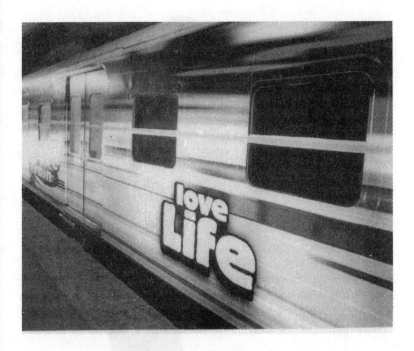

Plate 6.9 The loveTrain, as it Moved from One Location to Another, Helped Spur Talk about HIV/AIDS in South Africa

The loveTrain is a traveling sexual health center that moves across South Africa promoting the work of loveLife, an organization devoted to enhancing sexual responsibility among the South African youth. The train, which many call the world's largest movable HIV/AIDS billboard, provides clinical services, counseling, and HIV testing.

Source: loveLife.

destigmatization of the disease. A striking illustration of this is the pink ribbon groups of breast cancer survivors that began to march and organize in other ways in the United States in the 1970s. Susan G. Komen, a lawyer who survived breast cancer, founded an association of breast cancer survivors to lobby the U.S. government for more funding for women's diseases, and to raise private funding for such research. Today, the Susan G. Komen Foundation is an important funding source, and the pink ribbon of the Breast Cancer Survivors Association is the widely recognized symbol of breast

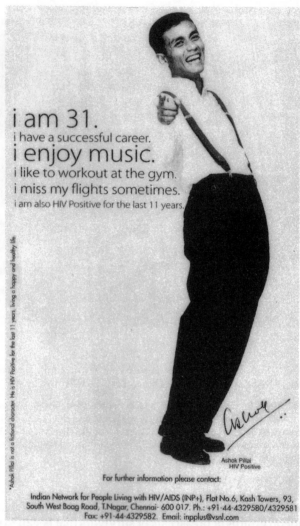

i am 31.
i have a successful career.
i enjoy music.
i like to workout at the gym.
i miss my flights sometimes.
i am also HIV Positive for the last 11 years.

*Ashok Pillai is not a fictional character. He is HIV Positive for the last 11 years, living a happy and healthy life.

Ashok Pillai
HIV Positive

For further information please contact:

Indian Network for People Living with HIV/AIDS (INP+), Flat No.6, Kash Towers, 93,
South West Boag Road, T.Nagar, Chennai- 600 017. Ph.: +91-44-4329580/4329581
Fax: +91-44-4329582. Email: inpplus@vsnl.com

Plate 6.10   The Late Activist Ashok Pillai in India

Pillai was president of the Indian Network for HIV/AIDS Positive People
(INP+). After INP+ was unable to find a movie actor or sports star to appear
on an anti-stigma poster in India, Pillai reluctantly agreed to serve as the role
model for young urban professionals with HIV. As a result of this disclosure,
Pillai was asked by his landlord to vacate his apartment in Chennai. Pillai died
in April 2002.

Source: INP+.

cancer concern. The U.S. Postal Service sells a pink ribbon stamp, with part of the cost going to breast cancer research.

People living with AIDS are gradually becoming more organized and are gaining power for their advocacy throughout the world. These groups encourage individuals to disclose publicly that they are HIV+, and provide social support to their members. In many countries, HIV-positive people play an important role in advocating for low-priced anti-retrovirals, and, at least in Thailand, PWA groups distribute information about the appropriate use of anti-retroviral drugs. They also advocate for alternative treatments, such as herbal medicines, which are far more affordable than the triple cocktail. These PWA groups have a unique ability to reach out to people with HIV/AIDS, wherever they are located, and to represent their concerns. Through the collective actions of PWA groups, individuals can accomplish objectives that are out of their reach when they act separately.

In Thailand, the organization of HIV-positive people was initiated in 1991 in Chiang Mai in the northern area of the country. Individuals with HIV/AIDS were greatly stigmatized at this stage, and most of them were afraid to disclose their HIV status. While a traditional health provider was "cooking up" a batch of herbal medicines, a group of PWAs gathered to await the drugs. With the encouragement of the traditional healer, the PWAs decided to form a support group. The Red Cross, Norwegian Church AID, World Vision, and other Christian organizations then provided assistance to PWAs in forming support groups in Thailand.

From one (in Chiang Mai) in 1991, the number of PWA groups in Thailand grew to 15 in 1994, 35 in 1995, 78 in 1996, 105 in 1997, 195 in 1998, and to 224 in 1999; and this just in the six northern provinces around Chiang Mai (Phusahat, 2000). Over 400 PWA groups existed in Thailand in 2001. This phenomenal growth of PWA groups was aided by government funding, which first became available in 1995. The PWA groups have interesting names, which hint at their functions: New Life Friends, Doi Saket Widows, White Sky, Warmly Love, and Tapestry of Friendship. An important function of the PWA groups in Thailand is to provide psychological support to HIV-positive individuals. These groups also provide vocational training and marketing assistance to HIV-positive people who learn to embroider and to produce other types of handicrafts.

The formation of PWA groups is an illustration of *organizing for social change*, defined as the process through which disempowered individuals form groups to gain control of their future. By forming local groups, people living with HIV/AIDS gain a feeling of collective efficacy, lobby for their civil rights, and defeat stigma. Over the long term, PWA groups are becoming an even more powerful force in the global struggle against the epidemic.

Nationally, the PWA groups in Thailand are networked as part of the AIDS ACCESS Foundation, led by Senator Jon Ungpakorn. AIDS ACCESS is an influential pressure group that seeks to protect the rights of PWAs, obtain lower-priced anti-retrovirals, and to expand assistance for AIDS orphans. Such organized activities by HIV+ people have done much to attack the stigma of HIV/AIDS in Thailand (Phusahat, 2000).

Within less than a decade, many HIV-positive people were able to lead fairly normal lives, mingling with a Thai society that had become relatively free from stigma. The battle is not won, however, says Senator Ungpakorn: "Many older attitudes still prevail today" (personal interview, 2 August 2001). Why is HIV/AIDS still stigmatized in Thailand, while individuals with cancer are not stigmatized? The answer, says Dr. Wiwat Rojanagithayakorn, former director of the Thai AIDS control program, is the nature of the disease: "Cancer is not infectious" (personal interview, Bangkok, 2 August 2001). So fear is a key ingredient in stigma.

In countries like India, organized efforts by PWA groups are at an early stage of development. The Indian Network for People Living with HIV/AIDS (INP+) was formed in 1997 by 12 PWAs in Chennai, and has since expanded to Delhi and other Indian cities. Anti-AIDS stigma is still very strong in India, and the INP+ faces a considerable struggle. At present, this PWA association has only about 1,000 members, in large part reflecting PWAs' caution about disclosing their status, wary of retribution from a stigmatizing society.

Organizations of PWAs in several nations are included in national-level policy-making bodies, although sometimes this is a sham. For example, the late Ashok Pillai, chairman of the INP+, told us of his futile participation in the National AIDS Committee, which meets once a year in New Delhi. The 2001 meeting occurred on a Friday afternoon from 3 to 6 P.M. (personal interview, Chennai, 24 December 2001). Of the 70 members of this advisory committee,

Pillai was the only person who had disclosed his HIV-positive status. India's minister of health gave a speech, followed by speeches by other prominent bureaucrats. The 90 minutes of discussion time remaining were mostly used up by committee members to request more resources, including an increase in their travel allowance and free telephone service. In the 2001 annual meeting, Pillai raised his hand four times to represent the PWA point of view. His comments were duly noted, but there was no response and no discussion. No minutes were distributed after the meeting, and no actions ensued. While such an experience was a big turn-off, Pillai noted that resigning from the committee would be worse. At least he represented a visible symbol of AIDS in India, although humanizing the issue in a useless national forum does little to tackle the epidemic.

The story of Ashok Pillai's life with HIV/AIDS is itself a commentary on the nature of stigma. Pillai joined the Indian Navy in 1988 when he was 17 years old. One day, in 1991, when he delivered a report to the medical officer, the latter noticed a rash on his skin, and ordered a blood test. Then followed a second test. The doctor called Pillai to his office and told him bluntly: "Your HIV test is positive."

"What is HIV?" asked Pillai.

"It's AIDS."

"What about the treatment? Will I get any medicines?" Pillai asked.

"There is no treatment as such," came the dispassionate answer.

"What am I supposed to do then?" he asked.

"You can eat good food, sleep well, exercise, and live."

"How long am I going to live?"

"We don't know. You might live for two years, three years, four years . . .."

"Okay, fine. At least I have four years to live." Pillai smiled and walked away.

Pillai actually went on to live for 11 more years, until his death at age 31.

Anti-stigma Campaigns: Anti-stigma campaigns have been mounted in various nations, using mass media and other intervention components. A *campaign* is intended to generate specific outcomes or effects in a relatively large number of individuals, usually within a specific period of time, and through an organized set of communication activities (Rogers & Storey, 1987). Confronting stigma means that communication campaigns must also be designed to reduce prejudice against gays, injecting drug users, and commercial sex workers. One relatively short-term campaign, however, is seldom enough to remove the powerful nature of AIDS stigma. Such campaigns need to be backed by national policies, and to be supported by the personal commitment of national leaders.

When Mechai Viravaidya served as a Cabinet minister in Thailand in charge of the national AIDS control program, he drank Coke out of the same glass as an HIV+ child. This act helped to show that sharing utensils was not a means of HIV transmission. Mechai's much-publicized action also showed that he accepted HIV-positive people on a personal basis. Actress Elizabeth Taylor has been a tireless spokesperson and fund-raiser for HIV/AIDS programs and research in the United States. Taylor was a personal friend of actor Rock Hudson, who died in 1985. The chief minister of Tamil Nadu state in India, Mr. Karunanidhi, held hands with children living with HIV/AIDS in a human chain on World AIDS Day in the late 1990s. This symbolic act of acceptance communicated an important message against stigma.

Policy Implementation: A national government can establish and implement policies intended to overcome stigma (Herek & Glunt, 1988). Preserving the confidentiality and privacy of an individual with HIV is essential. Stiff penalties should be attached to unauthorized disclosure of this information. Also, policies should prohibit discrimination on the basis of HIV status in offices, schools, and hospitals. In Thailand during the 1991–92 Mechai period, when so much was done in a few months to combat the epidemic, national policies were established to protect the privacy of people living with HIV/AIDS. AIDS education, including anti-stigma lessons, was instituted in every Thai school.

The Indian government was forced to drop the mandatory testing of people like CSWs (a policy that had been legalized in the 1989 AIDS Prevention Bill) by the World Bank as one condition for receiving the $84 million loan in 1994. In this case, an external influence forced a policy change in India.

Conclusions

AIDS is a disease of ignorance and intolerance, as well as a biological illness. When the mass media profile AIDS as a disease of gays, injecting drug users, and commercial sex workers, it perpetuates stigma. Fear, prejudice, injustice, and stigma are every bit as dangerous, if not more so, than the biological virus. An HIV-positive Brazilian writer, Herbert Daniel, said: "Prejudice kills during life, causing civilian death. . . . [Such a death] is worse than real death" (quoted in Daniel & Parker, 1993, p. 131). Further, taboos surrounding HIV/AIDS often prevent recognition, discussion, and acceptance of safer sex practices, and serve as a barrier to testing, counseling, treatment, and care. *Stigma is one of the major barriers to effective communication about AIDS.*

AIDS stigma evokes negative reactions — denial, shame, fear, anger, prejudice, and discrimination — that manifest themselves in interpersonal and group relationships. Hence, communication strategies need to be at the heart of all efforts to overcome the stigma of HIV and AIDS. Although useful lessons about combating stigma have been learned, few anti-stigma programs have been very effective, as they do not take into account communication theories. Wearing down the mountains of stigma requires repeated efforts over dozens of years.

Communication strategies can help break the silence about AIDS, and move the discussion of HIV/AIDS from the personal-private to the public-policy sphere, thus gradually overcoming taboo-ness. Tragic figures like Ryan White in the United States, and Little Sheila Cortopassi in Brazil, helped lessen the stigma which the public attached to HIV+ people. The AIDS Memorial Quilt Project, which began in San Francisco in 1986, reminds the public that people who died from AIDS were former friends, brothers, sisters, sons, daughters, parents, and lovers. A somewhat similar project in South Africa, memorializing people who died from AIDS, involves the use of memory boxes.

The stigmatized nature of HIV/AIDS in most societies is an important barrier to effective program interventions. An Indian wife, who fears that her husband and his family will reject her if she tests HIV-positive, is unlikely to seek a blood test. Likewise, in Thailand, many HIV-positive people, once their employers learn of their HIV status, are fired. This practice, an outcropping of stigma, naturally discourages testing for HIV. As a result, neither individuals nor their nations have the basic information that they need to fight the epidemic.

Someday, perhaps, we will live in a world without the stigma of AIDS. Until then, we all suffer.

Notes

1. This section draws on UNAIDS (2000b).
2. This section draws on UNAIDS (1999a, pp. 54–55).

7

Entertainment-Education

■

*I have listened to your program and understood that this
radio program* Twende na Wakati *will save my life and
that of my wife.*

A male letter-writer to the Tanzanian radio
soap opera in 1997.

*I learned that it is good to practice safe sex by using a
condom. As a result I have been using it ever since I
watched* Soul City. *And I always educate my friends
about condoms and advise them as they are for their
own safety. I sometimes provide them with condoms
because I always carry them.*

An avid male viewer of *Soul City* in 1997.

In the 1999 *Soul City* entertainment-education television series in
South Africa, a new collective behavior was modeled to portray
how neighbors might intervene in a domestic violence situation.
The prevailing cultural norm in South Africa was for neighbors,
even if they wished to help a victim, not to intervene in a domestic
abuse situation. Wife (or partner) abuse was seen as a private
matter, carried out in a private space, with curtains drawn and
behind closed doors.

In the *Soul City* series, neighbors collectively decided to break the ongoing cycle of spousal abuse in a neighboring home. When the next wife-beating episode occurred, they gathered around the abuser's residence and collectively banged pots and pans, censuring the abuser's actions. This prime-time entertainment-education episode, which earned one of the highest audience ratings in South Africa in 1999, demonstrated the importance of creatively modeling collective efficacy in order to energize neighbors, who, for cultural reasons, previously felt inefficacious. Evaluation research found that exposure to the Soul City E-E intervention was associated with willingness to stand outside the home of an abuser and bang pots (Soul City, 2000). After this episode was broadcast, pot-banging to stop partner abuse was reported in several locations in South Africa (Singhal & Rogers, 2002). Patrons of a local pub in Thembisa Township in South Africa exhibited a variation of this practice: They collectively banged bottles when a man physically abused his girlfriend (Soul City, 2000).

The entertainment-education strategy, as exemplified by the melodramatic pot-banging episode in South Africa, has been consciously applied to HIV/AIDS prevention in the form of: (a) radio and television soap operas, for instance, *Twende na Wakati* (Let's Go with the Times) in Tanzania, *Soul City* in South Africa, *Ushikwapo Shikimana* (If Assisted, Assist Yourself) in Kenya, *Tinka Tinka Sukh* (Happiness Lies in Small Things) in India, *Nshilakamona* (I Have Not Seen It) in Zambia, *Malhacão* (Working Out) in Brazil, *Sexto Sentido* (Sixth Sense) in Nicaragua, and *Kamisama Mo Sukoshidake* (Please God Just a Little More Time) in Japan; (b) talk shows such as *Good Times with DJ Berry* in Uganda and *Erotica* in Brazil; (c) popular music and celebrity concerts, for instance, Franco Luambo's hit song "Beware of AIDS" in the Democratic Republic of Congo and the Hits for Hope concerts in Uganda; (d) feature films such as *Philadelphia* in the U.S. and *It's Not Easy* in Uganda; (e) animation films like *Karate Kids* targeted to street children in over 100 countries; and (f) competitive events like bicycle rallies in Uganda, soccer matches in Cameroon, and condom-blowing contests in Thailand (Church & Geller, 1989; Piotrow et al., 1997; Rogers et al., 1999; Singhal & Rogers, 1999; Valente & Bharath, 1999).

Research evaluations of these programs suggest that the entertainment-education strategy—through its use of formative research, audience segmentation, a multimedia campaign approach, media celebrities, and other creative techniques such as humor, animation, and claymation, among others — can effectively promote HIV/AIDS prevention behavior (Church & Geller, 1989; Piotrow et al., 1997; Singhal & Rogers, 1999; Valente, 1997; Vaughan, Rogers et al., 2000). Entertainment-education is widely used to combat the epidemic throughout the world.

The present chapter analyzes the contributions of the entertainment-education strategy to HIV prevention, highlighting the use of popular, long-running television and radio soap operas to engage audiences emotionally, and to encourage public discussion. *Twende na Wakati* in Tanzania, *Soul City* in South Africa, and other noteworthy HIV/AIDS entertainment-education initiatives are documented here, and lessons about their effective use are distilled from these initiatives.

The Entertainment-Education Strategy

The entertainment-education (E-E) strategy in development communication abrogates a needless dichotomy in almost all mass media content: that mass media programs must be either entertaining *or* educational (Singhal & Rogers, 1999, 2002). *Entertainment-education* is the process of purposely designing and implementing a media message to both entertain and educate, in order to increase audience members' knowledge about an issue, create favorable attitudes, shift social norms, and change the overt behavior of individuals and communities. The larger purpose of entertainment-education programming is to contribute to the process of directed social change, which can occur at the individual, community, or societal level.

The entertainment-education strategy contributes to social change in two ways:

1. It can influence audience awareness, attitudes, and behaviors toward a socially desirable end. Here, the anticipated effects are located in the individual audience members. An illustration is provided by the radio soap opera *Twende na Wakati* in Tanzania that convinced several hundred thousand sexually active adults to

adopt HIV prevention behaviors (like using condoms and reducing their number of sexual partners) (Rogers et al., 1999).

2. It can influence the audiences' external environment to help create the necessary conditions for social change at the group or system level. Here, the major effects are located in the interpersonal and social-political spheres of the audience members' environment. Entertainment-education media can serve as a social mobilizer, an advocate, or agenda-setter, influencing public and policy initiatives in a socially desirable direction (Wallack, 1990). An Indian village, Lutsaan, rejected dowry as a result of community-based listening to a radio soap opera, *Tinka Tinka Sukh*. These system-level social changes resulted from entertainment-education (Papa et al., 2000).

The Rise of Entertainment-Education

The idea of combining entertainment with education is not new: It goes far back in human history to the timeless art of storytelling. For thousands of years, music, drama, dance, and various folk media have been used in many countries for recreation, devotion, reformation, and instructional purposes. However, while the concept of combining entertainment with education is not new, "entertainment-education" is a relatively new concept. Its use in radio, television, comic books, and popular music, at least when designed according to behavioral change theories, has largely developed over the past three decades (Singhal & Rogers, 1999, 2001b).

In radio, the earliest well-known illustration of the entertainment-education strategy dates back to 1951, when the British Broadcasting Corporation (BBC) began to air *The Archers*, a radio soap opera that conveyed educational messages about agricultural development (*The Archers* continued to be broadcast in 2002, addressing contemporary educational issues like HIV/AIDS prevention and environmental conservation). The entertainment-education strategy in television was discovered more or less by accident in Peru in 1969, when the television soap opera *Simplemente María* was broadcast (Singhal et al,, 1994). The main character, María, a migrant to the capital city, faced tragic setbacks, like becoming a single mother. María worked during the day, and enrolled in adult literacy classes in the evening. She climbed the socioeconomic ladder of success through her hard work, strong motivation, and through her skills with a Singer sewing machine. *Simplemente María* attracted very high audience ratings, and the sale of Singer sewing machines boomed in Peru. So did the number of young girls enrolling in adult literacy and sewing classes. When *Simplemente María* was broadcast in other Latin American nations, similar effects were produced. Audience identification with María was very strong, especially among poor, working-class women: She represented a role model for upward social and economic mobility.

Inspired by the audience success and the unintended educational effects of *Simplemente María*, Miguel Sabido, a television writer-producer-director in Mexico, developed a methodology for creating entertainment-education soap operas. Between 1975 and 1982, Sabido produced seven entertainment-education television soap operas (one each year), which helped motivate enrollment in adult literacy classes, encouraged the adoption of family planning methods, promoted gender equality, and so forth (Nariman, 1993). Sabido's entertainment-education soap operas were also commercial hits for Televisa, the Mexican television network, demonstrating that educational messages do not limit the popularity (and profitability) of entertainment programs.

These events of the past several decades led to the birth of the strategy of combining education with entertainment in the mass media. This strategy has since spread to over 100 projects in 50 countries, spurred by (*a*) Population Communications International (PCI), a non-governmental organization headquartered in New York city, and (*b*) Johns Hopkins University's Center for Communication Programs. The entertainment-education strategy has been widely recreated in television, radio, film, print, and theater, including the well-known, multimedia *Soul City* series in South Africa (discussed later in this chapter).

Why Entertainment-Education?

Entertainment-education programs represent a viable weapon in the worldwide war against HIV/AIDS (Piotrow et al., 1992). Such programs utilize the popular appeal of entertainment formats (such as melodrama) to consciously address educational issues (Piotrow et al., 1997; Singhal & Rogers, 1999). These interventions earn high audience ratings, involve audience members emotionally, and spur interpersonal conversations among audience members on various topics. The ability of E-E programs to stimulate conversation can bring taboo topics like HIV/AIDS into public discourse. While audience members are usually reluctant to discuss the details of their personal lives in public, they feel comfortable talking about the lifestyles of their favorite characters, and commenting on the accompanying consequences.

The appeal of E-E comes from its narrative approach, which is not perceived as didactic or preachy by audience members. Walter Fisher (1987) argued that humans are essentially storytellers (*homo narrans*) who employ a narrative logic in processing discourse. Entertainment-education soap operas, whether on television or on radio, or via some other channel, consist of highly complex narratives with various protagonists and antagonists, plots and subplots, and conflicts and resolutions. Such narratives, designed with the use of formative research, are perceived by audience members as more coherent, believable, and involving, than straightforward rational appeals. Green & Brock (2000) conducted experimental research indicating the ability of narratives to "transport" audience members from their real-life situations into a hypothetical situation. Thus, the Tanzanian radio soap opera *Twende na Wakati* transported listeners into the life of a truck driver, Mkwaju, who becomes HIV-positive.

Entertainment-education programs also appeal to audience members because exposure is a pleasurable activity. Viewers of E-E enjoy conflict-laden, suspenseful drama. Repeated empathic distress from seeing a favorite character in imminent danger often enhances the enjoyment of drama and the resolution of the threat (Zillman & Vorderer, 2000).

Entertainment-education programs appeal to the emotions of audience members. Affect from a media character is communicated to audience members, often through the process of *parasocial interaction*, the tendency of individuals to perceive a personal relationship with a media or public personality (Horton & Wohl, 1956; Sood & Rogers, 2000). Audience members perceive media characters as their personal friends, and welcome them into their homes at an appointed hour (through a television or a radio set), so as to have an ongoing relationship with them. Audience members often talk out loud to their favorite characters, laugh and cry with them. The characters "infect" the audience members with their feelings. Such is the power of entertainment-education in behavior change communication.

From Private Closets to Public Discourse*

In Japan, the number of HIV tests and requests for HIV/AIDS counseling more than doubled from July to September 1998, thanks to a popular melodramatic television series, *Kamisama Mo Sukoshidake* (Please God Just a Little More Time), which told the story of a high school girl who became infected with HIV from commercial sex work. This television program, broadcast for three months, addressed the issue of HIV/AIDS prevention, and that of teenage prostitution, in a culturally sensitive manner, breaking the media's silence on these topics.

Prior to broadcasts of *Kamisama Mo Sukoshidake*, which explored human emotions in confronting stigma, guilt, fear, and anger, public awareness of HIV/AIDS had declined in Japan for five years. The media were reluctant to address this taboo topic. Then NHK, the government television network in Japan, pioneered the broadcasting of *Kamisama Mo Sukoshidake*. The television series earned the second highest ratings of all television programs broadcast during the summer of 1998 in Japan. It moved a highly stigmatized topic into the domain of public discourse.

* This case draws upon Watts (1998).

Key Elements in Creating Entertainment-Education

The Values Grid

Prior to launching an entertainment-education intervention, a framework of the specific educational issues to be emphasized in the intervention, or a values grid for the educational messages, is created (Singhal & Rogers, 2001b). This framework can be derived from a nation's constitution, its legal statutes, or from documents such as the UN Declaration of Human Rights to which the country is a signatory. For instance, a constitutional right such as "All citizens will have an equal opportunity for personal and professional development" provides the basis for media messages about gender equality.

The values grid, often derived from formative research, is a chart of the educational issues to be tackled, and the positive and negative values to be encouraged and discouraged. It contains statements such as "All girl children have the right to attend school," and "It is a violation of a girl child's rights not to send her to school." A values grid specifies the behavior changes that are to be encouraged or discouraged in an entertainment-education project such as a soap opera. It may be a formal statement signed by government, religious, and media officials, pledging their support of the educational values promoted in the intervention. For example, Miguel Sabido asked Catholic church leaders in Mexico to help develop the values grid for his *telenovela* about family planning in the mid-1970s. The values grid contributes to the consistency of the characters and storyline with the intended goals of an entertainment-education intervention. The grid also helps to bring on board key stakeholders, providing credibility to the intervention, and blunting later attacks. The setting, characters, storyline, and subplots are based on the values grid.

When the Tanzanian radio soap opera *Twende na Wakati* was being planned in 1993, health, religious, and political leaders participating in a week-long workshop decided that the values grid should include HIV prevention, as well as family planning adoption. A research project by AMREF (1992) had just been completed on the alarmingly high rate of HIV infection among truck drivers and CSWs at truck stops. Accordingly, the entertainment-education soap opera centered on a negative role model, Mkwaju (literally, Walking Stick), who is infected with HIV and eventually dies of AIDS. The planning workshop also chose the name for the entertainment-education radio program, *Twende na Wakati* (Let's Go with the Times, in Swahili).

Formative Evaluation Research

Formative evaluation research is conducted with the intended audience to design the entertainment-education intervention. *Formative evaluation* is a type of research conducted while an activity, process, or system is being developed or is ongoing in order to improve its effectiveness (Singhal & Rogers, 1999). Research-based information about the characteristics, needs, and preferences of a target audience can fine-tune the values grid, and sharpen the design of entertainment-education. For example, a formative evaluation survey in Tanzania in 1992 found that many adults, including those using the rhythm method of contraception, did not know the days in the woman's menstrual cycle when fertilization was most likely. Correct information was then provided in *Twende na Wakati*. Pilot episodes of an entertainment-education intervention are typically produced, pre-tested with the intended audience, and then revised.

Blunder in South Africa*

In 1994, the South African Ministry of Health commissioned the award-winning producer of *Sarafina*, a musical play that became a worldwide hit, to produce a similar program on HIV/AIDS prevention. The resulting $2.5 million musical production scored highly on its musical content, but contained several pieces of inaccurate (and even dangerous) public health information. Subject-matter specialists on HIV/AIDS had not been consulted, and the production elements were not pre-tested. The ensuing scandal, prominently featured in the South African mass media, came close to unseating the minister of health. This expensive intervention did little to encourage HIV prevention.

* This case draws upon Singhal & Rogers (1999).

Theory-based Message Design

Messages for an entertainment-education intervention are designed on the basis of theories of behavior change communication. Human communication theories are seldom used in designing most media messages. At the heart of understanding the process of entertainment-education is Albert Bandura's social learning theory (1977, 1997), which states that human learning can occur through observing media role models. This vicarious learning can, under certain conditions, be even more effective than direct experiential learning. For instance, why should a couple have more children than they can afford, and suffer economic hardship throughout their lives, to realize eventually that it was a mistake not to adopt family planning? They could learn the same lesson by observing media role models, who face the realistic consequences of adopting or not adopting family planning in a television soap opera.

Media role models can also give individuals and communities self-efficacy and collective efficacy, leading to behavior change (Bandura, 1997). For instance, Suraj, a youth leader in the Indian radio soap opera *Tinka Tinka Sukh*, inspired young audience members in Lutsaan village to initiate various self-help activities, including planting trees, repairing village hand-pumps, and petitioning to open a high school in the village (so they would not have to travel to the neighboring town). Mkwaju's dutiful wife, Tunu, in *Twende na Wakati* becomes disgusted with Mkwaju's promiscuous sexual behavior, divorces him, and becomes economically self-sufficient so that she can support their children. Her life-story becomes a lesson in self-efficacy.

Multimedia Campaign Activities

Launching a multimedia broadcast with supportive activities is crucial for effective entertainment-education. The effects of entertainment-education are magnified when supplementary activities are included in an integrated communication campaign. In the mid-1980s, Johns Hopkins University's Population Communication Services utilized rock music songs to promote sexual responsibility among teenagers in the Philippines. Each song was accompanied by print and broadcast advertisements, personal appearances by the two singers, lapel buttons urging youth to "Say no to sex," posters, and a telephone hotline ("Dial-A-Friend"). These messages constituted a coordinated communication campaign, rather than just a popular song featuring lyrics with an educational message (Piotrow et al., 1997). While the cost and effort invested in a total campaign is greater than that required for just the entertainment-education message, the synergy of the communication campaign elements yields greater effects in changing human behavior. Multiple exposure to a variety of messages about the same educational topic leads to greater behavior change than does a single exposure.

Entertainment-education interventions have their strongest effects on audience behavior change when messages stimulate reflection, debate, and interpersonal communication about the educational topic among audience members (Papa et al., 2000), and when services can be delivered locally. One means of stimulating peer conversations is to broadcast to organized listening groups.

In 2002, All India Radio (AIR), the Indian national radio network, in cooperation with Population Communications International (PCI), New York, broadcast an entertainment-education radio soap opera *Taru* (the name of the female protagonist) in four Hindi-speaking states, Bihar, Jharkhand, Madhya Pradesh, and Chhattisgarh, which together have a population of about 180 million people. The ground-based partner in these four Indian states was Janani, an NGO that trained 20,000 rural medical practitioners (RMPs) and their spouses in reproductive health care services. Pre-program publicity about *Taru* was conducted on-air by All India Radio, encouraging people to listen, and also persuading prospective audience members to organize listening groups. On the ground, in the 20,000 villages where Janani operates, *Taru* was publicized by the rural medical practitioners through wall paintings, posters, stickers, and through folk media performance. Group listening was encouraged in villages, and its effects on audience members were carefully studied. In essence, All India Radio provided the message "air cover," and Janani provided the community-based "ground forces" to stimulate the message reception environment. Janani's RMPs provided service delivery locally, including condoms, pills, pregnancy dipsticks, vitamins, and other medications. One of the present authors (Singhal) is leading a research investigation of *Taru* to gauge the impacts of integrating entertainment-education media broadcasts with community-based listening and service delivery.

Process and Summative Evaluations

Entertainment-education campaigns can be strengthened through such process evaluation activities as the analysis of audience letters, monitoring of clinic data (to track the number of AIDS blood tests, for example), and content analysis of the entertainment-education messages (to determine if the scripts are consistent with the values grid). Feedback can thus be provided in a timely manner to entertainment-education producers for appropriate mid-course corrections. *Process evaluation* consists of gathering data about the effectiveness of an intervention program while it is underway.

Summative evaluation research measures the effects of an entertainment-education intervention on audience behaviors. Often, multi-method triangulation is employed to ascertain effects. For example, the entertainment-education radio soap opera *Tinka Tinka Sukh*, broadcast in Hindi-speaking northern India, was evaluated by a field experiment (using pre-post, treatment-control audience surveys), a content analysis of the episodes and viewers' letters, and a case study of one village in which the program had strong effects (Papa et al., 2000).

Twende na Wakati Versus HIV in Tanzania

The AIDS epidemic probably spread to Tanzania from neighboring countries in East Africa via long-distance truck drivers. They infected commercial sex workers at truck stops along Tanzania's Trans-African Highway (Plate 7.1). The first three AIDS cases in Tanzania were reported in 1983 (only two years after the identification of the first five AIDS cases in Los Angeles). A 1991 study at seven main truck stops found that 28 percent of the truckers and 56 percent of the commercial sex workers were HIV-positive (AMREF, 1992). The national AIDS control program in 1991 estimated the number of AIDS cases at about 400,000 (2.6 percent of the approximately 15 million adults on the Tanzanian mainland). In 1995, on the basis of blood donor data, the national AIDS control program estimated that 1.2 million Tanzanians were infected with HIV, about 8 percent of the 15 million adults. Clearly, the epidemic was taking off in Tanzania in the early 1990s, and at an alarming rate.

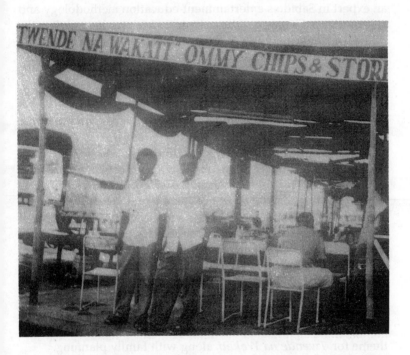

Plate 7.1   A Restaurant at a Main Truck Stop on the Trans-African Highway near Dar es Salaam, Tanzania, Changed its Name to the *Twende na Wakati* Café in 1993, Soon after the Broadcasts of the Radio Soap Opera Began

The restaurant owner reported that his sales jumped as a result of the name change, because of the popularity of the entertainment-education radio soap opera. Truck stops represent a major site for HIV transmission in Tanzania, and hence the storyline of *Twende na Wakati* centered on the life of a promiscuous truck driver, Mkwaju (Walking Stick in Kiswahili). Shown here is the director of Radio Tanzania and the actor who provides Mkwaju's voice.

Source: Personal files of the authors.

Twende na Wakati began broadcasting in Tanzania in mid-1993, and has continued through 2002. This soap opera is broadcast twice weekly in the evening hours. *Twende na Wakati* is produced by the staff of Radio Tanzania, the government radio network in Dar es Salaam, with technical assistance provided by Population Communications International (PCI) of New York. Dr. Kimani Njogu, an expert in Sabido's entertainment-education methodology and an experienced Kenyan radio soap opera scriptwriter, advises the Radio Tanzania staff as a PCI consultant. So *Twende na Wakati* represents an international collaboration, although the soap opera's scriptwriters and actors are all Tanzanians.

Extensive pre-production research was completed for *Twende na Wakati* in 1993, including 4,800 personal interviews and 160 focus group interviews with the target audience. The formative research provided the scriptwriters and producers of *Twende na Wakati* with: (*a*) a detailed understanding of the educational issues to be addressed; and (*b*) the nature of message content that would be appropriate for the audience. Based on formative research, representatives of religious, governmental, and educational organizations formulated a values grid to guide the content of *Twende na Wakati* at a workshop in February 1993. The values grid consisted of 57 statements, such as: "It is good for people to understand that mosquitoes cannot spread AIDS." These statements from the values grid formed the basis for the soap opera's storyline, and for the roles played by the main characters. The workshop also chose the name for the radio soap opera, *Twende na Wakati* (Let's Go with the Times). AIDS prevention was selected as an educational theme for *Twende na Wakati*, along with family planning.[1]

Based on formative research, three character types are featured in *Twende na Wakati*: positive and negative role models, who share or reject, respectively, the educational values promoted by the radio soap opera, and transitional characters, whose attitudes and behaviors change so that they eventually adopt the positive educational values. Positive role models are rewarded in the soap opera's storyline, while negative role models are punished. For example, the main character in *Twende na Wakati*, Mkwaju, is, as noted previously, a long-distance truck driver, who is promiscuous, contracts HIV, and eventually suffers from AIDS. As a negative role model, Mkwaju faces the consequences of his behaviors, and eventually dies in the radio soap opera's storyline. Mkwaju is also a negative role model for gender equality and family planning. He has a strong preference for male children. In *Twende na Wakati*, Mkwaju's wife and his three girlfriends deliver a total of five daughters, to his great disappointment. Thus, opposition to son preference, one of the 57 educational themes stated in the values grid, is conveyed by the radio soap opera to its listeners through positive, negative, and transitional role models who act out this educational value.

Tunu, Mkwaju's wife, plays the role of a compliant, submissive spouse during the early months of the soap opera's broadcast. After initially tolerating her husband's infidelity and alcoholism, Tunu becomes a positive role model for the educational elements in the values grid dealing with female equality, economic self-sufficiency, and HIV prevention. She separates from Mkwaju, and establishes a small business to support herself and her children. Tunu is positively rewarded by being spared from HIV infection, and by prospering economically. Thus she is a transitional character.

As these examples illustrate, the behavior change messages conveyed by *Twende na Wakati* are subtle. Negative role models like Mkwaju suffer the consequences of their socially undesirable actions in the soap opera's storyline, and positive role models who have made the "transition," like Tunu, are rewarded, as Bandura's (1977, 1997) social learning theory dictates. Some transitional characters never make the positive shift, and do not serve as role models for the audience members to imitate. In such interventions, no preaching about family planning or HIV prevention occurs. The role models provide the vehicle for getting the educational message across to the audience. The radio drama is involving, so that people are motivated to discuss it with peers. This interpersonal communication triggers behavior change, such as the adoption of HIV prevention behaviors.

The Tanzanian radio soap opera closely followed Miguel Sabido's "formula" for the entertainment-education strategy: (*a*) conducting formative research; (*b*) creating a values grid; (*c*) conveying the educational topics through positive, negative, and transitional role models; and (*d*) ending each episode with an "epilogue," a brief 20 to 30 second summary statement by a highly credible source. Often, the epilogues in *Twende na Wakati* asked rhetorical questions such as: "Here we saw how Mkwaju's alcoholism leads him to mistreat his devoted wife, Tunu. Do you know people like Mkwaju? What should society do to combat alcoholism and wife abuse?" Epilogues can stimulate reflection and elaboration on educational issues, sparking conversations between spouses, among community members, and moving certain audience members to action. Viewers of a popular Indian entertainment-education soap opera, *Hum Log*, responded enthusiastically to the epilogues delivered by the late Ashok Kumar, a famous Hindi film actor, launching village cleanliness drives, signing eye and organ donation pledge cards, and planting trees (Singhal & Rogers, 2001b).

"Don't be a Mkwaju!"

Insight into the effects of *Twende na Wakati* on its listeners is provided by the following letter, written to Radio Tanzania in 1995: "Mkwaju has a wife and children and yet decides to involve himself in extramarital sexual relations with three different girls and has fathered children by each of the three. When Mkwaju is infected with AIDS, he is going to involve even some innocent ones . . . . Who knows, for Tunu may also be infected with AIDS through Mkwaju . . . . You people with Mkwaju's behavior, what are you waiting for? Change now. You are many Mkwajus!"

Mkwaju (Walking Stick) became a part of everyday discourse in Tanzania during the 1990s. When a man boasted of his sexual exploits, a friend would say: "Don't be a Mkwaju!"

Mkwaju, the negative character for HIV prevention in the Tanzanian radio drama, became very well known. The annual survey interviews from 1993 to 1995 showed that listeners understood that he was a negative role model, and that his behavior was punished. The audience learned that they should do the opposite of what Mkwaju did.

The entertainment-education radio soap opera in Tanzania which was rigorously evaluated from 1993 to 1997 (discussed ii greater detail in the following chapter), was a turning point in the use of E-E interventions for HIV/AIDS prevention. Population Communications International entered into collaborative E-E projects in India, Pakistan, China, and the Caribbean (these projects are described later).

Soul City in South Africa

Soul City is a notable entertainment-education intervention that utilizes a multimedia campaign to promote HIV/AIDS prevention in South Africa. In 2002, almost five million adults (22 percent of the adult population) in South Africa were HIV-positive and an estimated 500,000 children had been orphaned by AIDS. So HIV/AIDS is a very high priority public health problem in South Africa.

Founding Soul City

The story of Soul City begins in the late 1980s when Dr. Garth Japhet, a young medical doctor, was assigned to a rural health clinic in South Africa's KwaZulu Natal province. While treating poor, rural patients, Japhet realized that South Africa harbored "developing" country health problems within a "developed" country (South Africa has one of the highest levels of per capita income of any African nation, although it is very unequally distributed). For children under 5 years of age, the largest single cause of death is diarrhea, a disease that is not difficult to prevent (such as with oral rehydration therapy). This dismal health record existed despite a highly developed mass media system in South Africa: About 98 percent of South Africans have access to radio, 65 percent watch television, and over 40 percent read newspapers and magazines.

In 1990, Japhet moved from KwaZulu Natal to serve at Alex Clinic, in Alexandra Township, a huge black township on the outskirts of Johannesburg. At Alex Clinic, which was a model clinic for the practice of community medicine, Japhet saw at close hand the wretched health conditions of South Africa's urban poor during the nation's Apartheid era: crime, overcrowding, alcoholism, wife and child abuse, and the gathering storm of the HIV/AIDS epidemic. Japhet launched several outreach activities in the community, including a Sunday school for Alexandra's delinquent youth, and wrote a health column for *The Sowetan*, a daily newspaper with a large black readership. The column, which stressed immunizations to prevent infant deaths, and explained how burns and accidents could be avoided, generated enthusiastic reader response, convincing Japhet of the mass media's potential in promoting public health.

Japhet noted that health promotion activities in the South African media were inadequate and mainly slogan-based. They included a Tuberculosis Day, an AIDS Day, a Malaria Day, and so on. Such health promotional efforts lacked sustainability. Research did not play a role in health communication. Although South Africa had a robust advertising industry, lessons from social marketing were not applied in health communication campaigns. Further, institutional partnerships between the media, the government, and the private sector did not exist for health communication. The health ministry usually implemented programs in a top–down manner. Japhet also realized that despite a wealth of mass media talent and resources, there was little indigenous drama on South African television or radio. Health information on television was limited to dull programs like "Sister Lydia gives the 3 P.M. health talk" (Japhet, quoted in McNeil, 2002, p. 6). Japhet wanted a format that would move health into prime time.

In 1991, Japhet traveled to the United States, Canada, the Netherlands, and England to learn about innovative communication approaches to address South Africa's health problems. His trip was funded by $10,000 in seed money from the South African Medical Research Council. Aggrey Klaaste, the highly respected editor of *The Sowetan* who coined the term "nation-building" during the demise of the Apartheid era, paid Japhet's salary for the three months of his study tour. Japhet returned to South Africa convinced that his "prime-time vehicle for health promotion would be an entertainment-education drama" (personal interview, 6 July 2000).

Japhet knocked on many doors in South Africa, bringing aboard partners from the entertainment and media industries, professionals, professors, medical doctors, and international agencies. In 1992, another young medical doctor, Dr. Shereen Usdin, a public health and anti-Apartheid activist, walked into Japhet's office at Alex Clinic and volunteered (only later, when funds allowed, could Japhet hire employees). Usdin was co-editor of *Critical Health*, a publication that examined the impact of Apartheid on the health of South Africans, and, like Japhet, Usdin believed in the power of the media in health promotion. Usdin, an avid consumer of media entertainment, remembers watching the feature film *Roots* (about black people's struggle against slavery) in school. Usdin remembers the film's powerful impact: "I came out of *Roots* in an altered state" (personal interview, 19 September 2000).

Japhet and Usdin founded Soul City in a one-room office of Alex Clinic (Plate 7.2). Its mission was to harness the mass media for promoting health. Both Japhet and Usdin realized that for media-based health promotion interventions to be sustainable, they had to be popular, attract the highest possible prime-time audiences, and be of top-notch quality. They also realized that government, media, private corporations, and donor agencies had to form a "win–win" relationship. Commercial and health interests both had to be honored. Entertainment-education was placed at the core of Soul City's health promotion strategy. Research, both formative and summative, undergirded this entertainment-education focus. Dr. Sue Goldstein, a project advisor during the organization's early years (now a senior manager), has played a key role in institutionalizing research at Soul City.

Entertainment-Education and Soul City

Soul City is a unique example of entertainment-education, in that it represents a series of integrated, ongoing mass media activities, year after year.[2] Each year, a series of mass media interventions are implemented, including the flagship *Soul City*, a 13-part prime-time television drama series, broadcast for three months, that promotes specific health issues. Simultaneously, a 60-episode radio drama series is broadcast daily (Monday through Friday) at prime time in nine South African languages. While the story in the radio drama is different, the health issues it addresses are the same as in the television series. Simultaneously with the broadcasting of the television and radio series, three million health education booklets, designed around the popularity of the television series' characters,

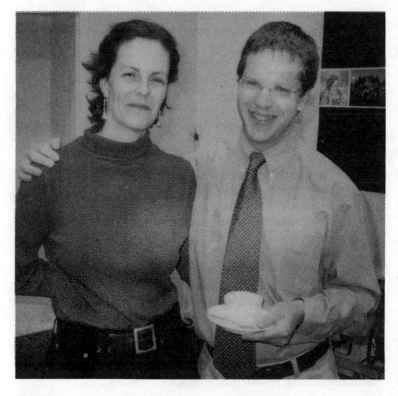

Plate 7.2   Drs. Garth Japhet (Right) and Shereen Usdin, Co-founders of Soul City in South Africa, while Attending an International Conference on Entertainment-Education in the Netherlands in 2000

Soul City is an ongoing, multimedia, entertainment-education initiative in South Africa that constitutes an exemplar of disease prevention and health promotion.

Source: Personal files of the authors.

are distributed free of cost to selected target audiences. The booklets are also serialized by 11 major newspapers in South Africa (Plate 7.3).

The first *Soul City* television series, broadcast in 1994, focused on maternal and child health, and on HIV prevention. The second *Soul City* series, broadcast in 1996, dealt with HIV, tuberculosis, tobacco control, and housing reform. The third series broadcast in

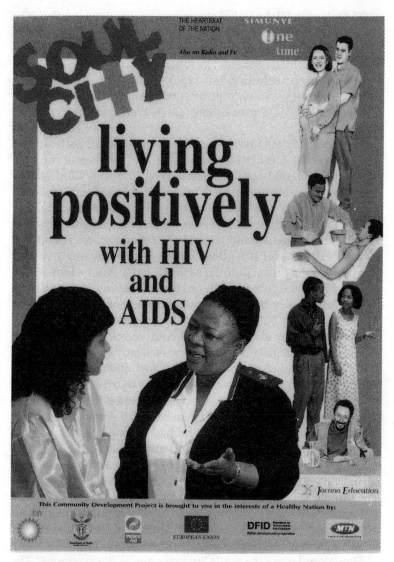

Plate 7.3   Cover of the Health Education Booklet that Accompanies the *Soul City* Television Broadcasts

Sister Bettina, a nurse at Masakhane Clinic in the *Soul City* television series, is shown here in the health education booklet, counseling a young girl about the results of her HIV test.

Source: Soul City Institute of Health and Development Communication.

1997 dealt with HIV, alcohol abuse, and energy conservation. The fourth *Soul City* series (in 1999) focused on violence against women, AIDS and youth sexuality, hypertension, and personal finance and small business management. The fifth series dealt with HIV/AIDS, youth sexuality (including date rape), coping with disability, and management of micro-enterprises. Only issues of national priority (such as HIV/AIDS prevention) are woven into the *Soul City* storyline.

The *Soul City* television storyline is set in an urban township (called Soul City), much like Alexandra, and revolves around the workings of Masakhane Clinic, patterned after Alex Clinic. Many of the health problems depicted in *Soul City*'s broadcasts are based on real-life cases that occur in townships like Alexandra. For instance, the fourth *Soul City* series began with a murder mystery. A subplot centered around 15-year-old Tebogo, whose friends tell him he will go mad if he does not have sex, warning him that pimples are the first symptom (McNeil, 2002). After a movie date with a classmate, Tebogo pulls out a condom, and insists that his date owes him sex because he paid for the movie, popcorn, and soda. She refuses, but Tebogo lies to his friends that he succeeded. When she finds out about Tebogo's empty boasting, the girl is livid, and Tebogo apologizes. Her girlfriends tell her "she is lucky — their boyfriends sometimes rape them" (McNeil, 2000, p. 6). Indeed, a national survey of 26,000 youth in South African schools showed that, by the age of 18, one in four males admitted to having forced sex without a woman's consent (Ncube, 2000). Further, one in six schoolboys thought a woman who had been raped enjoyed the ordeal; and twice as many thought that she had "asked" for it. A majority of women were "resigned to their fate and believed that sexual violence, or rough sex, was a fact of life" (Ncube, 2000, p. 15). The connection of *Soul City* s storyline with reality generates dramatic excitement in the broadcasts; sparks a public debate about power, masculinity, and sexuality; and provides alternative models of sexuality that are respectful of women's sexual rights.

How popular are the Soul City mass media interventions? The *Soul City* television series consistently ranks among the three top-rated television drama series in South Africa (Japhet & Goldstein, 1997a). The prime-time radio series (called *Healing Hearts*), broadcast in nine languages, also earns very high audience ratings. What is remarkable is that the lowest-status audience members in

South Africa give the highest ratings to *Soul City*. So this entertainment-education program is reaching the audience segment that most needs educational messages about health.

Soul City's Yearly Campaigns

By using a multimedia approach, Soul City helps build a campaign atmosphere that is sustained throughout the year. Each medium reinforces the popularity of the *Soul City* television series, while appealing to a somewhat different target audience: Television primarily reaches urban viewers, while radio broadcasts mainly reach rural listeners. Further, each medium reinforces the health messages of the other media, while carrying different aspects of the educational message. Booklets[3] and newspapers provide more detailed information on a health topic than is possible on television or on radio. Such a multimedia, synergistic strategy helps broker media partnerships: "Print wants to be involved because television is involved; radio wants to come aboard because print is on board" (Japhet & Goldstein, 1997a).

Soul City recognizes that overt behavior change is facilitated when audience members talk to one another about a health issue. Research evaluations show that the Soul City series stimulates interpersonal discussion (Figure 7.1). After the television and radio series are broadcast, several campaign activities are implemented to *keep* people talking. High-quality education and lifeskills packets, produced cooperatively by curriculum specialists and creative designers, are targeted to adult and youth populations nationwide. The adult packet includes the health education booklet (mentioned previously), comic books based on the story of the television series, audiotapes of the comic books, *Soul City* posters, and a facilitator's guide to maximizing impact. The youth packets, in keeping with its audience's needs, are geared toward building lifeskills competencies and consist of a comic book based on the television series as well as four workbooks that address issues of personal responsibility, self-identity, and personal relationships. They also include a facilitator's guide for use in high schools.[4]

The credibility of the Soul City brand name, and the popularity of its media programs, are harnessed by initiatives such as the "Soul City Search for Stars" (to recruit talent for the next year's

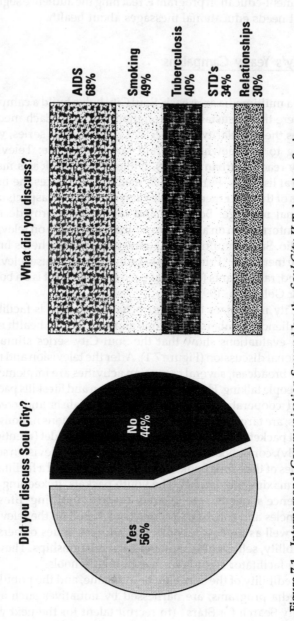

Figure 7.1 Interpersonal Communication Spurred by the *Soul City II* Television Series

Soul City stimulated person-to-person communication about the five health topics emphasized in that year's broadcasts.

Source: Soul City Institute of Health and Development Communication.

Did you discuss Soul City?

Yes 56%

No 44%

What did you discuss?

AIDS 68%

Smoking 49%

Tuberculosis 40%

STD's 34%

Relationships 30%

television and radio series), and the "Soul City Health Care Worker of the Year" (to recognize outstanding outreach workers). Additionally, Soul City has entered into partner relationships with 12 journalists, representing the most influential South African newspapers, who regularly publish health education features derived from Soul City's activities.

In 2000, Soul City launched *Soul Buddyz*, a prime-time television series aimed at children aged 8 to 12, which addresses substance abuse, race and xenophobia, and AIDS and sexuality, including a storyline on how children cope with the death of their parents from AIDS. The invisible nature of HIV transmission was not understood by many South African children. A 10-year-old boy said: "If you stand next to them [HIV-positive persons], they infect you. If they have it, then you'll get it also" (Goldstein et al., in press). Such misunderstandings were corrected in *Soul Buddyz* broadcasts. An audience survey showed that 81 percent of those exposed talked about HIV/AIDS with their peers.

By carrying out these multiple health promotion activities, Soul City has emerged as a highly recognized and trusted name in South Africa, an honor that they use to their advantage. The cornerstone of the Soul City health promotion strategy is the production of high-quality media materials. Only skilled scriptwriters, actors, producers, and directors are hired, including Darryl Roodt, the highly acclaimed South African director of films such as *Cry, My Beloved Country* and *Sarafina*. They are paid at the market rate or more. The *Soul City* television series is broadcast at 8:30 P.M., a prime-time slot when one-third of South Africa's population is tuned in.[5] "So our media materials have to not just compete with the best. . . . They have to *be* the best" (Japhet & Goldstein, 1997a).

The continuing, year-after-year nature of Soul City's health promotion activities has certain advantages. Various health and development groups in South Africa piggyback issues of national priority on Soul City's media interventions. More importantly, by broadcasting a recurrent television and radio series, Soul City avoids the problem of *audience lag*, the time needed to build a sizeable and dedicated audience for a new media program. A popular *Soul City* television series broadcast in one year ensures a large audience at the beginning of the next season of broadcasts. For instance, the fourth *Soul City* campaign series reached almost 80 percent of its target audience in South Africa (Soul City, 2001).

The Key Role of Research

Formative and summative research are key to designing and evaluating Soul City's mass media interventions. Formative research is conducted to identify health issues of national priority, and to ensure that the mass media interventions can be backed up at the ground level by the needed infrastructure.[6] Formative research activities include focus group discussions and in-depth interviews, participatory rural appraisals, archival research, and pre-testing. Formative research ensures that Soul City's television and radio series are realistic, and resonate among audience members. Dr. Sue Goldstein related to us how, in a *Soul City* television broadcast, an HIV-positive man took a health clinic hostage (personal interview, Johannesburg, 15 June 2001). The storyline was suggested by a real-world event in which an HIV-positive man committed this criminal act in order to be killed by the police. In the real world, and in the *Soul City* show, the man eventually became an AIDS activist.

Soul City has two full-time formative researchers, Thuli Shongwe and Agnes Shabalala. Shongwe grew up in Alexandra Township as the daughter of an unwed mother "who sold alcohol from home to support her 10 children" (personal interview, 7 July 2000). Married and a mother of two children at a young age, Shongwe studied at home to earn a high school certificate and to gain computer proficiency. She was hired at Alex Clinic as a research assistant, where she met Garth Japhet in the early 1990s, at the time that Soul City was getting underway. "She knows the health and community issues first-hand . . . she has lived through them . . . ", said Japhet about the invaluable formative research resource that Shongwe brings to Soul City (personal interview, 14 June 2001).

Summative research procedures include gathering ratings and viewership data, and conducting before–after national and regional sample surveys to determine the effects of the television, radio, and print interventions. Summative research reports show that the Soul City mass media interventions increase knowledge about health issues, promote more positive attitudes toward them, influence social norms, facilitate media and political advocacy, and contribute to behavior change (CASE, 1995; Japhet & Goldstein, 1997b; Soul City, 2000). Figure 7.2 shows that *Soul City* influenced viewers of all age groups to always use condoms in sexual encounters to prevent HIV.

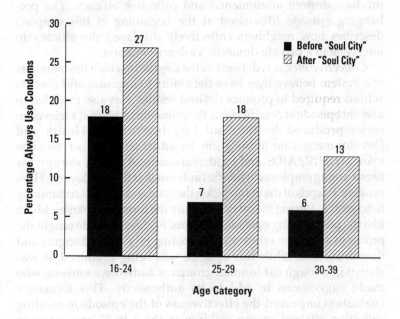

Figure 7.2   Influence of the *Soul City II* Television Series in Convincing Viewers in each Age Group to always use Condoms to Prevent HIV

A major increase in condom use occurred for each age group as a result of exposure to *Soul City*.

Source: Soul City Institute of Health and Development Communication.

Further, after watching *Soul City*, 75 percent of viewers reported being convinced that an HIV-positive person should not keep his/her HIV status secret from loved ones. Prior to the *Soul City* broadcasts, only 3 percent of respondents had supported this idea.

Raising Efficacy

Soul City models both individual *self-efficacy* (defined as an individual's perception of his or her capacity to organize and execute the actions required to manage prospective situations to produce desired attainments) and collective efficacy. The pot-banging episode (discussed at the beginning of this chapter) describes how neighbors collectively displayed the efficacy to intervene in a private domestic violence situation.

Collective efficacy, defined as the degree to which the members of a system believe they have the ability to organize and execute actions required to produce desired results, was also modeled in a recent episode of *Soul Buddyz*, the prime-time children's television series produced by the Soul City Institute for Health and Development Communication to address issues of teenage sexuality, HIV/AIDS, and accidental deaths. A grocery store owner fires a young employee when he finds out that the employee is HIV-positive. Friends of the youth picket the store and urge the community to boycott it, forcing the owner to rehire the former employee. Much like the pot-banging episode, this *Soul Buddyz* episode taught the power of collective efficacy in combating HIV-related stigma and discrimination. While this episode was being produced, it was shown in a rough cut to small groups of audience members, who made suggestions to add to its authenticity. This formative evaluation improved the effectiveness of the episode in creating collective efficacy among children in the 8 to 12 age group in South Africa.

Costs and Reach

The total annual cost incurred by Soul City for its multimedia materials, including production of the 13-episode *Soul City* television series, the 60-episode radio series in nine local South African languages, three million booklets, plus marketing, advertising, and public relations activities, is about U.S. $4 million. How is this money raised? Approximately 15 percent is provided by the South African government, 70 percent by international donor agencies such as DFID, the European Union, and UNICEF, and the remaining 15 percent by corporations such as British Petroleum, Old Mutual, and the broadcast media.[7] Japhet emphasizes that these partnerships with government, media, corporate, and donor agencies are the key reason for Soul City's effectiveness: "Partnerships make this intervention possible. . . . The more you work together, the more people understand the intervention, and the stronger the partnership gets. . . . Also the expertise of the technical production staff improves" (Japhet & Goldstein, 1997a). Japhet aptly calls this process "a cycle of positive reinforcement."

Soul City is mainly a research and management organization. It coordinates the activities of its various corporate, government, media, and donor partners. Its employees do not directly produce, direct, or publish its health communication materials. They commission professionals to perform these actions, and through research and hands-on management, they ensure high quality. Soul City owns the media product that is produced, and Soul City pays the bills. This role gives them the power to "veto" a media product if it does not meet their high standards.

The reach and influence of Soul City extend beyond South Africa. Soul City materials, through local, in-country partnerships, are being produced and distributed in neighboring Botswana, Zimbabwe, Lesotho, Swaziland, Namibia, and Zambia. Evaluations show that the materials are highly popular in these countries, where audiences find these messages culturally shareable (Japhet & Goldstein, 1997a; Singhal & Svenkerud, 1994). African countries like Nigeria, Ghana, and Malawi have also requested Soul City materials for local use.

Soul City has also inspired certain organizations in other developing countries to produce local, research-based, ongoing, multimedia entertainment-education initiatives. For instance, managers of Puntos de Encuentro (Issues We Encounter), a Nicaraguan NGO, educated themselves about the *Soul City* experience, including the general lessons learned about imple- menting entertainment-education, and produced a youth television drama series *Sexto Sentido* (Sixth Sense) in 2001. This highly popular television soap opera addresses teenage sexuality, gender rela- tions (including issues of date rape), and HIV/AIDS. The television series is complemented by a radio drama series (to reach rural audiences), by comic books (based on the storyline of *Sexto Sentido*), and by outreach activities (personal correspondence, Dr. Rafael Obregon, 16 March 2002). *Sexto Sentido*'s multimedia materials are developed through formative research and are extensively pre-tested. In 2002, the *Sexto Sentido* entertainment-education initiative was in its second cycle of broadcasts, emulating the ongoing nature of the *Soul City* campaign. Amy Banks, a former

AIDS activist in San Francisco, coordinates the Puntos de Encuentro's E-E initiative.

Soul City constitutes a unique entertainment-education campaign: (*a*) it is developed locally;[8] (*b*) it is targeted nationally; (*c*) it incorporates extensive formative research and theoretical vigor; (*d*) it is orchestrated as a continuing, multimedia E-E campaign; (*e*) it is based on "win–win" partnerships among various stakeholders (donors, government agencies, media organizations, development infrastructure, creative personnel, and communication researchers); (*f*) it is used to influence individual attitudes, boost self-efficacy and collective efficacy, change social norms, and put issues on the public agenda; (*g*) it forms part of a media advocacy initiative that promotes a policy and legislative agenda; and (*h*) it provides a "branded" image.

Today, Soul City is headquartered in an attractive office building in Parkstown, a suburb of Johannesburg, a far cry from its modest start in a small office at Alex Clinic. Its multimedia project budget for South Africa has grown from $10,000 in seed money in the early 1990s to $4 million in 2002.[9] From its two co-founders, Soul City has "grown into a large team [36 people] of highly talented and innovative people" (Dr. Shereen Usdin, quoted in www.comminit.com/interviews_archives5.html).

When we met with Soul City personnel in June 2001, we visited Alexandra Township and the Alex Clinic, where Soul City originated. When we parked our van in Alexandra Township, half a dozen schoolchildren surrounded the vehicle, pointing excitedly to the *Soul City* logo painted on its door. Then, without provocation, they sang the *Soul City* theme song for us!

Using Markers in Entertainment-Education Programs

During the production of E-E messages, multiple "markers" are often proactively incorporated in the E-E intervention. *Markers* are distinctive elements of a message that are identifiable by audience individuals (Singhal & Rogers, 2002). One way to introduce a marker in an E-E intervention is to "rename" an existing product so that the E-E message becomes identifiable with only that product. For instance, in the popular St. Lucia family planning radio soap opera *Apwé Plézi* (After the Pleasure), a new condom brand called "Catapult" was introduced. This new term was identified by 28 percent of the radio program's listeners, validating their claim of direct exposure to the program, and by 13 percent of the non-listeners, suggesting that the message was diffused via interpersonal channels (Vaughan et al., 2000).

Alternatively, a marker might consist of a creatively named character in an E-E program, like the skirt-chasing character Scattershot in *Nasebery Street*, a radio soap opera about sexually responsible fatherhood in Jamaica (Singhal & Rogers, 1999). Scattershot, a negative role model, became a common term in Jamaican discourse, as in "Oh, you Scattershot, you," providing an opportunity to trace the direct and indirect effects of listening to the radio program.

The most powerful markers model new, culturally appropriate realities to break oppressive power structures in society, exemplified by the collective pot-banging by neighbors in South Africa's *Soul City* so as to stop wife/partner abuse (Singhal & Rogers, 2002). Markers, which model new realities, not only enhance the message content of the E-E intervention, but also provide additional validation of whether or not audience members were directly or indirectly exposed to the E-E intervention.

Malhacão in Brazil

Brazil is the land of *telenovelas* (television soap operas). Not only are soap operas the most popular television fare in Brazil, *telenovelas* are exported by Brazilian networks to 60 other nations around the world. Thus, it is not surprising that a soap opera played an important role in putting the issue of HIV/AIDS on the national agenda, and also taught many individuals how to live as HIV-positive people taking the anti-retrovirals.

Malhacão began broadcasting in 1995 as the first youth soap opera in Brazil. Initially, the *telenovela* was set in a workout gym in Rio de Janeiro, where young people gathered to develop perfect bodies and to boast of their love conquests. *Malhacão* means "working out" in Portuguese. This Brazilian version of *Baywatch* earned low television ratings, and so *Malhacão* changed to a middle-class school setting and to a focus on social issues, particularly HIV/AIDS. The ratings jumped to an average of 30 points, rising to a spectacular peak of 37 when the teenage star of the show, Erica, learns that she is HIV-positive.

Erica wrestles with such dilemmas as whether or not she can have boyfriends, and whether she will be able to have children. When Erica dates her heartthrob, Touro, one of the continuing uncertainties of the *telenovela* is whether or not they should have sexual intercourse. *Malhacão* appeals to adults as well as youth, in part because audience members feel that the *telenovela* tackles real-life issues. After 1996, when the Brazilian government began to distribute free anti-retroviral drugs to HIV+ people, the *telenovela* dealt with how to live with HIV, a familiar situation for many members of the television audience.

Malhacão does not follow closely the Miguel Sabido formula for the entertainment-education strategy (with positive, negative, and transitional characters for the educational issue). Rather, it represents the social merchandizing approach of TV Globo, Brazil's largest national television network, in which *telenovela* scriptwriters are encouraged to incorporate contemporary social themes such as land reform, breast cancer, HIV, and democracy (Ruiz, 1995).

Participatory E-E Approaches for HIV Prevention

Several entertainment-education participatory approaches promote HIV prevention, care, and support. Brazilian theater director Augusto Boal founded the Theater of the Oppressed (TO) movement. Based on the Brazilian educator Paulo Freire's principles of dialogue, interaction, problem-posing, reflection, and conscientization, TO's techniques are designed to activate spectators ("spect-actors") to take control of situations, rather than passively allowing actions to happen to them (Boal, 1979).

The idea of a "spect-actor" first occurred to Boal when he encouraged audience members to stop a theater performance, and to suggest different actions for the actors, who then carry out the audience's suggestions. During one such performance, a woman in the audience was so outraged when an actor could not understand her suggestion that she stormed onto the stage to enact what she meant (Singhal, 2001b). From that day on, audience members were invited on the stage. Boal discovered that audience members became empowered not only to imagine change, but to actually — and collectively — practice it. Community organizers and facilitators have used TO's techniques, through a network of thousands of drama troupes all over the world, as participatory tools for democratizing organizations, analyzing social problems, and transforming reality through direct action.

Artists against AIDS in Brazil

Participatory strategies are driving a strong grassroots movement in the state of Ceará in Brazil, which in 1997 brought artists from all walks of life to join hands against AIDS. This movement is the brainchild of Ranulfo Cardoso, Jr., who was greatly influenced by Paulo Freire's participatory strategy, and worked closely with Betinho in founding ABIA (discussed in Chapter 2). When we met Cardoso in Brasília in March 2001, he told us of his dissatisfaction with the serious, fearful messages about HIV/AIDS that had characterized Brazil's early response to the epidemic, and of his wish to correct this situation: "Brazilians are happy people . . . serious messages were turning them off" (personal interview, Ranulfo Cardoso, Jr., 14 March 2001).

Beginning in Fortaleza, the capital of Ceará state, and supported by funds from the MacArthur Foundation, the Bricantes Contra a AIDS (Street Artists against AIDS) Project trained hundreds of artists to develop emotionally powerful scripts on HIV prevention, care, and support, and to perform them in schools, prisons, and street markets. Cordel, a popular, rhyming, storytelling folk form in Brazil's north-east, was coopted for this movement. The most effective theater scripts were turned into entertainment-education *radionovelas* (radio soap operas), launching another movement called Radialistas Contra a AIDS (Radio Broadcasters against AIDS). The most popular of these radio soap operas, *Radionovela da Camisinha* (Radio Soap Opera Condom), is broadcast in Ceará and in other states of Brazil. It tells the story of a couple preparing for their first night of love, and how the "macho" man, a stud, is creatively and erotically convinced by his lover to use a condom.

In 1999, Cardoso hosted a workshop to share the state of Ceará's participatory experiences in using theater, art, and radio to promote HIV prevention and to reduce AIDS-related stigma with artists from eight Brazilian states, including Rio de Janeiro, Bahia, Pernabuco, and others. The use of local folk media forms, coupled with radio, which reaches 90 percent of the low-income population in Brazil (both in rural areas and urban *favelas*), represents an innovative integration of E-E approaches to HIV prevention.

Participatory strategies are also utilized by Nalamdana (in Chennai, India) for audience involvement in street theater dramas about HIV prevention.

Community Street Theater in Zimbabwe*

The Chirumhanzu Home-Based Care Project in the Midlands Province of Zimbabwe grew out of an initiative by hospital health workers, including senior nurses, Dominican sisters, and expatriate doctors. The home-based care project was launched because of overcrowded hospital wards, the high costs of hospital care, and the desire of AIDS patients to receive home care from their families until their deaths.

The Chirumhanzu Project works closely with traditional village leaders, who are first invited to visit the local hospital or clinic to meet with the project staff. A video on home care and HIV/AIDS is shown during this visit. Then the Chirumhanzu staff visits the village, where the local chief calls a public meeting. The public meeting begins with a skit created by Chirumhanzu's drama troupe to entertain the public while providing relevant information about HIV/AIDS prevention, care, and support. The drama performance is followed by a discussion of the effects of HIV/AIDS on the local community, most often facilitated by a respected nurse practitioner. The meeting ends with the chief, his advisors, and local people beginning home care services for people living with AIDS.

> In a nation where hospital care is an extremely scarce
> resource, home care for people living with HIV/AIDS makes
> eminent good sense.
>
> * This case draws upon Singhal (2001b).

Nalamdana in India

Nalamdana means "Are you well?" in Tamil, and the street theater
and other entertainment-education interventions that Nalamdana
provides all deal with some aspect of health: HIV/AIDS, maternal
and child health (MCH), children's rights, suicide prevention,
cancer, women's empowerment (Plate 7.4). Since 2000, Nalamdana
has focused exclusively on HIV/AIDS and MCH issues,
establishing its core competence in these areas. Of the many types
of entertainment-education that the present authors observed on
their five-nation trip, Nalamdana was one of the most impressive.
We visited Nalamdana for two days while we were in Chennai in
December 2001. We learned a great deal from this intensive
workshop, and admire the dedication and ingenuity of the
Nalamdana troupe.

Nalamdana was begun in 1993. Four of its founders—Jeeva,
Sampath, Oyya, and Ravi—had been street theater enthusiasts
since the late 1980s, when they were college students in Madurai,
a temple town in the southern part of the state of Tamil Nadu (Plate
7.5). Active in the National Service Scheme, they began staging
local street theater plays about female infanticide, an important
social problem in India in recent years (in India, ultrasound
techniques are widely utilized to determine the sex of a fetus). In
1993, Jeeva had a chance meeting with Ms. Uttara Bharath, a
development activist in Chennai, who believed in participatory
approaches to health and education. Bharath and the four Madurai-
based college youths joined hands, and Nalamdana was established
in Chennai. The four Nalamdana founders moved to Chennai,
which has been their headquarters since. Bharath, who is now
deputy chief of party at the Zambia field office of Johns Hopkins
University Center for Communication Programs, plays the
"outsider" role, helping Nalamdana's activities from a distance

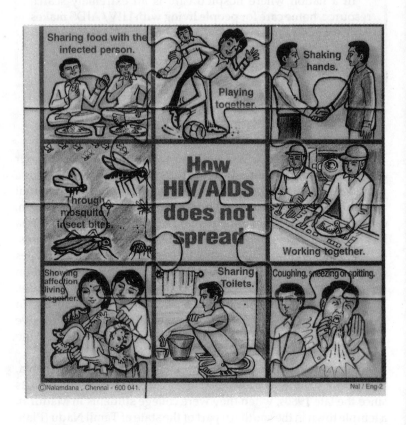

Plate 7.4 Entertainment-Education Can Take many Forms, Including this Puzzle Designed to Show how HIV is not Transmitted

Nalamdana, a non-governmental organization in Chennai, India, pioneered many types of entertainment-education, particularly street theater in villages. This puzzle not only teaches how HIV is not transmitted, but also serves to decrease the stigma of HIV/AIDS.

Source: Nalamdana. Designed by R. Jeevanandham.

and leaving the day-to-day management of the organization to the four founders and Nithaya Balaji, Nalamdana's executive trustee. While earning a Master's degree in Public Health at Johns Hopkins

University, Bharath collaborated with Professor Tom Valente in an evaluation research study of the effects of Nalamdana's street theater (Valente & Bharath, 1999).

A typical Nalamdana presentation takes place in the evening, in the open air of a village square or an urban slum, with several thousand audience members sitting on the ground. The performance takes place on an improvised stage, with blankets and clothes draped as a backdrop. Before the play begins, the actors announce

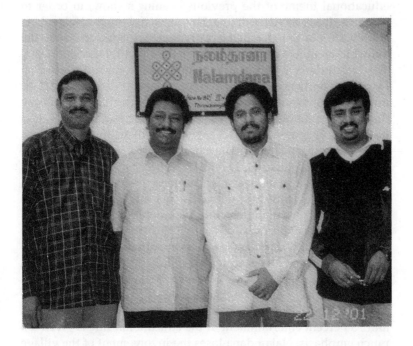

Plate 7.5 The Four Founders of Nalamdana, the Entertainment-Education NGO in Chennai, India, that Specializes in the use of Street Theater for HIV Prevention

The founders (left to right) are M. Raviraj, P. Oyya, R. Jeevanandham, and M. Sampath. Nalamdana presented over 1,000 street plays about HIV/AIDS in villages in Tamil Nadu state, each to an average audience of 1,000 people. Nalamdana's logo is a *kolam*, which is painted on the doorstep of a South Indian home with rice powder each morning, symbolizing health and hygiene. *Nalamdana* means (in Tamil) "Are you well?"

Source: Personal files of the authors.

that five individuals will be invited from the audience after the show to answer questions about its educational content. A theatrical performance on HIV/AIDS might be followed by questions about the means of HIV transmission. The two-hour show might end with an announcement providing the addresses and telephone numbers of nearby HIV testing and counseling centers, and brochures might be distributed.

The following day, the Nalamdana actors *return* to the same location for a series of small group "workshops" about the educational theme of the previous evening's show, in order to obtain feedback about the drama. Thus the scripts for the Nalamdana shows are continually being rewritten, with inputs from the audience members who participate in the day-after post-mortems. The Nalamdana acting troupe members are constantly learning from their audiences about what they like and dislike, and their other reactions to the dramas. In fact, the Nalamdana actors say that they see their main role as conducting research, rather than just acting. The continuing exchange with audience members keeps the acting fresh, and prevents burnout among the actors. Nalamdana prefers street theater to television or film, because this format allows the direct exchange of ideas with audience members. Nalamdana estimates that over the past nine years, their street theater audiences have totaled over a million people, mainly composed of audiences in urban slums and rural areas with little formal education (those most in need of Nalamdana's HIV prevention messages).

Audience members are highly involved in the street theater. From the stage, the audience looks like "a sea of eyeballs," says R. Jeevanandham, project manager of the Nalamdana group. The actors estimate that their typical drama is about 25 percent education and 75 percent entertainment. If the educational side is given too much emphasis, Nalamdana loses the involvement of the village audiences.

A scholarly journal article reporting an evaluation of Nalamdana's dramas says that they are particularly effective in correcting misconceptions about HIV/AIDS (Valente & Bharath, 1999). For instance, when a sample of the audience was asked whether mosquito bites could transmit HIV, the rate of correct answers increased from 42 percent pre-test (before the performance) to 98 percent post-test. Individuals with the lowest levels of formal education increased their knowledge of HIV transmission the most as a result of Nalamdana's shows. Self-reported attitudes toward people living with HIV/AIDS improved, showing that the Nalamdana drama decreased stigma.

In short, Nalamdana provides a cost-effective type of behavior change communication about HIV prevention, and reaches those individuals who need it most. The world needs hundreds of Nalamdanas.

Culturally Shareable Entertainment-Education Programs

Cultural shareability of a media program is the extent to which it can appeal to heterophilous (dissimilar) audience groups (Sthapitanonda-Sarabol & Singhal, 1999). In the global society of today, people in different parts of the world are frequently exposed to media programs produced in other countries. The popularity of certain entertainment programs in diverse cultural contexts inspired media practitioners to produce entertainment-education programs that promoted literacy, gender equality, and HIV/AIDS prevention, and then to broadcast such programs across diverse sociocultural contexts (Singhal & Svenkerud, 1994; Singhal & Udornpim, 1997; Svenkerud et al., 1995). Culturally shareable entertainment-education programs can address the common health problems of different countries, reducing the redundancy of production effort and the duplication of costs.

Several notable examples of culturally shareable entertainment-education programs in the past decade may be cited. For example, Johns Hopkins University's Population Communication Services launched two highly popular rock music videos, *Cuando Estemos Juntos* (When We Are Together) and *Detente* (Wait) in over a dozen countries of Latin America to promote sexual responsibility among young adults (Piotrow et al., 1997). Since the mid-1980s, Zimbabwe-based film-maker John Riber has produced films such as *Consequences, It's Not Easy*, and *Yellow Card*, dealing with teenage pregnancy, sexual responsibility, and HIV/AIDS prevention respectively. These films have been highly popular with audiences in a dozen African countries (Singhal & Svenkerud, 1994).

The UNICEF-sponsored *Meena* and *Sara* animation films, and Street Kids International's *Karate Kids* animated film, are examples of culturally shareable entertainment-education products. *Meena* (named after the young girl who serves as the film's role model) was designed for use in various countries in South Asia; *Sara* (also a young girl role model) was designed for use in various countries of eastern and southern Africa (Plate 7.6) (McKee et al., in press). Both programs focus on gender equality in raising children, and on reducing the vulnerability of the girl child to health and sexuality problems. For instance, *Sara* attacked female genital cutting in certain parts of Africa, a practice which increases the risk of HIV infection. Both *Meena* and *Sara* are multimedia projects, which include several episodes of the animated film (each dealing with a specific educational issue, for example, female literacy), radio drama series, comic books, school books, posters, short stories, music, and puppetry. *Meena* games, dolls, and textiles were also developed to commercially brand this South Asian symbol of an empowered child. *Karate Kids* has been shown in dozens of countries to combat the vulnerability of street children to prostitution and the threat of HIV infection (Sthapitanonda-Sarabol & Singhal, 1998, 1999).

We conclude that *if entertainment-education messages are designed to be shared across cultures, a tremendous cost-saving can be realized*. In the past, too many entertainment-education interventions have been limited to a single nation.

The Global Institutionalization of Entertainment-Education

Population Communications International (PCI) headquartered in New York, Johns Hopkins University's Center for Communication Programs (JHU/CCP) in Baltimore, and Soul City in Parkstown, South Africa, are some of the leading organizations that implement HIV/AIDS entertainment-education interventions. Both PCI and JHU/CCP were established in the early 1980s, and their E-E programming is global in scope (covering the countries of Asia, Africa, and Latin America), whereas Soul City was established a decade later (in the early 1990s) to operate mostly in South Africa (although it is now expanding to other African countries).

Other organizations also utilize the entertainment-education strategy to address HIV/AIDS. The Centers for Disease Control and

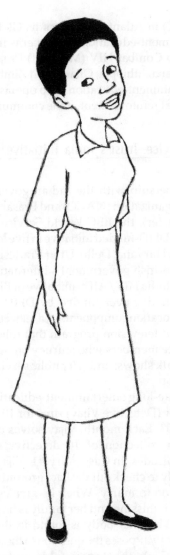

Plate 7.6   Sara, the Girl who Serves as a Media Role Model for Gender Issues in Eastern and Southern Africa

The UNICEF-sponsored *Sara* animation films, comic books, and lifeskills materials are examples of culturally shareable entertainment-education products.

Source: UNICEF.

Prevention (CDC) in Atlanta, as part of its Global AIDS Program, utilizes entertainment-education soap operas in its Modeling and Reinforcement to Combat HIV (MARCH) Project in four African countries: Botswana, Ethiopia, Ghana, and Zimbabwe (Galavotti et al., 2001). Entertainment-education soap operas are supplemented with interpersonal reinforcement at the community level.

BBC World Service Trust's India Initiative[10]

In 2002, in partnership with the Indian government's National AIDS Control Organization (NACO) and Prasar Bharati (the Indian national broadcaster), the BBC World Service Trust (BBC WST) launched a major DFID-funded initiative in five low HIV-prevalence states: Rajasthan, Haryana, Delhi, Uttar Pradesh, and Uttaranchal. The DFID is the British government's international development aid ministry. The India HIV/AIDS initiative of BBC WST, the largest media health initiative ever funded by DFID, includes a strong entertainment-education component: (*a*) a television detective series; (*b*) a reality-based television program that follows the lives of 80 youthful audience members who journey on buses across the five states; (*c*) radio talk shows; and (*d*) public service announcements on HIV prevention.

The 120-episode-long entertainment-education detective series titled *Jasoos Vijay* (Detective Vijay) runs for 10 months from June 2002 to April 2003. Each month, Vijay solves one case; so *Jasoos Vijay* is really a collection of 10 detective case stories, each comprising 12 episodes. In Case Story #1, Vijay is commissioned by an urban family to check out the background of a rural girl, who they wish their son to marry. When he arrives in the village, he discovers the girl is missing and her family is trying to cover up her disappearance. When her body is found in the village well, the epilogue in *Jasoos Vijay* poses the question to the audience members: "How did she die?" As the story unfolds, audience members find out that the dead girl was a childhood friend of a village outcast, who was ostracized by the community because he was HIV-positive.

Jasoos Vijay is an interactive, fast-paced drama series in which episodes end on a cliffhanging note and an epilogue is delivered by Om Puri, a famous film celebrity. The epilogue summarizes plot developments, focuses viewers' attention on the key HIV/AIDS dilemmas, and urges viewers to write in responses to the central question posed. Audience members with the most interesting answers take part in a studio discussion with a key character of *Jasoos Vijay* who is placed "In the Hot Seat." The invited viewers can then ask the character (for instance, an "unfaithful husband") a range of questions regarding his behavior, motivations, and feelings.

Complementing *Jasoos Vijay* is the youth reality television show, *Haath Se Haath Milaa* (Hand in Hand Together), set aboard two buses (one for boys, one for girls) that, over a 10-month period, journeys in the five Indian states. Each bus, at any given time, carries two *humsafars* (co-travelers), with each pair of *humsafars* spending no more than two weeks on the bus. The buses, equipped with bunk beds, cooking facilities, television cameras, and a presenter, visit cities, villages, college campuses, ancient forts, farms, and temples, signifying the youth journey of a lifetime. During this journey, the *humsafars* learn the skills to live life to the fullest, to protect themselves from HIV/AIDS, and to have more compassion for those living with AIDS. Each week, the presenters provide the *humsafars* with a creative, entertaining challenge: for instance, who among them is least embarrassed buying a condom; a role-playing game wherein each repulses the advances of the opposite sex; and so forth.

The boys' and the girls' buses take different routes, but come together at various locations for interactions between them. While on separate-sex buses, boys will be asked questions about girls, and girls about boys. Each week, the reality-based sequences are filmed, edited, and broadcast, in a total of 40 episodes, each episode 30 minutes long, during the 10-month period overlapping with *Jasoos Vijay*'s broadcast. The bus-based reality television presentation will be complemented with a *Haath Se Haath Milaa* media fair, including performances by local musicians, village poets, and celebrities of the Bombay film industry. Celebrity endorsements on HIV/AIDS will also be included in each week's episode, and prize competitions will be held for audience members on the issues of AIDS, health, and lifeskills. Finally, after 40 weeks, the buses, carrying all 80 *humsafars* (40 boys and 40 girls), arrive in Delhi to meet with the prime minister of India.

As the BBC World Service Trust's India project testifies, entertainment-education is increasingly at the center of most media-based HIV/AIDS interventions.

"On the Edge": A Warrior Vanquishes the Demon

As noted in Chapter 4, soldiers represent a group at especially high risk for contracting HIV. In 2002, Professor William J. Brown of Regent University, an expert on entertainment-education, and his colleagues collaborated with the Tanzanian military to produce an entertainment-education film, *On the Edge*, to increase adoption of HIV/AIDS prevention behaviors by Tanzanian soldiers. Some 15 percent of Tanzanian soldiers are HIV-positive, and several thousands have died of AIDS in the past decade.

The storyline for *On the Edge* was created on the basis of extensive formative research, including numerous in-depth interviews with soldiers and military personnel on Tanzanian military bases, and an understanding of soldiers' use of local bars and brothels. The plot centers on Tesha, a soldier who contracts HIV, and who tries to save his friend, Paulo, from contracting the virus. Tesha tells Paulo the traditional Masai folktale about Ngulpa, the handsome warrior, and Ogre, the demon, to symbolize how AIDS can be vanquished (Ngulpa killed the demon). The film is currently being pre-tested in Tanzania, after which it will be duplicated in several hundreds of copies, and used in military training programs on different military bases.

Entertainment-education films such as *On the Edge* can reach a large number of high-risk individuals who agglomerate in multiple locations: prisoners, commercial sex workers, and soldiers.

PCI's Entertainment-Education Interventions

HIV/AIDS initiatives undertaken by Population Communications International (PCI) reflect the role of E-E in addressing the epidemic. Established in 1985, PCI works with in-country partner organizations to implement entertainment-education for radio and television interventions in Asia, Africa, Latin America, the

Caribbean, and the United States. Headquartered in New York City, PCI's entertainment-education soap operas promote sexual and reproductive health, including HIV prevention; gender equality; education and literacy; and protection of the environment. Since 1998, PCI has greatly strengthened the HIV/AIDS education component in its roster of international programs in China, the eastern Caribbean (produced in Grenada for broadcast there as also in Antigua, Dominica, and St. Vincent and the Grenadines), Kenya, Mexico, Pakistan, South India, and Tanzania. The U.S. initiatives of the PCI, based in Los Angeles, added HIV/AIDS prevention messages through its Soap Summits, an annual meeting of Hollywood soap opera professionals.

In 1999, PCI added a unit to its E-E training workshops that explained the ways HIV can and cannot be transmitted. All scriptwriters, directors, and producers are exposed to this information at PCI's methodology and scriptwriting workshops. Only if they are knowledgeable themselves about HIV/AIDS can they write authentic and accurate stories that include life-saving messages.

In China, PCI's television mini-series, *Bai Xing* (Ordinary People), is currently preparing scripts for episodes 39 through 58 that will air in 2003. This third set of 45-minute dramas includes a character that has been distinguished by his promiscuity, arrogance, and lack of consideration for others. Ershui contracts HIV and by the end of the show is suffering with AIDS. His story is used as a vehicle for informing the public about modes of transmission (mainly unprotected heterosexual relations with multiple partners, in his case). The female protagonist, Lü Ye, already loved by the audience, is a model of positive behavior. She leads the villagers to accept Ershui and to treat him with compassion, regardless of his HIV status (Singhal et al., 1999). Viewers are thus reassured that caring for an HIV-positive person and treating him kindly entail no risks of transmission.

In the eastern Caribbean, the nations of Antigua, Dominica, Grenada, and St. Vincent and the Grenadines were chosen as the site for a regional soap opera. These four island nations were selected for their relative homogeneity of language, lifestyles, and health problems. Working in partnership with the RARE Center for Tropical Conservation, Grenada was selected, through a competitive process, as the island from which to produce and broadcast the show *Coconut Bay*. Building on knowledge gained in producing St. Lucia's successful *Apwé Plézi*, Grenada's scriptwriters from the Heritage Theater Company constructed a story that boldly tackled the risks of HIV for the characters in authentic island life. Having multiple sexual partners and not following safer sex practices lead to transmission of HIV in this story. The soap opera's main purpose is to provide life-saving messages about HIV prevention in the Caribbean, a region second only to Sub-Saharan Africa in its high rate of HIV incidence.

In Pakistan, a certain E-E radio program is ideally placed to address HIV/AIDS in South Asia, where the epidemic threatens to escalate. The program raises questions that are usually not spoken aloud – questions of access to reproductive health care for women, family planning, protection from STDs, and open communication about sexual issues. The Pakistani program is breaking new ground, paving the way for open discussion of HIV/AIDS transmission and prevention. The program, called *Dukh Sukh Apney* (Our Sorrows and Happinesses), creates a climate in which accurate information about HIV/AIDS is accepted.

Population Communications International's radio soap opera broadcasts in four states of South India – Andhra Pradesh, Karnataka, Kerala, and Tamil Nadu – also promote open communication about subjects traditionally considered inappropriate and taboo. In Tamil Nadu, the storyline included the revelation that a male character, whose marriage had been arranged to a young woman in a local village, was HIV-positive. This news was received with horror, but later on, the soap opera's compassionate treatment of the HIV-positive individual showed that a community can be educated to respond with sympathy. This narrative represents PCI's recent move, from simply including information about HIV/AIDS in E-E interventions, toward also promoting destigmatization.

In addition to PCI's international programs, reproductive health, gender equality, and sustainable development are encouraged for its U.S. audiences. An annual meeting of soap opera professionals includes writers, directors, producers, and actors from the 10 prominent U.S. daytime television soaps. The keynote speaker, U.S. Congressman Ronald Dellums, addressing Soap Summit V in 2000 in Los Angeles, sounded the alarm about the staggering statistics of the worldwide HIV/AIDS burden. His talk was a call to arms, challenging the talented professionals gathered in the room to educate the public about the HIV/AIDS pandemic.

Ushikwapo Shikamana in Kenya

In Kenya, PCI's 15-minute radio soap opera *Ushikwapo Shikamana* (If Assisted, Assist Yourself) has been on the air since 1998. It is broadcast by the Kenyan Broadcasting Corporation (KBC) twice a week on Mondays and Wednesdays, with a 30-minute omnibus on Saturdays. The language of the soap opera is Kiswahili, Kenya's national language. *Ushikwapo Shikamana* has a crackerjack scriptwriting team, headed by Dr. Kimani Njogu, a specialist in Kiswahili literary criticism. Njogu served as PCI's trainer in over half a dozen countries, including in the popular Tanzanian radio series *Twende na Wakati* (discussed previously). *Ushikwapo Shikamana* is sponsored by Unga Limited, a Kenyan company that manufactures nutritional products, and is thus able to recover some of its production costs.

The story of *Ushikwapo Shikamana* is about life's struggles. It begins when the elders of two prominent families, Gogo and Mchikichi, decide to marry off their school-aged children, Kinga (a boy 18 years old) and Pendo (a girl of 14). Once this decision is made, the bride-to-be, Pendo, has to be initiated into womanhood according to prevailing cultural practice. Everyone supports Pendo's circumcision ceremony except Pendo, the village school teacher, Tatu, who herself escaped this brutal practice of female genital mutilation in her home village, and Kinga, the groom-to-be.

The decision to circumcise Pendo leads to a protracted struggle between the younger and the older generations, a struggle that is painful and bitter, leading Kinga to leave the village. After Pendo is circumcised, she learns that her marriage is being arranged with Konga, an old man, and she runs away to the city. Eventually, Pendo finds true love in Sulubu, who shares the value of being monogamous, and they both undergo premarital testing for HIV/AIDS. The couple provides care for the growing number of AIDS orphans in their community. Pendo and Sulubu work closely with the local school teacher, Tatu, who organizes women in the local community to take care of AIDS orphans. HIV/AIDS is a major theme in *Ushikwapo Shikamana*. The story conveys information on risk factors, means of transmission and prevention, testing, informing partners, debunking myths surrounding HIV, coping with illness, compassion for the sick, and death and dying.

The fictitious Kanyageni Boarding School in *Ushikwapo Shikamana*, where girls resisting female circumcision are enrolled, is modeled after an actual school, the AIC Kajiado Boarding School. The show's creative team visited the school to gather first-hand impressions so they could better portray the girl students as characters in the soap opera. Through the years that *Ushikwapo Shikamana* has aired, the headmistress, Mrs. Nankurai, has encouraged her students to listen to the radio program for the positive messages it provides.

Ushikwapo Shikamana Comics

To strengthen the impact of the educational issues addressed in the popular radio program, PCI, in conjunction with Twaweza Communications, created a comic strip titled *Ushikwapo Shikamana*. First published in 1999, the comic strip continues to be featured three times a week in the national Kiswahili newspaper *Taifa Leo*. Although the strip does not follow the radio program episode by episode, its characters and storyline mirror those of the serial drama (much like Soul City's serialized story in 11 South African newspapers). Readers are encouraged to respond to the storyline and to ask questions about the issues raised. This information is monitored by PCI researchers, and used to clarify the messages relayed in the radio program.

The character Tatu is a catalyst for positive HIV/AIDS messages in the comic strips. One of her students, Dimba, approaches her with what he thinks may be symptoms of HIV/AIDS. Tatu advises him to practice responsible sexual behavior and to get tested for HIV (Plate 7.7). Dimba agrees, and the results show that he has a curable STD. He is, however, strongly advised that although he may have escaped HIV infection this time, he must act responsibly and use protection every time that he has sex in the future. The comic book reaches a young audience facing the critical challenge of growing up in a world ravaged by HIV/AIDS.

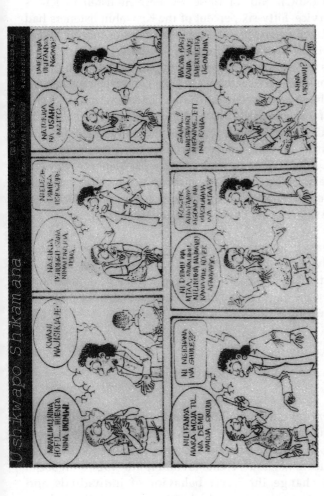

Plate 7.7 The Comic Book Version of *Ushikwapo Shikamana*, an Entertainment-Education Radio Soap Opera in Kenya

Ushikwapo Shikamana (If Assisted, Assist Yourself) is a popular, long-running soap opera broadcast in Kiswahili, the national language of Kenya. This comic strip appears in a widely circulated newspaper, and also as a comic book. The frames shown here deal with HIV/AIDS. Teacher Tatu advises Dimba, a student, to practice responsible sexual behavior and to get tested for HIV

Source: Kimani Njogu.

Program Effects

A 1999 survey showed that 99 percent of all Kenyans who are exposed to the radio regularly listen to the Kenyan Broadcasting Corporation (KBC), and, of these, 90 percent listen to KBC's Kiswahili service. Fifty-six percent of the Kiswahili listeners had tuned in to *Ushikwapo Shikamana* in the previous month, and of these, 61 percent listen to the program regularly.

Epilogues are used to heighten the impact of the radio drama and to call on audience members to take concrete steps toward addressing the issues raised in the drama. Telephone numbers and addresses of organizations that provide relevant services are mentioned after each episode. A list of these organizations was compiled during the formative research for the radio series.

Ushikwapo Shikamana generates hundreds of letters each week in response to the epilogues and the newspaper comic strip. Listeners write to convey their impressions of the entertaining and educational nature of the radio series. For example, one listener wrote:

> The program in both the radio and the *Taifa Leo* newspaper have really brought an awakening to most of us. The threat posed by the HIV scourge is worrying. With a program like this one, the message reaches many people and thereby makes them more aware.

Conclusions

Entertainment-education is defined as the process of purposely designing and implementing a media message to both entertain and educate, in order to increase audience members' knowledge about an educational issue, create favorable attitudes, shift social norms, and change the overt behavior of individuals and communities. The entertainment-education strategy, through the use of formative research, role models, epilogues, a multimedia campaign approach, and other creative techniques, such as humor and animation, can be highly effective in promoting HIV/AIDS prevention. The effectiveness of E-E in this regard has been proven in Tanzania, South Africa, India, and dozens of other countries.

When entertainment-education interventions are properly planned and implemented, experiences in many countries show that this strategy can be very effective in stimulating public discourse about HIV, thus breaking the silence surrounding this issue. Entertainment-education has the capacity to stimulate interpersonal peer communication, such as between an individual and his/her sexual partner. Such interpersonal communication has the unique ability to bring about behavior change, such as HIV prevention.

Entertainment-education interventions are only one of many competing messages. Audience members expose themselves selectively to E-E messages, perceive them selectively, recall their content selectively, and use it selectively for purposes they value. In this sense, entertainment-education is a "democratic" intervention, stimulating individual audience members to form their own actions, based on talking with peers.

Notes

1. The radio soap opera in Tanzania may be one of the first entertainment-education projects focusing on *both* family planning and HIV prevention. In most nations, family planning and HIV prevention projects are conducted separately, although both promote the use of condoms and are usually organized as programs in the national ministry of health.

2. Five *Soul City* television series were broadcast in 1994, 1996, 1997, 1999, and 2001. The intent is to broadcast one new 13-episode television series each year. In years when the television series was not broadcast, for instance, in 1995, 1998, and 2000, other health campaign activities were underway in South Africa.

3. Audiences are encouraged to keep the printed booklets and to refer to them. Each booklet has comic sections and activity-inserts, helping the audience members integrate health improvement into their daily lives.

4. Although they have been effectively used by other non-governmental organizations in South Africa.

5. In contrast, educational programs on South African television earn dismal ratings of 2 to 3 percent.

6. If a health issue is not a "national" priority, it is not included in the *Soul City* television series. It may be treated in the more localized radio broadcasts, the booklets, educational packets for adults and the youth, and serialized newspaper pages. Before addressing any health issue, whether national or local, field research is carried out to ensure that local infrastructure exists to support the message. For instance, if HIV testing were promoted in a particular mass media intervention, Soul City would ensure that the local infrastructure could meet the increased demand for that health service.

7. With respect to the media's contribution, the national television network in South Africa contributes significantly to the cost of producing the *Soul City* television series; the national and regional radio stations carry out the production and translations of the nine language radio series (from a common script) at very little cost to Soul City, and newspapers provide the space for serializing the booklets at no cost to Soul City.

8. As opposed to being implemented with technical assistance from an international aid agency.

9. In addition, Soul City has a budget of $6 million per year for its eight-country Africa roll-out program currently underway in Botswana, Swaziland, Namibia, Lesotho, Zimbabwe, Zambia, and other countries.

10. This section draws upon conversations with Peter Gill, Lori McDougall, Sangeeta Sharma Mehta, and Jyoti Mehra of the BBC World Service Trust in New Delhi in December 2001, January 2002, and March 2002. Arvind Singhal participated in the message design workshop for this HIV/AIDS media initiative in New Delhi in January 2002.

8

Monitoring and Evaluation

∎

Give me the lone ethnographer any day over multi-million dollar [HIV prevention] team projects. It takes only one person to be insightful, whereas it takes many to crunch numbers, to compress the garbage being produced.

Ralph Bolton (1995, p. 299).

The problem with qualitative researchers is that they don't see things as things they are. Rather, they see things as they are.

A comment made by a quantitative researcher at a health communication conference at Athens, Ohio.

During our December 2001 India visit, we were impressed with how quantitative research procedures, in the form of annual behavior surveillance surveys (BSS), were being strategically utilized by the AIDS Prevention and Control (APAC) Project in the Indian state of Tamil Nadu to plan, monitor, and evaluate targeted HIV/AIDS interventions. The annual rounds of BSS serve as an early warning system for APAC, inform HIV/AIDS program design, and help to evaluate targeted intervention programs by tracking behavior changes. For instance, the fifth BSS survey, conducted in

2000, showed that knowledge about prevention of STDs was high among all intervention subgroups (over 90 percent) except female factory workers, among whom it was only 53 percent. Knowledge that condoms can prevent STDs was even lower among the female factory workers (only 33 percent) (APAC, 2001a). The targeted interventions in 2001 were fine-tuned accordingly, with a special focus on female factory workers in Tamil Nadu state.

The present chapter describes how HIV/AIDS programs are monitored and evaluated, highlighting donor and programmatic exigencies, as well as the treatment of respondents as "objects" of research in what represents a dominant focus in measuring individual behavior change. Alternative conceptions of respondents as "subjects" of research, community involvement and participation in data collection and analysis, and social change indicators of HIV/AIDS are also highlighted. The strengths, limitations, and contingencies associated with these monitoring and evaluation approaches are stressed, including the lessons learned about implementing a more pluralistic evaluation of HIV/AIDS initiatives.

Ideally, large investments in HIV prevention in developing countries would be guided by adequate data about the number of HIV-positive people in a nation, their characteristics and geographical location, their adoption of condoms and other safe sex behaviors, their level of stigmatization, and other relevant variables. Ideally, every HIV prevention program would be evaluated, and then the intervention's implementation would be modified based on its tested effectiveness. Ideally, each program, as it is carried out, would be monitored to ensure that it is implemented in the most effective way.

In reality, much of the data just described are not available or are not utilized by HIV/AIDS control programs. However, several HIV prevention interventions are firmly grounded on sound data and their conduct is guided by process evaluation. This chapter describes certain of these interventions, and the quantitative and qualitative research on which they are based.

Field Experiments

A *field experiment* is an experiment conducted in the real world, rather than in a laboratory, with before and after surveys utilized to measure the outcome variables. In biomedical and behavioral research, the randomized control field experiments represent the "gold standard," in which members of a target population are recruited and randomly assigned to receive an experimental intervention, allowing for comparisons with a control group which does not receive the intervention (Kalichman, 1998).

The Opinion Leadership Field Experiment in Gay Bars

In Chapter 1, we described the concept of *opinion leadership*, defined as the degree to which certain individuals are sought by others for information and advice. We mentioned Kelly et al.'s (1997) field experiment with opinion leaders in gay bars in U.S. cities. This investigation determined the effects of using an opinion leader strategy in promoting HIV prevention in four U.S. cities and compared them with four other paired cities in which opinion leaders were not used.

Participants in Kelly's field experiments were men who patronized gay bars in the eight U.S. cities. In the gay bars in the four control sites, high-quality wall posters, graphics, and brochures about HIV prevention were prominently displayed. In the intervention sites, the same materials were displayed, but, in addition, popular opinion leaders, through conversations, spread endorsements of safer sex practices with their peers. To identify opinion leaders, bartenders in the gay bars of the intervention city were asked to rate people they judged to be the most popular with other men: those who were most often greeted, who greeted others, and who seemed well liked (Kelly et al., 1997). Opinion leaders went through a two-hour training session once a week, for five weeks, to learn conversational strategies about safer sex practices and HIV risk reduction.

Gay men completed survey questionnaires about their sexual behavior when they entered the bars before the intervention and in the impact evaluation a year later. Several behavioral risk indicators were gauged in the surveys: frequency of unprotected anal intercourse during the previous two months, the percentage of all anal intercourse acts in the previous two months in which condoms were used, and the number of sexual partners during the previous two months.

Results suggested that risk behavior decreased significantly in the intervention sites, as compared to the control sites: frequency of unprotected anal intercourse decreased, and the percentage of anal intercourse protected by condoms increased. Increased numbers of condoms taken from dispensers in intervention city bars corroborated risk behavior self-reports. The findings suggested that popular and well-liked members of a community, who systematically recommended risk reduction behaviors, could positively influence the sexual risk practices of others in their social networks (Kelly et al., 1997). Community members perceived such peer-based networking approaches to HIV prevention as credible and trustworthy. The conversational styles utilized by peer opinion leaders were perceived as non-threatening by the gay bar patrons.

This randomized controlled field experiment points to the promise of using the opinion leadership strategy with other populations at high risk for HIV, for instance, injecting drug users, adolescents, or commercial sex workers. Illiterate populations can be reached by these peer conversations.

The Field Experiment in Chennai

The next step was to conduct a series of field experiments on the effects of the opinion leader strategy in five developing countries. The National Institute for Mental Health (NIMH), a U.S. government agency, funded this five-year investigation in India, Peru, Russia, China, and Zimbabwe. Jeff Kelly is a technical consultant to the five-country study. The India field experiment is carried out by the Y.R.G. Center for AIDS Research and Education (Y.R.G. CARE) in Chennai, under the direction of Dr. Suniti Solomon, an eminent AIDS expert. Her special hospital ward for HIV/AIDS patients is described as "the biggest AIDS clinic in southern India, and it is probably the best one in the country" (Specter, 2001, p. 80). The ward receives about five new HIV+ cases per day, cares for many AIDS patients (including certain of the rich and famous people of India), and looks after 75 HIV-positive children. Dr. Solomon has treated 6,000 individuals with HIV/AIDS since identifying the first

HIV-positive commercial sex workers in India in 1986, something of a Guinness record for health providers.

The experimental treatment in the NIMH-funded project is to identify opinion leaders in 30 of Chennai's 945 slums, train them about HIV transmission and prevention, and encourage them to pass this information along informally to their peers. The opinion leaders, called "C-POLs" (community popular opinion leaders), are expected to be about 15 percent of the population in the 30 slums. Each of the slums in Chennai is very compact, with approximately 300 households, and more than 1,000 people, residing in a total area of 2,000 to 3,000 square feet (about the size of the typical American house). Many of the slums are in out-of-the-way places, such as under an overpass, along a road, or near a construction site. Often the slum consists of squatters who have simply moved onto a plot of available urban land.

One of the first steps in the NIMH project in Chennai was to map each of the 30 slums of study, identify each household with a unique number, and then randomly sample 65 of the households in each slum containing a woman aged from 18 to 40. Personal interviews were conducted using a laptop computer on which to record the data, which was transmitted directly to the Research Triangle Institute (RTI) in North Carolina for analysis. Each female respondent was asked to take a vaginal swab, so that STDs could be measured; many women refused this procedure, although they allowed a nurse or doctor to take the swab.

A high percentage of the intended respondents cooperated in providing data; in return, Y.R.G. CARE agreed to provide health care in each slum. The researchers found that the interviewers had to be a different set of people than the health care providers, in order to protect the privacy of the respondents (personal interview, A.K. Srikrishnan, Chennai, 22 December 2001). The C-POLs are selected in each slum, and then the field experiment's treatment intervention begins. In a set of control slums, no C-POLs are identified and trained. The difference between the effects of the intervention in the treatment slums and its effects in the control slums accounts for the contemporaneous changes that occur. A main dependent variable in the Chennai slum experiment is the rate of HIV and STD infection, before and after the C-POL intervention.

The Field Experiment in Tanzania to Evaluate
Twende na Wakati

In the previous chapter, we discussed the Tanzanian experience with *Twende na Wakati*, a radio soap opera that, since 1993, has promoted HIV/AIDS prevention, small family size, and other development issues.

The effects of *Twende na Wakati* were measured in a field experiment[1] in which most of Tanzania was exposed to this entertainment-education radio soap opera (the treatment), while the broadcasts were blocked from a large central region of the country (Dodoma) for two years from 1993 to 1995 (the control, or comparison, area). Eight types of evaluation data were gathered, including personal interviews with about 3,000 respondents in the control and treatment areas each year for five years, point-of-referral data on family planning adoption at 79 clinics in the treatment and control areas, focus group discussions and in-depth interviews with new family planning adopters in the control and treatment areas, and a content analysis of audience letters received in response to *Twende na Wakati* (Rogers et al., 1999). The evaluation study was carried out by one of the present authors (Rogers), Dr. Peter Vaughan at the University of New Mexico, and by Population Family Life Education Program (POFLEP), a research center headquartered in Arusha, Tanzania, led by Ramadhan Swalehe and Verhan Bakari. Funding for this evaluation research came from the Rockefeller Foundation and the United Nations Population Fund.

Closing the KAP-Gap: *Twende na Wakati* was very popular. By 1994, some 55 percent of Tanzanians were listening to the radio soap opera, and about half of these individuals listened regularly (that is, to at least one or both of the episodes that were broadcast each week). By 1997–98, about 72 percent of the people in the Dodoma area were listening to the radio soap opera.

When broadcasts of *Twende na Wakati* began in 1993, almost everyone in Tanzania had already heard of AIDS, and many people perceived that they were at risk for AIDS. However, only a small percentage of sexually active Tanzanians practiced safer sex. So the main effect of the radio soap opera was expected to be that of closing the KAP-gap (the gap between knowledge and favorable attitudes, on the one hand, and overt behavior, or practice, on the other) by encouraging the adoption of HIV prevention methods.

Exposure to *Twende na Wakati* produced a strong effect upon HIV prevention behavior. Some 72 percent of the listeners in 1994 said that they had adopted an HIV prevention behavior because of listening to *Twende na Wakati*. This percentage increased to 82 in the 1995 survey after a second year of broadcast (Figure 8.1).[2] Seventy-seven percent of these individuals who adopted HIV prevention methods reduced their number of sexual partners, 16 percent began using condoms, and 6 percent stopped sharing razors and/or needles. The percentage of listeners who believed that they could avoid being infected with HIV by using insect repellents decreased from 24 percent in 1993 to 14 percent in 1995 in the treatment area, while it remained constant at 9 percent in the comparison area (Dodoma) from 1993 to 1995 (the incorrect belief that the virus could be transmitted by mosquitoes was debunked in the episodes of *Twende na Wakati*).[3]

Stimulating Interpersonal Communication: *Exposure to the radio soap opera influenced individuals to adopt safer sex by stimulating interpersonal communication about HIV* (this process also occurred in the case of family planning). Listeners of *Twende na Wakati* who talked with others (61 percent of the listeners in 1995) reported talking to: (*a*) friends, 55 percent; (*b*) spouse, 37 percent; and (*c*) other individuals, 8 percent (Figure 8.2). Listeners who talked with others about HIV prevention were much more likely to adopt an AIDS prevention method (92 percent) than were listeners who did not talk with others (69 percent). Adoption of condom use and other safe sex behaviors was more likely if audience individuals who listened to *Twende na Wakati* then discussed these behavioral changes, acted out and encouraged by the characters in the radio soap opera, with their sexual partners. Again, *interpersonal communication with peers motivates behavior change.*

Male respondents with multiple sexual partners, who perceived that they were at higher risk for AIDS, were much more likely to use condoms from 1993 to 1995, than were monogamous men. Some 21 percent of the 204 episodes of *Twende na Wakati* broadcast from

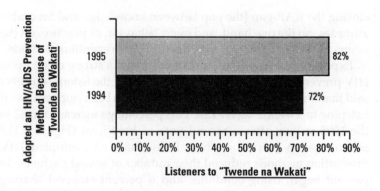

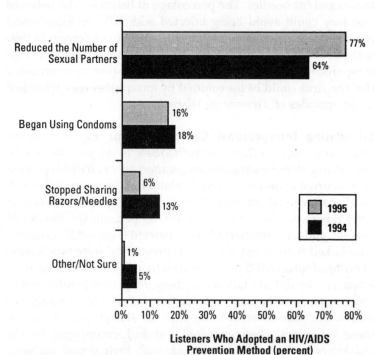

Figure 8.1   Self-reported HIV/AIDS Behavior Change by *Twende na Wakati* Listeners

After two years of broadcasts, this radio soap opera in Tanzania led to widespread adoption of HIV prevention behaviors.

Source: Singhal & Rogers (1999).

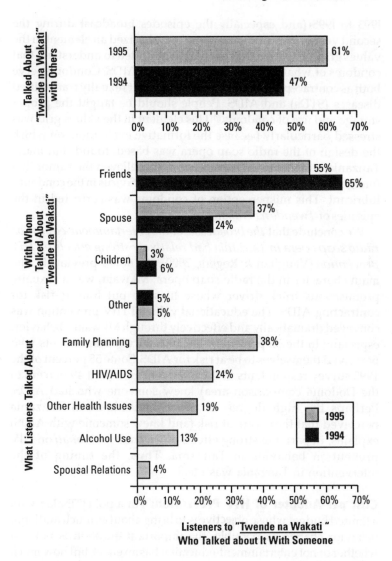

Figure 8.2 *Twende na Wakati* Stimulated Interpersonal Communication with Friends and Spouse

One of the main ways that an entertainment-education program influences human behavior change is by stimulating peer communication about an educational topic like HIV prevention.

Source: Singhal & Rogers (1999).

1993 to 1995 (and especially the episodes broadcast during the second year of the radio soap opera) emphasized an element in the values grid: "It is good that people are educated to understand that condoms of whatever brand do not spread AIDS. Condoms serve both as contraceptives and protection against sexually transmitted diseases (STDs) and AIDS. People should be taught the proper storage and use of condoms." This element in the values grid was stressed particularly because the formative evaluation, on which the design of the radio soap opera was based, found that many Tanzanians at that time (November 1992) believed the rumor that foreign brands of condoms contained the AIDS virus in the condom's lubricant. This misperception of condoms was corrected in the episodes of *Twende na Wakati*.

We conclude that *the broadcasts of the entertainment-education radio soap opera in Tanzania had relatively strong effects on HIV prevention* (Vaughan & Rogers, 2000). As noted previously, the main character in the radio soap opera, Mkwaju, was a sexually promiscuous truck driver whose lifestyle put him at risk for contracting AIDS. The educational value of HIV prevention was conveyed dramatically and effectively through Mkwaju's behavior, especially to the 58 percent of the 1995 survey respondents who perceived themselves to be at risk for AIDS. Some 58 percent of the 1995 survey respondents in the treatment area (and 49 percent in the Dodoma comparison area) knew someone who had AIDS. Perhaps the high degree to which individuals in Tanzania perceived that they were at risk (and knew someone with AIDS) explains, in part, the strong effects of *Twende na Wakati* on HIV prevention behavior in Tanzania. Thus, the timing of the intervention in Tanzania was ideal.

Cost per Adopter of HIV Prevention: For a policy-maker with a limited budget whose objective is to bring about as much audience behavior change as possible, the important question is not just whether or not entertainment-education has an effect, but how much each individual behavior change costs, compared to alternative approaches. For this reason, several entertainment-education projects have been evaluated in terms of their cost per adopter.

The cost-effectiveness of *Twende na Wakati* was impressive: less than 10 cents (U.S.) per adopter of HIV prevention (Singhal & Rogers, 1999). These figures are very important in a desperately poor nation like Tanzania, where the per capita income was only $150 per year in 1997.

A Quantitative Approach to HIV/AIDS Research

While randomized control field experiments can serve a very useful purpose, there exists an overwhelming reliance on quantitative methods in investigating HIV interventions. Institutional and donor agendas championed such behavioral and biomedical studies, while generally de-emphasizing and sidelining qualitative methodologies.

The Centers for Disease Control's AIDS Community Demonstration Project (ACDP) is a case in point. The ACDP was a multi-million-dollar, multi-site project evaluating HIV interventions in five U.S. cities: Dallas, Denver, Long Beach, New York, and Seattle. The ACDP evaluated the effectiveness of using community volunteers to increase the use of condoms and/or bleach (to clean drug needles) among hard-to-reach, high-risk population groups: gays, injecting drug users, CSWs, and youth in inner-city neighborhoods. The findings of the ACDP showed that high-risk individuals could be influenced to form intentions to perform, and adopt, protective behaviors (Fishbein et al., 1997). However, by focusing primarily on influencing individual-level behavior, such studies tend to overlook the sociocultural complexities that mediate the adoption or rejection of protective behavior. Methodological pluralism in designing, implementing, and evaluating HIV interventions will not be achieved until donors and institutions, dominated by biomedical expertise, are willing to consider alternative methodological approaches, and back them with adequate resources.

Quantitative methods can be useful in describing, monitoring, and evaluating HIV prevention programs. Such methods can describe human behaviors that are known risk factors for spreading HIV, monitor changes in these behaviors, understand what caused these behavior changes, and evaluate the effects of these interventions. While quantitative methods play an important role in meeting these objectives, they are often insufficient to capture the complexity of AIDS.

As it is difficult to directly observe the private behaviors related to sex and drug use, quantitative studies use indirect proxy measures to gauge the effects of HIV interventions. These proxy measures can be either self-reports or biological markers (such as the incidence of STDs). The relative validity of these measures is sometimes questionable (Auerbach & Coates, 2000). Self-reports are usually initiated around questions that gauge the number of sexual partners, rates of protected and unprotected occasions of vaginal and anal sex, and the percentage of safe acts in which condoms are used. A problem with self-reports is that respondents may deny (or lie about) their behavior, especially socially unacceptable behavior (Brody, 1995). Self-reports, especially about stigmatized behaviors like anal sex, may not be trusted, because of the tendency of respondents to provide socially desirable responses. Social desirability biases can lead to the over-reporting of condom use, for example.

Minor variations in the wording of survey questions can negatively impact a measurement. For instance, in a knowledge–attitude–practice (KAP) survey conducted in six Mexican cities in 1988, gay men and female CSWs were asked about the number of sexual "partners" they had had in the past month. The response from the CSWs showed an average of "four" partners per month. Later, researchers discovered that the CSWs had interpreted the question as asking about their "steady" partners. Wording and language issues can become problematic when measures and instruments developed with white participants, for instance, are administered to African American respondents in the United States. The English language spoken by African Americans, in terms of metaphors, phrases, and colloquial expressions, is quite different from that spoken by the mainstream white populations (Rogers & Steinfatt, 1999). Both linguistic and ethnic validation of instruments is critical in quantitative research.

Randomized controlled field experiments are susceptible to the limitations just discussed (self-reports, socially desirable responses, etc.). Critics argue that the sociocultural undercurrents of HIV/AIDS may not lend themselves to quantification. There may be problems in recruiting and retaining participants, leading to attrition. Further, programs developed, implemented, and evaluated in a relatively controlled situation may perform differently when scaled up for community-wide implementation.

Quantitative research focuses on measuring individual-level behavior changes (as discussed in Chapter 5). Investigations of HIV/AIDS interventions can benefit from an understanding of various types of desired behavior changes: (a) individual versus collective; (b) one-time (for example, disclosing one's HIV status) versus recurring (for example, trying to hide one's HIV status); (c) self-controlled (for example, abstaining from sex) versus other-dependent (for example, seeking counseling and testing); (d) private (for example, using a condom) versus public (for example, voluntee-ring to work in an AIDS hospice); (e) preventive (for example, using clean needles) versus curative (for example, seeking STD treatment); (f) costly (for example, taking anti-retroviral drugs) versus low-cost (for example, taking herbal treatments); and (g) high involvement (for example, community activism on behalf of PWAs) versus low involvement (for example, maintaining silence about the epidemic).

HIV/AIDS research would benefit from a broader understanding of individual-, group-, and social-level changes. It is a dangerous oversimplification to think of the adoption of a behavior change like safe sex as entirely an individual action. The individual's partner may be involved in the decision, along with peers, family elders, the community, and even national health policies.

Social Change Indicators

Evaluators of HIV prevention programs need to develop indicators for measuring social and organizational change in the community that go beyond the measurement of individual-level changes. Social change indicators for HIV/AIDS communication interventions might include changes in the degree (frequency, reach, intensity, and quality) to which:

1. workplaces in the community implement HIV/AIDS prevention programs;
2. the community initiates home-based care programs;
3. local health services offer HIV/AIDS testing and counseling;
4. local health services ensure, and provide access to, a safe blood supply;

5. local brothels insist on condom use, and an HIV testing policy;
6. local prisons and military establishments institute HIV/AIDS prevention programs;
7. local schools adopt an HIV/AIDS education curriculum;
8. the dropout rate among AIDS orphans at local schools decreases;
9. people living with HIV/AIDS are part of "mainstream" society (employed in regular jobs, working as counselors, etc.);
10. individuals living with HIV/AIDS are protected by laws designed to uphold their rights;
11. the quality of life of those living with AIDS, and those caring for them, is enhanced;
12. community members openly discuss HIV/AIDS issues in public meetings;
13. new community-based programs are launched to address HIV/AIDS prevention, care, and support;
14. new coalitions emerge among community organizations to address HIV/AIDS issues;
15. community members collectively make decisions or pass resolutions to combat HIV/AIDS;
16. grassroots leadership emerges from within the community to tackle HIV/AIDS issues;
17. religious organizations and spiritual leaders are involved in HIV prevention, care, and support programs;
18. the community engages in acts of mobilization and activism for HIV/AIDS-related issues;
19. the community engages with the local administration, service delivery organizations, non-governmental organizations, and others on HIV/AIDS issues;
20. the community's cultural activities (sports, folk media, festivals, celebrations, songs, etc.) engage with HIV/AIDS issues;
21. the most vulnerable groups at risk for HIV/AIDS in the community are empowered to take greater control of their external environment;
22. media coverage and media advocacy for HIV/AIDS increases;

23. the overall rate of STDs and new HIV infections decreases;
24. the community becomes AIDS-competent in terms of prevention, care, and support;
25. multi-sectoral involvement exists at the national level for HIV/AIDS control.

Imirim in São Paulo, Brazil, with its population of 30,000, among whom Padre Valeriano founded the AIDS hospice for children (discussed in Chapter 6), exemplifies several of the social change indicators outlined above. Three children's AIDS hospices exist in Imirim. HIV-positive children regularly attend the local school without stigma. Padre Valeriano, the parish preacher, integrates AIDS messages in each of his weekly sermons. Community members volunteer in the neighborhood's AIDS hospices, and contribute funds for medicines and hospital care. An HIV counseling and testing center exists in Imirim, and AIDS drugs are available free of charge to HIV-positive individuals through local public health services. When children die of AIDS in the neighborhood hospices, hundreds of community members attend their funerals to mourn their passing away.

Behavior Surveillance Surveys in Tamil Nadu

The AIDS Prevention and Control (APAC) Project in the Indian state of Tamil Nadu conducts annual behavior surveillance surveys (BSS) to plan, monitor, and evaluate targeted HIV/AIDS interventions. *Behavior surveillance surveys* measure behavior changes among targeted groups over a period of time. Begun in 1996, APAC is supported by the U.S. Agency for International Development, and operated by Voluntary Health Services, a Chennai-based NGO. The APAC Project implements a range of highly targeted interventions for STD/HIV/AIDS prevention in Tamil Nadu through a network of 35 NGOs. With the proliferation of HIV/AIDS intervention programs in Tamil Nadu, APAC aptly fulfills the role of a coordinating organization. It provides technical and financial support to its partner NGOs through a "lean and mean" organizational structure, comprising half a dozen technical personnel and a dozen support staff members. The APAC Project in Tamil Nadu also developed partnerships with NGO support organizations (NSOs), which offer NGOs development training and support services (APAC, 1999). The project's NGO partners work with various subpopulations like truckers and their helpers, CSWs, and youth in urban slums. The APAC Project's intervention strategy for HIV/AIDS centers on behavior change communication, quality STD care, promotion of condoms, and the use of research to make strategic decisions.

The Tamil Nadu APAC Project pioneered in collecting quantitative information on sexual behavior in India. Biomedical indicators for HIV/AIDS are difficult to gauge over a short time, so APAC collects data annually to track changes in prevention behaviors by targeted groups. It conducted six annual waves of BSS in Tamil Nadu, beginning in 1996. The annual BSS are a planning, designing, and monitoring tool for APAC. Technical expertise in designing the BSS was provided to APAC by Family Health International (FHI), a North Carolina-based agency. Family Health International had gained valuable experience in conducting BSS in Thailand in the early 1990s, and in Cambodia in the late 1990s.

The APAC Project works in tandem with the Tamil Nadu State AIDS Control Society (TANSACS) that undertakes an HIV sentinel surveillance (HSS) annually to understand trends in HIV prevalence among various high-risk and vulnerable groups, truckers and helpers, antenatal mothers, tuberculosis patients, and STD patients. *HIV sentinel surveillance* measures HIV prevalence trends over time in a sentinel site through biomedical markers, such as STD rates, percentage of HIV-positive women in antenatal clinics, and others. The behavior surveillance survey undertaken by APAC complements TANSACS's HSS by collecting additional data on the sexual behavior of vulnerable population groups.

BSS Methodology

The BSS involves "annual" waves of data collection from the *same* populations in the *same* sample areas in Tamil Nadu, using the *same* survey questionnaire. Unlike a general population sexual behavior survey, BSS captures behavior changes among the targeted groups. The annual BSS conducted by APAC gathers data from a sample of 13,000 respondents, divided into eight subgroups (female CSWs, truckers and helpers, male STD patients, male factory workers, female factory workers, male students, female students, and male youth in urban slums), in 13 selected towns in the state of Tamil Nadu. The survey collects data on 12 indicators under four broad headings (APAC, 2001b, pp. 10–11):

Knowledge Indicators:

1. Proportion of respondents who cite two acceptable ways of preventing STDs.
2. Proportion of respondents who know that condoms prevent STDs.
3. Proportion of respondents who cite two acceptable ways of preventing HIV/AIDS.
4. Proportion of respondents who know that condoms can prevent HIV/AIDS.

Behavior Indicators:

5. Proportion of respondents who report having had heterosexual intercourse with a non-regular partner in the last year.
6. Proportion of respondents who report condom use during their last sexual intercourse with a non-regular partner.
7. Proportion of male respondents who report having had sex with men in the last year.
8. Proportion of male respondents who report having had anal sex with a male sexual partner.
9. Proportion of male respondents who report condom use during their last anal sex encounter with a sexual partner.

Health-Seeking Behaviors:

10. Proportion of male respondents who reported symptoms of urethritis in the past year.

11. Proportion of male respondents who sought treatment from qualified medical doctors for urethritis in the past year.

Perception of Risk:

12. Proportion of respondents engaging in risk behavior who perceive that they are at risk for contracting HIV/AIDS.

Quality control is maintained by APAC over issues of sampling, interviewer training, data collection, data analysis, and other research protocols. The A.C. Nielsen Company conducts the annual rounds of data collection. The key is to conduct the first wave of BSS correctly, so that comparative data can be generated in succeeding years. The BSS has limitations, including its reliance on self-report data. However, these biases are present in all the annualized BSS waves, making the trend lines comparable. To supplement the quantitative data, APAC conducts focus group interviews with each of the targeted groups in order to gain qualitative insights into that group's sexual behavior. For instance, interviews with college students, both male and female, suggested how difficult it was for young people to buy condoms, for fear of others watching them. Interviews with youth living in urban slums showed the reasons why they liked to have sex with married women: no "burden" of marriage, pregnancy, and long-term commitment. Such qualitative insights can inform the designs of programs.

Peer-based Interventions

The APAC intervention strategy, targeted to subpopulation groups, centers on the training of peer outreach educators through partner NGOs. A Chennai-based NGO, CHES (discussed in Chapter 4), is part of APAC's network. This NGO uses commercial sex workers as peer educators to reach out to other commercial sex workers. Peer educators' conventions are organized by APAC to encourage ownership of the prevention program in their communities. The peer educators trained by APAC organized themselves into an association, which had 8,000 members by 2001.

One of APAC's interventions, directed at the population of truckers and their helpers, is called Prevention Along the Highway (PATH). Eleven NGOs work with APAC to implement this intervention. The 1996 baseline BSS showed that 94 percent of the truck drivers and their helpers were between 15 and 40 years of age; 50 percent were unmarried; and almost all of them were sexually active. The baseline BSS also showed that almost half the truck drivers and their helpers acknowledged having sex on the road with a non-regular partner (non-spouse), and only 44 percent had used condoms during their last sexual encounter. Data collected by Tamil Nadu's AIDS Control Society (TANSACS) during its HIV sentinel surveillance (HSS) suggested an alarming upward trend in seroprevalence among truck drivers and helpers: from 2.6 percent in 1994 to 9.4 percent in 1997. The 1996 BSS data further showed that 64 percent of the truckers and helpers who had not used a condom in their last non-regular intercourse were not aware of the risk of contracting HIV. Even among those who had used a condom, 74 percent had low or no risk perception for contracting HIV. Further, risk perception among commercial sex workers on the highway, who are the truckers' main sexual partners, was very low, as was the use of condoms. The 1996 BSS baseline data thus helped prioritize these problems in designing the PATH intervention.

The NGO partners of APAC in PATH had rich experience in implementing social welfare and community development projects, and possessed a rapport with the target community, transportation associations, and industries. Each NGO operated on a pre-determined stretch of the main highway, ranging from 20 kilometers to 70 kilometers, with field strength in that operational area (APAC, 1999). Participating NGOs, at the project's initiation, identified all major truck stops and hotspots for sexual activities.

Five years of intervention work, gauged by five rounds of BSS data, showed that as a result of PATH's activities, condom use among commercial sex workers and truckers had steadily increased in Tamil Nadu. However, condom use among male factory workers declined, suggesting the importance of reinvigorating this intervention (Figure 8.3).

What lessons has APAC learned from the BSS experience?

1. Behavior surveillance surveys help APAC to set priorities among subpopulation groups to be addressed

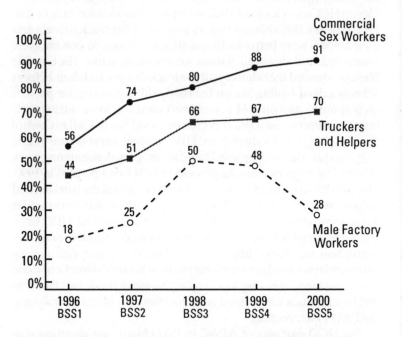

Figure 8.3   Condom usage among Commercial Sex Workers, Truckers and Helpers, and Male Factory Workers in Tamil Nadu, as Tracked by Five Annual Waves of Behavior Surveillance Surveys (BSS)

The AIDS Prevention and Control (APAC) Project in Tamil Nadu state utilizes longitudinal BSS data to identify problems, design program interventions targeted at various high-risk groups, and to monitor and evaluate their progress.

Source: APAC (2001a).

for HIV/AIDS interventions. The BSS helped obtain several rounds of comprehensive information on sexual risk behavior and condom usage by various population groups in Tamil Nadu state, which was not previously available. The BSS helped identify indicators of program effectiveness, as well as problem areas, informing the direction of the program design, and leading to mid-course corrections.

2. The BSS findings are disseminated by APAC to various partner NGOs, state AIDS control societies, the national government, and donors. These data serve as a tool for advocacy, raising the awareness of policy-makers (in the state of Tamil Nadu and at the national level) about the need for targeted interventions, and the importance of framing program strategies on the collected data. When the health minister of Tamil Nadu claimed there were no women in prostitution in his constituency, APAC arranged for 2,000 commercial sex workers from his hometown to meet with him.

3. Once the annual waves of BSS begin, there is momentum to continue. So BSS is an important way of initiating and maintaining political action.

Monitoring through Information Technology

In Brazil, the national AIDS control program of the federal government is linked with the AIDS control programs of Brazil's 27 states and 150 municipalities through several computer-based information systems that track behavioral indicators (gathered in the BSS), HIV-prevalence indicators (gathered in the HSS), and the free countrywide distribution of anti-retroviral drugs.

Over 425 institutions distribute free anti-retroviral AIDS drugs in Brazil, and the information system (called SICLOM) tracks *who* is giving *what* drug to *whom* and *when*. Thus, SICLOM ensures that the drugs are dispensed according to therapy guidelines, and helps manage the supply of drugs in Brazil's vast geographical area. Over 75 percent of Brazil's 800,000 HIV-positive individuals are covered on-line by SICLOM. The state of Amazonas, located in the Brazilian rainforest, provides such information via river boat, airplane, and mobile telephone.

Other computer systems, SICEL, SINAN, and SIM, track the CD4 counts of HIV-positive individuals, new HIV cases, and AIDS death rates, respectively. The CD4 count of each person who receives anti-retroviral drugs is checked every three months. These computer systems help in reporting new HIV cases, and identifying geographical areas where HIV prevalence may be rising, so that the necessary action may be taken speedily. These monitoring systems also serve important planning, monitoring, and advocacy purposes for HIV/AIDS in Brazil, akin to the role played by APAC's behavior surveillance surveys in Tamil Nadu.

A Qualitative Approach to HIV/AIDS Research

As noted previously, quantitative methods, shaped by the biomedical approach and by epidemiological questions, have dominated the design and implementation of HIV/AIDS interventions. Qualitative research is especially suited to unraveling the complexities of local knowledge, social and cultural peculiarities, and power and control issues (Parker, 1995). However, relatively few such qualitative studies are conducted. One exception is Farmer's (1995) study of the patterns of HIV transmission in rural Haiti, which showed how sociocultural, economic, and political factors influenced HIV transmission. Farmer found that poverty, sexism, lack of culturally appropriate prevention tools, and lack of political will were key reasons for the spread of HIV in Haiti.

Qualitative research is open-ended, and, unlike quantitative research, is unbound by predetermined variables. Qualitative research can be contextual, and is summarized by narratives rather than numerical statements. Sample sizes are often quite small, and the qualitative method is characterized by observations and in-depth interviews. Qualitative research traditions such as ethnography, case study, biography, grounded theory, and phenomenology are holistic, inductive, context-based and narrative-driven (Airhihenbuwa, 2002). They describe and interpret. The AIDS epidemic dramatizes what we do not know about sexuality, emphasizing the need for qualitative research. For instance, in Brazil, young people make a distinction between sex for "love" and sex for "release." In Mexico, there is usually a high degree of stigma attached to an individual who engages in receptive anal intercourse, but there exists cultural approval of "macho" males who play an active inserter role. Such cultural aspects of sexual behavior are important in planning effective HIV prevention programs, but difficult to gather with quantitative methods.

HIV/AIDS is reshaping the role of qualitative researchers, especially anthropologists, who study culture. Anthropologists now often go beyond the anthropology dictum "to not change the culture that you are studying." They may act as a change agent. Anthropologists and other qualitative scholars can suggest how to use culture for more effective HIV/AIDS interventions.

Qualitative research, like quantitative research, has its limitations. It runs the risk of researcher bias; that is, a person researching sexual behavior may encounter behaviors that are personally distasteful. Researchers may also be tempted to generalize from qualitative research.

Ideally, future research on HIV/AIDS behavior should combine quantitative and qualitative methods in a triangulation approach, so as to gain the benefits of both.

Participatory Evaluation

Most HIV intervention studies conducted in the 1980s and early 1990s did little to involve community members in designing local interventions, such as by eliciting information about community norms, social perceptions, and so forth (Fisher & Fisher, 1992). The community was seldom involved in evaluating these intervention programs. Brazilian educator Paulo Freire (1970, p. 73), a champion of participatory approaches, noted: "Any situation in which some men prevent others from engaging in the process of inquiry is one of violence. To alienate men from their own decision-making is to change them into objects."

Participatory evaluation involves building a community's capacity to track the progress of its own social change. These research methods can be used in designing, monitoring, and evaluating HIV/AIDS intervention programs. Participatory research is primarily community-based and is devoted to engaging local people in planning their own change processes (Jacobson, 1993). Local self-reflection and education facilitate an action orientation toward social change.

Participatory research regards traditional, indigenous, and local knowledge as being of primary importance. Participatory research methods include participatory rural appraisal (PRA), rapid rural appraisal (RRA), participatory action research, and action research. Participatory research involves interactive learning instead of expert-dominated social research (Jacobson, 1993). Essentially, the audience for communication interventions is involved in designing and conducting the research. On the ground, participatory facilitators use a variety of approaches, tools, and methods to gather information about the community and its problems, and to work closely with community members to prioritize problems and solutions.

Using Participatory Tools in Uganda[4]

Rakai AIDS Information Network (RAIN), a Ugandan NGO, designed several participatory tools to gather data about a community in order to prioritize community problems, and to generate a community action plan. The goal of RAIN is to reduce the rate of HIV infection in Rakai district. Managed by health care providers, health educators, counselors, and trainers from Uganda's Rakai District, RAIN's strategy is to provide integrated AIDS prevention interventions in a community-based health care framework. Because of its strong emphasis on community participation, RAIN facilitated participatory learning and action (PLA) workshops in two rural areas with high HIV prevalence. The workshops helped community members assess factors that put them at risk for HIV infection. Community members from several villages participated.

The first PLA activity was mapping. The participants divided themselves into groups by village, and each group drew a map of its village on the ground, using locally available materials (such as beans, corn, and stones). The participants drew physical landmarks, such as hills, swamps, and roads, and then added social markers such as homes, churches, schools, and farms (Plate 8.1). Participants identified the number, age, and sex of inhabitants, and the number of deaths that had occurred in each house during the previous year. The PLA facilitators asked community members how many of the deaths had been the result of AIDS, but the

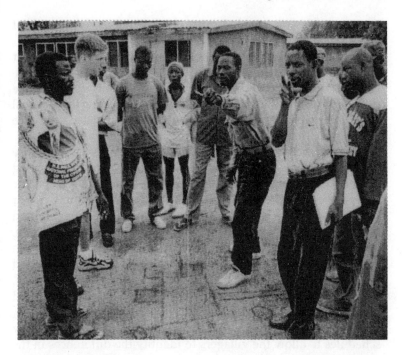

Plate 8.1   Villagers Drawing a Map of their Local Surroundings on the
Ground in Implementing a Participatory Action Research Project

Participatory research is primarily community-based and is devoted to
engaging local people in planning their own change processes.

Source: United Nations.

villagers did not want to reveal this information because of the
stigma associated with the disease.

The village maps were transferred to paper, and then presented
to the community at large. By identifying the number of deaths in the
past 12 months, participants realized that there had been at least one
death in each home. Although the causes of death were not identified,
participants knew that it was often AIDS. The number of deaths
helped the participants realize how widespread AIDS was in their
community. The epidemic threatened the community's very survival.

Next, participants identified specific locations where they might
be at risk of HIV infection. For example, they identified bars where
men met casual sex partners. They also identified isolated areas,

such as wells and wooded lots, where women were at risk of being raped.

After mapping, community members created a seasonal calendar on the ground in order to examine the patterns of various diseases. For each of the 12 months of the year, participants identified the prevalence of malaria and diarrhea. After transferring the seasonal calendar to paper, some educated participants related the occurrence of the two diseases to the occurrence of rain or sunshine.

Many participants were surprised by this relationship, because they had previously associated malaria and diarrhea with eating certain foods (maize and mangoes) that were available at specific times of the year. The PLA facilitator asked the participants whether HIV had a transmission season. Surprisingly, the villagers said that HIV transmission was highest during the harvest season (June, July, and August), when men had more money. The men could then drink more alcohol and pay for casual sex. Villagers also pointed out that HIV transmission was higher in December and in March, when men sold their stored crops to prepare for the Christmas and Easter holidays.

The final exercise involved the creation of 24-hour daily schedules to allow the villagers to identify the differences in the amount of work performed by men and women, and to identify leisure time activities that led to risky behaviors. The men and women conducted the exercise separately, and members of each group discussed what they did for each hour of the day. The exercise revealed that women engaged in many more activities than men during the day, and that men had more leisure time than women. The exercise also revealed that women were frequently asked by their husbands to have sex (sometimes as many as three times a day), and that women were often too tired to comply. Because of their extra leisure time and their tired wives, many men took on additional sexual partners. Both sexes realized that this behavior put men and their wives at risk for contracting HIV.

After completing each of these research activities — mapping, seasonal calendars, and daily schedules — participants were asked to think of solutions to the problems that were uncovered. After the mapping activity, participants realized that men were at risk of contracting HIV at bars (where they picked up casual sex partners), and that women were at risk of being raped in certain isolated places. As solutions, the men proposed that all drinking be done before sunset, and that the men come home early in the evening. To protect themselves from attack, the women decided to go in groups to collect firewood and water; and some men insisted that they accompany their wives.

It became evident that HIV transmission was highest at the times of year when men had the most disposable income. The RAIN staff decided to increase its condom distribution efforts and health education activities during these months. Women also realized that they needed to protect themselves particularly during the harvest season, and that they needed to encourage their husbands to take extra precautions during this period.

Creation of the 24-hour daily schedules led villagers to propose that husbands and wives should together decide how to share the workload better. They realized that this change would make women less tired and keep the men more occupied.

The Rakai project in Uganda shows how participation in the research process led people in the villages to greater self-awareness of their HIV/AIDS situation, aiding the identification of culturally appropriate solutions. Participatory research can be empowering for the local community.

Harvesting Questions

During our 2001 visit to Kenya, we met with officials of the Program for Appropriate Technology in Health (PATH) who run a highly participatory program on youth sexuality and HIV/AIDS prevention. In youth meetings, PATH facilitators consciously provoke questions, as opposed to providing answers (Gopinath, 2000). Their premise is that youth are more likely to "own" the answers, if *they* ask the questions. The nature of the questions asked provides clues about the knowledge, attitudes, and behaviors of the youth with respect to HIV/AIDS. Once the youths' "continuum of inquiry" is mapped, interventions can be tailored accordingly (personal interview, Michelle Folsom, 19 June 2001).

In Kenya, PATH is in the participatory business of provoking and harvesting questions!

Media Monitoring of AIDS

Why did Legionnaires' Disease, which claimed some 40 lives in the U.S. in the 1980s, get front-page news coverage, while the issue of AIDS languished with very little coverage for four years? Can the media be proactively monitored to influence the agenda-setting process for HIV/AIDS in a country?

During our March 2001 visit to Brazil, we met with ANDI, an organization that proactively monitors media coverage of children, with a special emphasis on HIV/AIDS. To gauge how HIV/AIDS is covered, ANDI, whose logo is a little bird (Plate 8.2), regularly content analyzes some 40 Brazilian magazines and newspapers. A report is then published which details what the media *are* doing with respect to HIV/AIDS, what the media are *not* doing, and what the media *should* be doing. Next, ANDI conducts training sessions for journalists on AIDS reporting, and provides them with a manual, *Os Jovens na midia o desafio de AIDS*, which includes contact information for HIV/AIDS officials at the federal, state, and municipal levels, plus a list of NGOs working in this field. Reporters are trained to compassionately report on PWAs, stimulate public debate, and reduce stigma and homophobia.

In this way, ANDI has created a cadre of 200 child-friendly journalists in Brazil who regularly report on children's issues in an accurate and compassionate manner (personal interview, Geraldinho Veira, executive director of ANDI, 14 March 2001). Cynthia Garda, a child-friendly journalist (an honor bestowed on her by ANDI), recalls how she went about doing her first story on AIDS orphans in Brazil: "When I got in touch with ANDI; they told me which NGOs and government offices to possibly contact in the local area. . . . They also made available to me, through their clipping service, all previous articles published in Brazil on AIDS orphans" (personal interview, 15 March 2001). Garda also told us how ANDI helped change the face of AIDS in the Brazilian media: "Previously HIV-positive children were not shown in Brazilian newspapers. Their faces were hidden or covered. And yesterday, there were six smiling children on the cover page of the national newspaper, and the headline said 'We are positive.'"

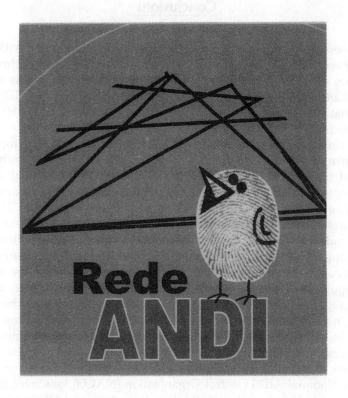

Plate 8.2   The Logo of ANDI, a Brazilian Organization that Monitors Media Coverage of Children, Including HIV/AIDS

The ANDI logo is a little bird, formed out of a thumbprint, which is appropriate, given that ANDI analyzes media content in Brazil and advocates children's and HIV/AIDS issues.

Source: ANDI.

Media coverage of children and HIV/AIDS is monitored by ANDI on a regular basis, so that it can track the quantitative and qualitative changes in AIDS reporting in Brazil. By feeding back these results to journalists, and training them in accurate HIV/AIDS reporting, ANDI helps to reframe the public and policy debate about the epidemic in Brazil.

Conclusions

Assessing the impacts of communication programs in HIV/AIDS prevention, care, and support is often a complicated task. How does one compute the impact of communication programs in enhancing the quality of life of individuals afflicted by HIV/AIDS? What are the best measures of program effects in preventing HIV infection?

Unfortunately, evaluation of HIV/AIDS programs is often top-down, in which participants are seen mainly as objects of study, and not as participants who can contribute to the evaluation process (Gumucio, 2001; Jacobson, 1993; Servaes, 1999). Quantitative studies are emphasized over qualitative insights. The objectives of such evaluations usually serve donor and institutional agendas, but may not benefit the people's agenda. Longitudinal, people-centered, qualitative methods and social change measures (in contrast to individual behavioral change measures) have an important place in HIV/AIDS research, given the centrality of quality-of-life measures for individuals, families, and communities.

In an earlier chapter, we saw how the Healthy Highways Project in India faced initial difficulties, but with pre-testing and mid-course corrections the project officials and evaluators learned to think like truck drivers. Then the project got back on course. Next, the National AIDS Control Organization (NACO) took over the project and appropriated it institutionally to state-level AIDS control societies. The project then petered out, a victim of institutional agendas. In this ownership change, no one seemed to be concerned about what was best for the truck drivers.

Monitoring and evaluation of HIV/AIDS intervention programs should be guided by the following principles:

1. Interventions should be both internally and externally evaluated, utilizing multiple methods that are both quantitative and qualitative.
2. Community members should be actively involved in assessing what kind of impact the HIV/AIDS intervention has had on the quality of community life. Communities should be encouraged to propose their own indicators of social change.

3. Evaluation research should be conducted before, during, and after the period of operation of a communication intervention for HIV prevention.
4. Skills in conducting evaluations of communication programs need to be strengthened so that the evaluations are useful, timely, relevant, and cost-effective. The key is to have a research agenda that is not just pluralistic, but is also practical and affordable. As a rough rule of thumb, many health programs devote 10 percent of their total budget to evaluation research.
5. Evaluation should serve evidence-based advocacy. Evaluation should articulate what role communication programs can play in promoting HIV/AIDS policies.

Notes

1. *Twende na Wakati* may not be the first entertainment-education project to include a control group in its research design: A JHU/CCP radio soap opera in The Gambia, *Fakube Jarra*, included a control group. However, the eight types of data gathered for *Twende na Wakati* (including data from a control group) make it an unusually rigorous research evaluation of the effects of entertainment-education.
2. This self-report by the 1995 respondents, that 82 percent had adopted HIV prevention because of listening to *Twende na Wakati*, is undoubtedly an overestimate, as was determined when this response was cross-classified with answers to another question in the survey interview (in which we also asked which specific method of HIV prevention the respondent had adopted).
3. The values grid that guided the design of *Twende na Wakati* included this element: "It is good that people are educated to understand that mosquitoes cannot spread AIDS. The AIDS virus cannot survive in mosquitoes."
4. This material draws upon Ssembatya et al. (1995, cited in de Negri et al., 1998).

9

Lessons Learned about Combating HIV/AIDS

■

A world that spent an estimated $500 billion to tackle the elusive Y2K bug on our computers must be able to do more to tackle a tragedy [AIDS] that has already blighted hundreds of millions of lives.

> Mark Malloch Brown, administrator of the
> United Nations Development Program (2001,
> p. 4).

AIDS Is Everybody's Business.

> Tag-line on an ACT UP poster, 1990.

What is the worst plague that the human race has ever experienced? One might think of the Black Death (bubonic plague) of the Middle Ages that wiped out 25 million people, one-third of Europe's population, between 1347 and 1352. In the next 150 years, the bubonic plague killed another 40 million people as it spread across the globe (DeNoon, 2002).

Reported first in China in the 1330s, the Black Death (which caused black spots on the skin and "buboes" or swellings of the lymph nodes) arrived in Europe on Italian merchant ships that docked in Sicily after conducting trade in China. Then it spread like wildfire in Europe and western Asia, decimating families, communities, and nations. The terrified residents of Europe believed the Black Death was a scourge from God. Individuals suspected of having the plague were ostracized, isolated, and stigmatized.

In the past two decades, AIDS has killed 25 million people, and another 40 million carry the virus, an almost certain death sentence for the 38 million who cannot afford anti-retroviral drugs. The Black Death occurred 700 years ago, when science as we know it today was just beginning (Lamptey, 2002). Despite the power of science today in solving many social problems, the AIDS epidemic continues to escalate.

Here we review what we have learned about the worldwide AIDS epidemic in the past 20 years, as we look toward an improved future.

Looking Backward

For 20 years, the world has been fighting the AIDS epidemic in a series of predominantly losing battles. Each year, more people become HIV-infected, and more die from AIDS in more countries. The two largest countries in the world in terms of population were spared from the epidemic until recent years. But now HIV/AIDS is spreading rapidly in India, and the epidemic is making inroads in China. Former Soviet republics, also relatively late in encountering AIDS, represent present-day hotspots for HIV infection.

A UNAIDS map of the world shows the severity of the epidemic in different colors, with red indicating nations in which more than 20 percent of the adult population is HIV-infected. In Africa, some 18 nations south of the Equator (which passes through Kenya) are colored red, indicating that HIV/AIDS is spreading rapidly through the general population. Today, this vast area of Sub-Saharan Africa is the worldwide center of the epidemic (Beresford, 2001). But the world center will soon shift to India, which, the World Bank predicts, will have 20 million HIV-positive people by 2005 (Ramasundaram, 2002).

Only five developing nations have been able to control the epidemic: Thailand, Uganda, Senegal, Cambodia, and, through a unique approach centering on anti-retrovirals, Brazil. These five countries were each able to halt the increasing rate of HIV infection.

The case of Thailand is illustrative. After several years of denial and do-nothing, the Thai government finally placed a high priority on controlling HIV/AIDS in 1991–92. The highest official in the nation led the AIDS control program, lending political will to the battle. HIV prevention thus became the concern of every government official. Targeted intervention programs such as the 100 Percent Condom Program were directed to high-risk populations like commercial sex workers, in an attempt to keep the epidemic from spreading further into the general population. In a relatively short time, the galloping rate of HIV infection plateaued, and Thailand's AIDS control program was deemed a success. Nevertheless, about one million Thais had been infected, and 55,000 of these individuals are dying every year. So this "success" came at a high cost in terms of human life. The main accomplishment of the Thai AIDS control program was to blunt the further spread of the epidemic. Can other developing nations learn useful lessons from Thailand's successful AIDS control program, and those of other "success" nations?

The HIV/AIDS epidemic today is predominantly a developing country phenomenon, with 95 percent of the 14,000 new HIV infections per day occurring in developing nations. Further, the sections of the population hardest hit by the epidemic within every country are the poorest people, those living in rural villages and urban slums (Mann & Tarantola, 1998). The high expectations from anti-retroviral drug therapies, when they were announced in 1996, have not been fulfilled, mainly for economic reasons. Even though the cost per person per year dropped tremendously during 2001, the price of the drugs ($350 per year) is still completely unaffordable for most people living with HIV/AIDS.

Despite their obvious benefits, anti-retrovirals are a harsh therapy, with powerful side-effects that make the drugs inappropriate for 20 to 30 percent of people living with HIV/AIDS. It is difficult for health providers to administer the anti-retrovirals correctly, as they involve a complicated regimen. In every country, individuals are turning to traditional herbal therapies, and these treatments may prove to be helpful to people living with HIV/AIDS. Perhaps the cost of the triple cocktail will drop to such a level that more developing nations will be able to provide them to those living with HIV/AIDS. But for tens of millions of poor people in developing countries of Asia, Africa, and Latin America, anti-retrovirals will forever be out of reach. As one HIV program manager in Brazil noted somberly: "Even if the cure for HIV/AIDS was a glass of clean drinking water, 75 percent of the individuals in developing countries would not have access to it."

Ignoring Culture

Everywhere in the world, cultural variables are important in understanding the AIDS epidemic. Culture explains, in part, why the disease is so much worse in certain nations than in others. Culture can be a barrier or a facilitator in controlling the epidemic. Insufficient attention has been paid to cultural factors in the spread of HIV infection and in its control, although UNAIDS in recent years has focused on cultural, spiritual, and other contextual factors in HIV prevention. When culture is the focus, it is often for its limitations but almost never for its strengths in encouraging HIV prevention (Airhihenbuwa, 1995).

A basic problem with national AIDS control programs is that the epidemic has been overdefined as a biomedical problem. Consequently, adequate attention has not been given to culturally anchored approaches to behavior change. This situation seems strange for a disease without a medical cure. The possibility of finding an AIDS vaccine in the foreseeable future, say a decade, seems remote. Such a vaccine, if it is developed, will probably be a therapy that lowers viral loads, similar to the present anti-retroviral drugs, but without the need for an individual to take 35 pills per day for the rest of his or her life. HIV/AIDS is not a medical problem; it is a behavioral change problem, as Mechai recognized in the successful Thai program that he led a decade ago. As long as the epidemic is mentally constructed as a biomedical problem, cultural factors will be shortchanged.

Islamic countries are generally absent from the list of developing nations plagued by the AIDS epidemic. Noteworthy because of their absence from the UNAIDS map of high-prevalence countries is a large group of countries, from Malaysia to Bangladesh and Pakistan, to Iran, across the Middle East, to North Africa. What, if any, is the apparent connection between Islamic religion, sexual behavior, and HIV/AIDS? Is AIDS largely under-diagnosed and unreported in Islamic countries? For instance, Yemen, a Middle Eastern country of 19 million people, officially reported only 1,000

HIV-positive cases. However, the World Health Organization estimates that for each reported case, at least 15 are not reported (Al-Qadhi, 2001). Yemen may be squandering the short window of opportunity in which to check the disease, before it spreads into the general population. Several nations in Sub-Saharan Africa, like Tanzania and Uganda, have considerable Islamic populations. Here, however, religion does not seem to be related to lower levels of HIV infection.

In addition to the puzzle of low rates of infection in almost all Islamic nations, some neighboring pairs of countries in the world have strikingly different experiences with the epidemic. For instance, Nicaragua had only 700 reported cases of HIV/AIDS in 2002. Meanwhile, its next-door neighbor, Honduras, had the highest rate of HIV/AIDS in Central America. How can this stark difference be explained? Not by religious contrast, as both nations are Catholic. Perhaps cultural and political factors are involved. Honduras does not yet perceive that the epidemic represents a real emergency, so little is being done to control the further spread of HIV/AIDS.

One instance of how culture limits effective HIV interventions in many nations is provided by widespread restrictions on needle exchange programs, which scientific evaluations show can be highly effective in limiting infection among injecting drug users. Many governments completely prohibit such needle exchange programs, on the mistaken assumption that providing clean needles encourages drug use. Here, cultural and political concerns block needle exchange programs.

Slow Political Action

Almost all countries have been slow in taking political action to stem the tide of HIV/AIDS. *One of the most important lessons of the past two decades has been the need for early and sustained political action to tackle AIDS head-on, before it begins to rage unchecked in the general population.*

In 2002, Botswana had the highest HIV seroprevalence levels of all nations: Thirty-eight of every 100 adults in this diamond-rich southern African country were HIV-positive (Stucky, 2001). A 15-year-old in Botswana has a one in two chance of dying of AIDS. Almost no family in Botswana is unaffected by AIDS. In 2002,

Botswana's president Festus G. Mogae led the charge on HIV/AIDS, chairing all meetings of the National AIDS Council, which coordinates a multi-sectoral and multi-ministerial approach to HIV/AIDS. While Mogae's political patronage of HIV/AIDS interventions is laudatory, it is too late for the half a million adults in Botswana who have died of AIDS or are now living with the virus. Similarly, in 2001, President Jean-Bertrand Aristide of Haiti launched the 2001–2006 National Strategic Plan with a speech that declared HIV/AIDS as "Public enemy number one" (quoted in Chantal, 2001, p. 17). While Aristide's political commitment to HIV/AIDS is commendable, it has come too late for over 300,000 Haitians who have died of AIDS over the past two decades, more than 160,000 children who are AIDS orphans, and the 260,000 Haitians who are currently living with HIV/AIDS. Mogae and Aristide are brave, committed national leaders. But many of their people's lives would have been saved had their actions, and the actions of their predecessors, been more timely. Each hour that passes can be expensive in the case of national HIV/AIDS prevention policies and programs.

One of the most important, yet unanswered, questions about HIV/AIDS in the past 20 years has been: *How can we produce the political action necessary to implement early and sustained HIV intervention programs?* Unfortunately, while tens of millions of dollars are spent studying the efficacy of biomedical interventions, little or no research is being conducted to answer this fundamental question (Bolton, 1995).

Political action for HIV/AIDS, or the lack of it, needs to be deconstructed in light of other political choices facing policy-makers. President George W. Bush plans to spend hundreds of billions of dollars on a missile defense shield to protect the United States from rogue nations. But when it came to developing a global shield against a rogue disease, the U.S. government contributed a paltry $200 million to the Global AIDS Fund, demonstrating the politicization of strategic priorities. Bono, the lead singer of U-2, a popular band from Ireland, acted as a one-man lobby against President Bush in 2002. One result was a much-expanded U.S. budget ($500 million) for HIV/AIDS prevention. Former U.S. President Jimmy Carter and Bill Gates, Sr., President of the William and Melinda Gates Foundation, toured Africa together in 2002 in order to identify needs for expanded funding of HIV/AIDS programs. So various celebrities are pitching in, to push for greater funding for HIV/AIDS interventions, including Brazilian soccer star, Ronaldo (Plate 9.1).

One of the main lessons, emphasized in the chapters of this book, is the importance of political will in controlling the epidemic. A national government is uniquely capable of mounting a program to deal effectively with HIV/AIDS in a developing nation. *If the issue of HIV/AIDS rises in the agenda-setting process to a high priority on the national agenda, and if real political commitment is mustered, the epidemic can be controlled.* That is the hopeful message of this book. Unfortunately, adequate political will has only been expressed in five developing nations thus far.

When the Lion Comes, Shout!

Yoweri Museveni, president of Uganda since 1986, has personally led Uganda's war against AIDS, since his first day in office (Madraa & Ruranga-Rubaramira, 1998). At a 2001 meeting of African heads of state to discuss the role of political leadership in combating AIDS, Museveni noted: "When a lion comes to the village, you don't make a small alarm. You make a very loud one. When I knew of AIDS, I said we must shout and shout and shout and shout" (quoted in Mutume, 2001, p. 21).

Born into a family of cattle-keepers in Ankole, western Uganda, Museveni has a long-standing record of fighting political and social injustices. When military dictator Idi Amin Dada came to power in Uganda in 1971, Museveni established the Front for National Salvation, a rebel group that, backed by Tanzania, ousted Amin. A decade later, Museveni's National Resistance Army (NRA), a guerilla rebel force, fought for five years to oust the oppressive regimes of Milton Obote and Tito Okello, paving the way for his rise to political power. During this guerilla struggle, hundreds of soldiers in Museveni's army succumbed to AIDS, including several close friends. Museveni vowed to "shout." The lion was decimating his stock.

Museveni believes that the top national leadership needs to confront AIDS each day at every opportunity. Anything less is unpardonable. As Museveni told his fellow African leaders: "When a district health officer comes to address a village meeting, 20 people show up. When Museveni addresses a rally, 20,000 show up. That's the time to pass the AIDS message. The top leadership needs to supervise the AIDS war" (quoted in Mutume, 2001, p. 21).

Museveni inspired several African leaders to speak out against AIDS. Former Ghanaian President Jerry Rawlings now serves as the United Nations's Eminent Campaigner for AIDS. Rawlings's successor, John Kufour, talked passionately about Ghana's tryst with AIDS during his 2002 New Year's address to the nation.

Lack of Business Involvement

Recently, Population Communications International approached Mexican business corporations about sponsoring *Ombligos al Sol* (Bellybuttons to the Sun), an entertainment-education program about HIV/AIDS, teenage pregnancy, and domestic values targeted to youth. The Mexican business leaders declined because, they said, their companies wanted to be associated with happiness and the good life, not with a social problem like the AIDS epidemic, which they perceived in a very negative light.

Business leaders throughout the world have been apathetic about HIV/AIDS, despite the devastation that the epidemic is wreaking in workplaces through absenteeism, loss of productivity, and rising health care costs. Both government and business, working in unison, are needed to confront the pandemic. Global businesses, barring certain exceptions, have either maintained silence on HIV/AIDS, or have been tightwads in providing resources for HIV interventions. The CDC sought to involve private U.S. corporations in a Business Responds to AIDS Program in the mid-1990s. Most companies did not respond.

When we visited Brazil in March 2001, we saw hundreds of ads on public buses promoting Johnson & Johnson's Jonex condoms. Johnson & Johnson timed its condom billboard campaign with the

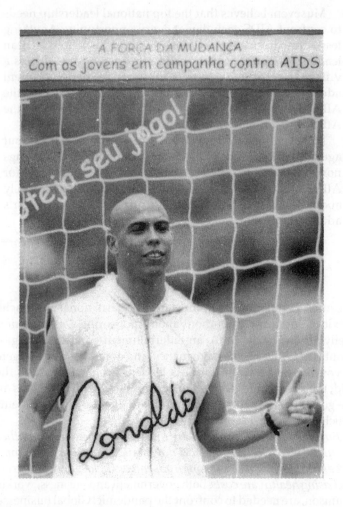

A FORÇA DA MUDANÇA
Com os jovens em campanha contra AIDS

oteja seu jogo!

Ronaldo

Plate 9.1 Brazilian Soccer Star Ronaldo on a UNAIDS Poster Urging HIV Prevention among the Youth

Ronaldo, an international sports celebrity, serves as UNDP's Goodwill Ambassador on Poverty. In a recent UNDP publication, Ronaldo (2001, p. 26) noted: "As a soccer player, I have the duty to tell my fans to protect themselves. As a young person, I can speak on the issue of HIV/AIDS to my generation. As a father, it is my duty to be prepared to talk about AIDS with my children."

Source: United Nations.

2001 Carnival celebrations, when high-risk sexual activity peaks in Brazil. Volkswagen de Brazil implemented a comprehensive HIV prevention, training, and treatment program for its workers that led to a 90 percent reduction in hospitalizations of its employees, boosting employee morale and productivity. Coca-Cola, the largest private sector employer in Africa with 100,000 employees, recently launched several new HIV/AIDS prevention projects, some in cooperation with UNAIDS (M. Brown, 2001). Coca-Cola's vast distribution network for soft drinks could easily transport condoms and AIDS drugs to rural and remote corners of the world. As the AIDS epidemic continues to wipe out employees and customers, business leaders might increasingly realize the wisdom of keeping their employees healthy and their markets alive (Neary, 2001). Nevertheless, the number of corporations actively involved in HIV prevention is discouragingly small. But there are bright spots.

William Roedy, president of Music Television (MTV) Networks International, has been perhaps the most strident business advocate for controlling HIV/AIDS. Roedy, who chaired the Global Business Council on AIDS, knows, perhaps better than any other business leader, the mindsets of sexually active youth worldwide. Roedy offers MTV, which reaches a global audience of one billion youth, as a vehicle for educating them through its entertaining broadcasts, thus reducing HIV prevalence and the accompanying denial, apathy, and stigma surrounding AIDS.

Erotica, MTV Brazil's most popular program, a one-hour, weekly, youth call-in show, daringly addresses questions about sex and HIV/AIDS. Hosted by a 36-year-old medical doctor, Jairo Bouer, *Erotica* is in its fourth year of broadcasting, and has brought sexuality issues "out of the closet" (personal interview, Eliane Izolan, 13 March 2001). Several years ago, Dr. Bouer, who is now a celebrity in Brazil (*Playboy* carried a four-page story on Bouer in a recent issue), wrote a syndicated column in a leading Brazilian newspaper in which such hitherto sensitive topics as masturbation, homosexuality, and drug use were discussed. Dr. Bouer's youth columns were adapted by MTV into a television format, in recognition that he provided young people with straight talk in a language they could understand. Bouer's website, www.caliente.com.br (*caliente* means "hot" in Portuguese), gets several thousand hits per day.

Stigma

Stigma makes the consequences of the AIDS epidemic much worse than they would otherwise be. India is one nation in which stigma is particularly strong. In our five-nation study, we learned of individuals who had been killed by a mob when it became known, or suspected, that they were HIV-positive. In each country, we learned of many individuals who had killed themselves when they learned they were seropositive. Communication interventions can decrease the stigma with which the disease is perceived. In some countries, like Thailand, for example, people living with HIV/AIDS (PWAs) organized for social change so as to combat stigma. When banded together in local groups and organized in a national association, empowered PWAs can bring about social changes that would be impossible for separate individuals to accomplish. Such social organizing strategies, along with medical drugs and doctors, can be important resources in fighting HIV/AIDS. Decreasing stigma is almost entirely a matter of organizing and communicating. Like any deep-seated prejudice, the stigma of HIV/AIDS is difficult to overcome, at least in the short range. Years of effort will be required.

Stigma blocks the effectiveness of many HIV intervention programs. For example, many Indians are reluctant to be tested for HIV because they so fear the stigma attached to being seropositive. A variety of communication strategies are being used to fight the stigma of HIV/AIDS: symbols (like the red ribbon), culturally appropriate humor, the support of religious leaders, safe and comfortable spaces (including the virtual space provided by anonymous telephone hotlines), memory boxes, and the AIDS memorial quilt. *Much greater effort should be made to decrease the stigma of HIV/AIDS throughout the world.* It will not be an easy battle.

Looking Forward

What would be needed to control the AIDS epidemic in the developing world? Led by Secretary General Kofi Annan, the United Nations established the AIDS Global Fund in April 2002, calling for $7 to 10 billion annually (for at least 10 years) to fight the epidemic.

To date, this objective has not been achieved. Much greater resources are needed to stem the tide of HIV, and these resources must also be used more strategically.

Communication Strategy

The world needs more effective HIV prevention programs. Our review of selected prevention programs (Chapter 4) in the present book concluded that even the most effective interventions leave much to be desired in achieving their goal of preventing the spread of HIV from specialized groups into the general population. What is wrong here?

HIV prevention programs lack adequate resources, so they can seldom be scaled up to make a strong impact. Further, *HIV prevention programs in developing nations seldom make very effective use of communication strategies.* As a consequence, the resources available for HIV prevention are not used judiciously. Even when such strategies as opinion leadership (based on diffusion of innovation theory) or entertainment-education (based on social learning theory) are utilized, the translation from theory into practice is sometimes flawed, resulting in interventions that are not always effective. But the main problem here is that HIV prevention programs are not guided by communication strategies.

Behavior change communication for HIV prevention is more effective when it is based upon a multidisciplinary approach that draws upon social psychology, anthropology, epidemiology, sociology, and public health, as well as communication. Seldom can any one of these disciplines alone provide the basis for an effective intervention program. So it is no wonder that biomedically dominated programs often fail. These interventions are just too narrow in their approach.

The epidemic spreads mainly through sexual relationships, which implies that feelings of romance and desire are usually involved. Transmission of the virus is not just a rational process in which an individual's knowledge of consequences guides that individual's actions. The role of emotions in HIV prevention is suggested by an observer of the audience for a theater play written and performed by students in a U.S. high school:

> In the course of the performance, the audience usually gets quieter and quieter. Not only do they laugh at jokes, many kids in the audience are crying. In the end, many want more information. Teachers have also told us that the kids do not stop talking about the play for weeks (Glick et al., 2002).

Given that HIV prevention involves emotions as well as knowledge, entertainment-education interventions would seem to be particularly appropriate. Coupled with other campaign activities, many E-E interventions have had strong effects in motivating preventive action. *Entertainment-education achieves its main effects by stimulating peer communication about HIV prevention.* For example, many individuals who adopted condoms, or who decreased their number of sexual partners in Tanzania in the 1990s, did so not only as the result of direct exposure to the entertainment-education radio soap opera *Twende na Wakati* (Let's Go with the Times), but also as a result of the peer communication that this intervention stimulated (Rogers et al., 1999; Vaughan, Rogers et al., 2000).

Many past E-E programs have been nationwide in scope. We feel that "bicycle-type" E-E interventions, as well as the "Cadillac-style" programs of the past, are needed. An example is the street theater by Nalamdana (see Chapter 7) in Tamil Nadu state in South India. Nalamdana's village presentations on HIV/AIDS prevention, night after night, each to an audience of several thousand, add up to millions of people. Their ever-changing, flexible, and localized entertainment-education street theater appeals to their audiences' emotions, while also conveying knowledge about the virus's transmission. The world needs many Nalamdanas.

Sometimes, an entertainment-education intervention stimulates collective action by a set of individuals. For example, this occurred in an episode of *Soul City* in which the neighbors of a battered woman gathered around the couple's home to bang pots and pans in unison to indicate their displeasure with the husband's behavior. As a result, the police arrived to take the husband away to jail. One effect of this *Soul City* episode was that pot-banging became a technique through which neighbors could oppose wife-beating in

South Africa. The vulnerability of individuals who are affected or afflicted by HIV/AIDS can be addressed through the solidarity of their community. The entertainment-education strategy can encourage collective efficacy to combat the epidemic. Here the system is activated, going beyond just individual action.

The epidemic begins in every developing nation in one or more high-risk populations, such as commercial sex workers, injecting drug users, or gay men. These high-risk audiences may be concentrated in a geographical space in an urban center. Examples are red-light districts like Patpong in Bangkok, Sonagachi in Kolkata, and Kamathipura in Mumbai. HIV prevention interventions are targeted to these high-risk populations in the initial era of the epidemic in a country in order to prevent HIV infection from spreading through interpersonal sexual networks to the general population. We argued in this book that *HIV spreads mainly through sexual networks, so HIV prevention programs should also utilize an interpersonal network approach.*

The relatively more effective of these targeted programs use peer educators (who are often selected from among opinion leaders) with commercial sex workers (Jha et al., 2001). The peer educators are themselves experienced CSWs, and are thus homophilous with their targeted audience individuals. When such peer education programs also provide free or subsidized condoms, health clinic services, and other needed resources, as the intervention in Kolkata does, the rate of HIV infection can be restricted to a small percentage (see Chapter 4). However, most intervention programs with high-risk populations did not begin soon enough, or lacked adequate resources, or were not implemented effectively. The epidemic then spreads into the general population, and poses a major threat to everyone in the society. One problem is that most interventions with high-risk populations are based on intuition, rather than on behavior change communication theories. When based on sound theories and grounded in the local sociocultural context, targeted interventions can be effective, as the experience of the STOP AIDS program in San Francisco suggests.

The rise of the Internet has opened up new possibilities for HIV/AIDS intervention programs, but this potential has not been fully exploited. A soap opera on the Internet was utilized to target older Hispanic women in the United States for mammography screening (Jibaja et al., 2000). Each woman's stage-of-change was determined, and then an appropriate message about mammography screening was delivered to her. Such tailoring through the Internet can be used for HIV prevention. One might expect that older Hispanic women in the United States would be unlikely to have access to the Internet. On the contrary, five million Spanish-speaking individuals (many of them older Hispanic women) sent e-mail messages to television soap opera characters in the previous year, encouraged by Univisión, the main Spanish-language television network in the United States. As the Internet continues to diffuse in developing nations, especially in the better-off countries of Asia, its potential for HIV prevention will become more important.

The Internet can also be used to advocate policy. For example, in 2000–01, Doctors Without Borders (MSF) organized a worldwide campaign for lower-priced anti-retrovirals via e-mail.

PWA Power

Over the long term, the empowerment of PWAs can change the face of efforts to fight the AIDS epidemic. For example, the coordinator of Colombia's national AIDS program in the national ministry of health is a medical doctor who is HIV-positive! His self-disclosure a few years ago helped decrease stigma in Colombia. Many, many of the volunteer leaders in NGOs involved in prevention or treatment of PWAs are themselves PWAs. Their seropositive status accords them a natural credibility that they could not have earned in any other way. When one of the authors (Rogers) was investigating the relative effectiveness of HIV/AIDS prevention programs in San Francisco in the early 1990s, a standard greeting from the director of a program was: "Hi, my name is Ralph. I am positive." Thus, an individual's HIV status was a crucial part of his/her identity. Sadly, almost all of the program officials interviewed by Rogers in 1993–95 are no longer with us.

Another fundamental question for PWAs, HIV/AIDS program managers, and scholars, which has not been tackled systematically to date, is: *How can HIV/AIDS intervention programs capitalize more fully on the high credibility attached to PWAs regarding HIV/AIDS?* Several proposals have been made in recent years to employ people living with HIV/AIDS in a worldwide Peace Corps (an "AIDS Corps") to fight the epidemic by working in prevention, treatment, and care programs (Bolton, 1995). This approach seems eminently sensible and would end the current exploitation of PWAs by paying them for the volunteer work that they now contribute for free. Such AIDS Corps employees would be homophilous with their audiences, and would help bring seropositivity out into the open.

The third decade of the AIDS epidemic will feature the growing political power of people living with HIV/AIDS, as they continue to grow in numbers and in organization. In nations like Thailand, PWAs have already flexed their muscles to gain increased access to anti-retrovirals. In the years ahead, PWAs will not only staff HIV prevention programs, but they will also direct national AIDS control agencies.

Recognizing Heroes

In previous chapters, we described individual heroes of the worldwide war on the AIDS epidemic. People like Mechai Viravaidya, who led the 1991–92 AIDS control program in Thailand, and turned an out-of-control epidemic around, come to mind. So do people like Ms. Pimjai Intamoon of the Don Kaew Community Health Project in a village near Chiang Mai, in northern Thailand. Father Valeriano created three homes for AIDS orphans in a Saõ Paulo suburb, despite strong initial resistance from the community. S. Ramasundaram, a member of the elite Indian Administrative Service, deserves credit for leading an effective intervention program in Tamil Nadu in the 1990s, which then became the model for AIDS control in other Indian states. Dr. Yusuf Hamied, managing director of the Mumbai-based drug company Cipla, is heroic for his role in precipitating a drastic reduction in anti-retroviral drug prices in 2001.

These are but a few of the many individuals that we encountered in writing this book, who demonstrated effective leadership in fighting for HIV prevention. *Heroes of the worldwide AIDS epidemic need greater recognition, and their actions need analysis, so that their contributions can be magnified.* Certain organizations also deserve credit for crucial contributions. Doctors Without Borders is everywhere, providing prevention and treatment services, and advocating for appropriate prevention and treatment policies. In recent years, UNAIDS has sought to redefine the epidemic and the HIV prevention interventions designed to control it.

It is such individuals and organizations who have provided the needed leadership in the world's battle against HIV/AIDS, even when it has not been to their individual advantage to do so. Altruism is an important quality of those who battle the epidemic, motivated in part by the enormity of this staggering problem.

Programmatic Synergy

In the past, HIV/AIDS prevention programs were kept completely separate from those for other health issues. Each occupied an isolated corner of a national ministry of health. Thus, HIV/AIDS programs competed with family planning, with maternal and child health, and even with health programs designed to deal with malaria, tuberculosis, and other opportunistic infections caused by AIDS. Such compartmentalization is dysfunctional. Useful synergies can be achieved, such as when HIV-positive mothers are delivering babies (Rosenfield & Meyer, 2001). Programs in several countries are geared to reducing mother-to-child transmission (MTCT) by administering AZT or Nevirapine (Plate 9.2). Here is an opportunity to combine maternal and child health programs with HIV prevention. The advantages of doing so would seem obvious.

A similar opportunity exists in most countries to combine family planning programs with HIV prevention interventions. After all, both promote condom use. However, family planning and AIDS control are usually organized as two different units in a national ministry of health. They compete for funds and attention. Under these circumstances, not much collaboration occurs.

The next decade of the AIDS epidemic should see increased integration of HIV/AIDS prevention programs with other health programs, and with other development programs, in order to achieve synergies of effort.

Sorting Ethical Dilemmas

Olympic swimmer Greg Louganis announced in the mid-1990s that he had AIDS. A debate erupted as to whether all Olympic competitors should be tested for HIV, and whether Louganis should

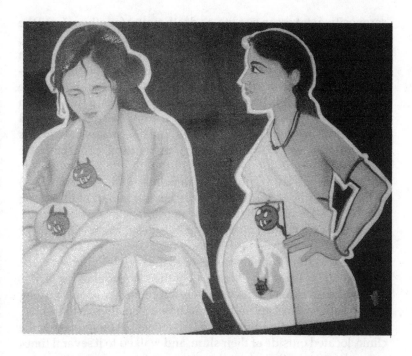

Plate 9.2   A Cloth Poster used by PSI Peer Educators to Educate Commercial Sex Workers at the Cotton Green Truck Stop in Mumbai about the Risk of Mother-to-Child HIV Transmission

Maternal and child health (MCH) programs should be integrated with HIV prevention and treatment programs by incorporating HIV testing, the use of AZT or Nevirapine at the time of delivery for HIV-positive mothers, and follow-up treatment of the mother with anti-retroviral therapy.

Source: Personal files of the authors.

have disclosed his seropositivity during the 1988 Seoul Olympic Games, when he struck his head on a diving board and received a scalp wound that required several stitches. Louganis's case illustrates the dilemma between preserving the confidentiality of an individual's HIV status versus the risk posed to other people.

More generally, the role of HIV/AIDS in sports competitions, as the case of the former basketball star Magic Johnson suggests, is far from settled. More attention must be given to clarifying the ethical dimensions of HIV/AIDS. Knowledge of an individual's seropositive status can be a life-or-death matter for others. Until the confidentiality of the results of an HIV blood test can be assured, relatively few individuals will come forward for such testing. Even if HIV testing is carried out anonymously, an individual's HIV-positive status can often be identified if anti-retroviral drugs are distributed through the public health system (as is the case in Brazil). HIV prevention programs cannot be designed and implemented without knowing which, and how many, individuals are seropositive. Without testing, prevention programs are flying blind.

Dr. Adriana Mauro Nunes (personal interview, 16 March 2001) of Doctors Without Borders in Rio de Janeiro told us of the strong anti-HIV/AIDS stigma that exists in many Brazilian *favelas* (slums). The *favelas* are located on the steep hillsides that circle the city of Rio de Janeiro. A drug lord in one *favela* demanded that a local clinic provide him with the names of all the people living with HIV in his area. He intended to force all of the PWAs out of his *favela*. We also heard about PWAs who were apprehensive about carrying their plastic sacks of anti-retrovirals home from their health clinic, for fear of being killed. Some *favela* dwellers left their drugs at the clinic, located outside of their slum, and walked to it several times every day to take their drug therapy.

In Kenya in recent years, tuberculosis has come to be perceived as an AIDS opportunistic infection by many people. Tuberculosis rates are much higher than before, due to the AIDS epidemic. The HIV/AIDS epidemic raises a host of ethical issues, including the confidentiality of individuals' seropositivity, the rights of unborn children, mandatory HIV testing, and protecting the rights of PWAs (Sweat et al., 2000). The ethical dimensions of the epidemic have scarcely been identified to date, let alone solved.

Redefining the Problem

The fight against AIDS is not just a fight against a biological virus, but a battle against bigotry, fear, denial, and ignorance. The enemy is winning in most nations. Communication strategies can help stop the epidemic, and certainly, they can slow it down. A fundamental step is to realize that the HIV/AIDS epidemic is not just a biomedical and health problem. It represents a political problem, a cultural problem, and a socioeconomic problem, one which behavior change communication can help address, and possibly solve.

One encouraging sign of the redefinition of the nature of the epidemic emerged during the 14th International AIDS Conference, held in Barcelona, Spain, on 7–12 July 2002. Past international AIDS conferences had emphasized biomedical research, with prevention and policy advocacy shoved into back rooms. The 1996 Vancouver Conference, with its theme of "One World, One Hope," focused on the announcement of the triple cocktail. The 13,000 delegates to the 2000 Durban Conference centered their attention on Brazil's daring program to provide free anti-retroviral drugs to every citizen who was HIV-positive. The biannual conferences are tremendously influential in defining the problems posed by the AIDS epidemic.

Jordi Casabona, director of the Center for Epidemiological HIV/AIDS Studies in the Catalan Health Department of Barcelona, and co-chair of the 2002 International AIDS Conference, stated that a biomedical approach was not enough to end the epidemic. The program of the Barcelona Conference focused equally on "science" and on "action." The science track included "prevention science" because, as Casabona explained, prevention studies are conducted as vigorously as clinical trials of new drugs. The "action" component of the Barcelona Conference included tracks on both intervention program evaluations and on policy advocacy. Obviously, what is really needed to change the world is an integration of biomedically based scientific findings with communication-science-based interventions and advocacy. The 2002 Barcelona Conference marked the emergence of intervention and policy from the shadows of biomedical science. Only 14 biannual international AIDS conferences were required to reach this obvious conclusion.

Once the worldwide epidemic is redefined more accurately, then its solution can be realized.

Glossary

∎

Agenda-setting is the process through which a news issue climbs to a higher priority in a system.

AIDS stands for Acquired Immune Deficiency Syndrome. It occurs when an HIV-positive individual has such lowered immune levels that he/she falls prey to a variety of opportunistic infections.

Anti-retroviral drugs combat HIV by disrupting various stages in the life cycle of the virus in the human body.

Behavior surveillance surveys measure behavior changes among targeted groups over a period of time.

A campaign is intended to generate specific outcomes or effects in a relatively large number of individuals, usually within a specific period of time and through an organized set of communication activities.

A champion is a charismatic individual who throws his/her weight behind an idea, thus helping it to gain acceptance.

Collectivistic cultures are those in which the collectivity's goals are valued over those of the individual.

Collective efficacy is the degree to which the members of a system (a community, a group, or an organization) believe they have the ability to organize and execute the actions required to produce desired attainments.

A communication strategy is a formula for behavior change, based on communication theories, that provides the basis for designing and implementing communication interventions.

Credibility is the degree to which a communication source is perceived as expert and trustworthy.

Cultural shareability of a media program is the extent to which it can appeal to heterophilous (culturally dissimilar) audience groups.

Effectiveness is the degree to which a program intervention fulfills its objectives.

Empowerment is the degree to which individuals perceive that they can control a situation.

Entertainment-education is the process of purposely designing and implementing a media message to both entertain and educate in order to increase audience members' knowledge about an educational issue, create favorable attitudes, shift social norms, and change the overt behavior of individuals and communities.

A field experiment is an experiment conducted in the real world, rather than in a laboratory, with before and after surveys utilized to measure the outcome variables.

Formative evaluation research is a type of research conducted early in a communication process so as to aid in designing messages that are relatively more effective with the intended audience.

HIV is an abbreviation for Human Immunodeficiency Virus, an organism that causes an infection that depletes white blood cells and leads to lessened immunity.

HIV sentinel surveillance (HSS) measures HIV prevalence trends over time in a sentinel site through biomedical markers, such as STD rates, percentage of HIV-positive women in antenatal clinics, and others.

Homophily is the degree to which two or more individuals who communicate are similar.

Individualistic cultures are those in which the individual's goals are valued over those of the collectivity.

Intervention refers to actions with a coherent objective to bring about behavioral change in order to produce identifiable outcomes.

The media agenda consists of the hierarchy of news issues ranked according to the amount of news coverage they receive.

Opinion leaders are individuals who are sought by others for information and advice about some topic.

Organizing for social change is a theoretical approach combining certain elements of organizational communication and development communication to understand the process through which a group of disempowered individuals gain control of their future.

Parasocial interaction is the tendency of individuals to perceive themselves as having a personal relationship with a media or public personality.

Participatory evaluation involves building the community's capacity to track the progress of its own social change.

The policy agenda is the set of issues that public officials consider as they allocate funding, pass laws, and make policies.

The public agenda is the priority that the public gives to issues that it perceives as important.

PWAs are people living with HIV or AIDS ("PWA" is the usually adopted convention, rather than the clumsier "PLWHA").

Real-world indicators are variables that measure more or less objectively the degree of severity or risk of a social problem.

Self-efficacy is the degree to which an individual believes in his/her capacity to organize and execute the actions required to manage prospective situations to produce desired attainments.

A seropositive individual is someone who has been infected by HIV and whose blood has tested positive for the antibodies to the virus or for the virus itself.

Social change is the process through which alterations take place in a system.

Social marketing is the use of strategies adapted from for-profit marketing to the non-profit marketing of condoms, oral contraceptives, oral rehydration therapy (ORT), and other means of improving health.

Stigma is prejudice and discrimination against a set of people who are regarded and treated in a negative way.

A taboo topic is one that is so sensitive that it cannot be discussed.

Targeting is the process of customizing the design and delivery of a communication program on the basis of the characteristics of an intended audience segment.

The triple cocktail is a cocktail of three anti-retroviral drugs (see also **anti-retroviral drugs**).

Uniqueness is the degree to which an audience of relatively homophilous individuals differs from the larger population of which it is a part.

References

■

Adam, Barry D. (1997). Mobilizing around AIDS: Sites of struggle in the formation of AIDS subjects. In Martine Levine, Peter M. Nardi, and John H. Gagnon (eds.), *In changing times: Gay men and lesbians encounter HIV/AIDS* (pp. 23-38). Chicago: University of Chicago Press.

Adelman, Mara B. (1992). Healthy passions: Safer sex as play. In Timothy Edgar, Mary Anne Fitzpatrick, and Vicki S. Freimuth (eds.), *AIDS: A communication perspective* (pp. 69-89). Mahwah, NJ: Lawrence Erlbaum Associates.

African Medical Research and Education Foundation (AMREF) (1992). *Tanzania: AIDS education and condom promotion for transport workers: Strengthening STD services.* Dar es Salaam, Tanzania: African Medical Research and Education Foundation.

AIDS Prevention and Control Project (APAC) (1999). *Prevention of STD/HIV/AIDS along the highway.* Chennai: Voluntary Health Services, AIDS Prevention and Control Project.

——— (2001a). *HIV risk behavior surveillance survey in Tamil Nadu.* Chennai: Voluntary Health Services, AIDS Prevention and Control Project.

——— (2001b). *Management of behavior surveillance survey experience of Tamil Nadu.* Chennai: Voluntary Health Services, AIDS Prevention and Control Project.

Ainsworth, Martha, Chris Beyrer, and Agnes Soucat (2000). *Thailand's response to AIDS: Building on success, confronting the future.* Bangkok: World Bank.

Airhihenbuwa, Collins O. (1995). *Health and culture: Beyond the western paradigm.* Thousand Oaks, CA: Sage Publications.

——— (1999). Of culture and multiverse: Renouncing "the universal truth" in health. *Journal of Health Education,* 30(5), pp. 267–73.

——— (2002). Qualitative research traditions. Unpublished manuscript, Department of Bio-behavioral Health, Pennsylvania State University, University Park, PA.

Airhihenbuwa, Collins O., and Rafael Obregon (2000). A critical assessment of theories/models used in health communication for HIV/AIDS. *Journal of Health Communication,* 5, pp. 5–15.

Al-Qadhi, Mohammed Hatem (2001). A silent threat in Yemen. *Choices,* 10(4), pp. 12–13.

Altman, Lawrence (1997). AIDS surge is forecast for China, India, and Eastern Europe. *The New York Times,* 4 November, p. A10.

Arguelles, Lourdes, and Anne Rivero (1997). Spiritual emergencies and psycho-spiritual treatment strategies among gay/homosexual Latinos with HIV disease. In Martine Levine, Peter M. Nardi, and John H. Gagnon (eds.), *In changing times: Gay men and lesbians encounter HIV/AIDS* (pp. 83–99). Chicago: University of Chicago Press.

Auerbach, Judith D., and Thomas J. Coates (2000). HIV prevention research: Accomplishments and challenges for the third decade of AIDS. *American Journal of Public Health,* 90(7), pp. 1029–32.

Baleta, Adele (2001). South Africa's stance on Nevirapine on trial. *Lancet,* 358, p. 1521 (3 November).

Bandura, Albert (1977). *Social learning theory.* Englewood Cliffs, NJ: Prentice-Hall.

——— (1986). *Social foundations of thought and action: A social cognitive theory.* Englewood Cliffs, NJ: Prentice-Hall.

——— (1997). *Self-efficacy: The exercise of control.* New York: Freeman.

Barnett, T., and P. Blaikie (1992). *AIDS in Africa: Its present and future impact.* New York: Guildorm Press.

Barouch, Dan H., Jennifer Kunstman, Marcelo J. Kuroda, Jorn E. Schmitz, Sampa Santra, Fred W. Peyerl, Georgia R. Krivulka, Kristin Beaudry, Michelle A. Lifton, Darci A. Gorgone, David C. Montefiori, Mark G. Lewis, Steven M. Wolinsky, and Norman L. Letvin (2002). Eventual AIDS vaccine failure in a rhesus monkey by viral escape from Cytotoxic T Lymphocytes. *Nature,* 415, pp. 335–39 (17 January).

Bartholemew, Courtenay (2002a). The Durban International AIDS Conference. *Trinidad Express* (Port of Spain, Trinidad & Tobago), 14 January, p. 1.

——— (2002b). Testing the AIDS vaccine. *Trinidad Express* (Port of Spain, Trinidad & Tobago), 19 January, p. 1.

——— (2002c). Safe, yes. Efficacious. *Trinidad Express* (Port of Spain, Trinidad & Tobago), 18 February, p. 1.

Beresford, Belinda (2001). AIDS takes an economic and social toll. *Africa Recovery*, 15(1-2), pp. 19-22.

Bergman, Andrew (2002). Aide de Camp. *Holland Herald*, 37(3), pp. 40-41 (March).

Bermingham, S., and S. Kippax (1998). HIV-related discrimination: A survey of New South Wales general practitioners. *Australian and New Zealand Journal of Public Health*, 22, pp. 92-97.

Beyrer, Chris (1998). *War in the blood: Sex, politics and AIDS in Southeast Asia*. New York: Zed Books/Bangkok: White Lotus.

Blair, C., D. Ojakaa, S.A. Ochola, and D. Gogi (1997). Barriers to behavior change: Results of focus group discussions conducted in high HIV/AIDS incidence areas of Kenya. In D.C. Umeh (ed.), *Confronting the AIDS epidemic: Cross-cultural perspectives on HIV/AIDS education* (pp. 47-57). Trenton, NJ: Africa World Press.

Boal, Augusto (1979). *The theater of the oppressed*. New York: Urizen Books.

Bolton, Ralph (1995). Rethinking anthropology: The study of AIDS. In Han ten Brummelheis and Gilbert Herdt (eds.), *Culture and sexual risk: Anthropological perspectives on AIDS* (pp. 285-314). Amsterdam: Gordon & Breach.

Bond, Katherine C., David D. Celentano, and Chayan Vaddhanaphuti (1996). "I'm not afraid of life or death": Women in brothels in northern Thailand. In Lynellyn D. Long and E. Maxine Ankrah (eds.), *Women's experience with HIV/AIDS: An international perspective* (pp. 123-49). New York: Columbia University Press.

Bond, Katherine C., David D. Celentano, Sukanya Phonsophak, and Chayan Vaddhanaphuti (1997). Mobility and migration: Female commercial sex work and the HIV epidemic in northern Thailand. In Gilbert Herdt (ed.), *Sexual cultures and migration in the era of AIDS: Anthropological and demographic perspectives* (pp. 185-215). New York: Oxford University Press.

Brody, S. (1995). Heterosexual transmission of HIV. *New England Journal of Medicine*, 331, p. 1718.

Brown, Mark Malloch (2001). The challenge of HIV/AIDS. *Choices*, 10(4), p. 4.

Brown, William J., and Michael D. Basil (1995). Media celebrities and public health: Responses to "Magic" Johnson's HIV disclosure and its impact on AIDS risk and high-risk behaviors. *Health Communication*, 7(4), pp. 345-70.

Brummelhuis, Han ten, and Gilbert Herdt (1995). *Culture and sexual risk: Anthropological perspectives on AIDS*. Amsterdam: Gordon & Breach.

Bultreys, Marc, Mary Glenn Fowler, Nathan Shaffer, Pius M. Tih, Alan E. Greenberg, Etienne Karita, Hoosen Coovadia, and Kevin De Cook

(2002). Role of traditional birth attendants in preventing perinatal transmission of HIV. *British Medical Journal*, 324, pp. 222-25 (26 January).

Burns, John F. (1996). The AIDS highway. *The New York Times*, 22 September, p. A1.

Celentano, David C., Katherine C. Bond, Cynthia M. Lyles, Sakol Eiumtrakul, Vivian F.-L. Go, Chris Beyrer, Chainarong na Chiangmai, Kenrad E. Nelson, Chirasak Khamboonruang, and Chayan Vaddhanaphuti (2000). Preventive intervention to reduce sexually transmitted infections: A field trial in the Royal Thai Army. *Archives of Internal Medicine*, 160, pp. 535-40.

Chandiramani, Radhika (1998). A view from the field: Phone help line in India helps identify HIV risk behaviors. *SIECUS Report*, June-July, pp. 4-6.

Chantal, Roromme (2001). Haiti battles both poverty and HIV/AIDS. *Choices*, 10(4), p. 17.

Church, C.A., and J. Geller. (1989). Lights! camera! action! Promoting family planning with TV, video, and film. *Population Reports*, J-38. Baltimore, MD: Johns Hopkins University, Population Information Program.

Cohen, Bernard (1963). *The press and foreign policy*. Princeton, NJ: Princeton University Press.

Community Agency for Social Inquiry (CASE) (1995). *Let the sky to be the limit: Soul City evaluation report*. Johannesburg: Jacana Education.

Crawford, Anne M. (1996). Stigma associated with AIDS: A meta-analysis. *Journal of Applied Social Psychology*, 26(5), pp. 398-416.

D'Agnes, Thomas (2001). *From condoms to cabbages: An authorized biography of Mechai Viravaidya*. Bangkok: Post Books.

Daily Nation (1999). Break the silence: Talk about AIDS through sports. *Daily Nation*, 6 November, p. 20.

Daniel, Herbert, and Richard Parker (1993). *Sexuality, politics, and AIDS in Brazil*. London: Falmer Press.

Dearing, James W., and Everett M. Rogers (1996). *Agenda-setting*. Thousand Oaks, CA: Sage Publications.

Dearing, James W., Everett M. Rogers, Gary Meyer, Mary K. Casey, Nagesh Rao, Shelly Campo, and Geoffrey M. Henderson (1996). Social marketing and diffusion-based strategies for communicating health with unique populations: HIV prevention in San Francisco. *Journal of Health Communication*, 1, pp. 343-63.

de Negri, B., E. Thomas, A. Illinigumugabo, I. Muvandi, and Gary Lewis (1998). *Empowering communities: Participatory techniques for community-based programme development*. Nairobi: The Center for African Family Studies, in collaboration with the Johns Hopkins

University Center for Communication Programs and the Academy for Educational Development.

DeNoon, Daniel (2002). AIDS worse than Black Death. *WebMD Medical News*, 25 January, p. 1.

de Waal, Shaun (1999). Judge who lives with AIDS. *Mail and Guardian*, 23–29 April, p. 1.

Diaz, Rafael Miguel (1997). Latino gay men and psycho-cultural barriers to AIDS prevention. In Martine Levine, Peter M. Nardi, and John H. Gagnon (eds.), *In changing times: Gay men and lesbians encounter HIV/AIDS* (pp. 221–44). Chicago: University of Chicago Press.

DiFrancisco, Wayne, Jeffrey A. Kelly, Laura Otto-Salaj, Timothy L. McAuliffe, Anton M. Somlai, Kristin Hackl, Timothy G. Heckman, David R. Holtgrave, and David J. Romero (1999). Factors influencing attitudes within AIDS service organizations toward the use of research-based HIV prevention interventions. *AIDS Education and Prevention*, 12(1), pp. 72–86.

Dionisie, Dan (2001). HIV/AIDS counseling for teens in Romania. *Choices*, 10(4), p. 19.

Diop, W. (2000). From government policy to community-based communication strategies in Africa: Lessons from Senegal and Uganda. *Journal of Health Communication*, 5, pp. 113–18.

Dube, Siddharth (2000). *Sex, lies, and AIDS*. New Delhi: HarperCollins.

Duesberg, Peter (1994). *Inventing the AIDS virus*. New York: St. Martin's Press.

Dugger, Celia W. (1999). Calcutta's prostitutes lead the fight on AIDS. *The New York Times*, 4 January, p. A1.

Durban Declaration (2000). *Nature*, 406, pp. 15–16.

Elwood, William N. (ed.) (1999). *Power in the blood: A handbook on AIDS, politics, and communication*. Mahwah, NJ: Lawrence Erlbaum Associates.

Fabj, Valeria, and Matthew J. Sabnosky (1993). Responses from the street: ACT UP and community organizing against AIDS. In Scott C. Ratzan (ed.), *AIDS: Effective health education from the 90s* (pp. 91–109). London: Taylor & Francis.

Farmer, Paul (1995). Culture, poverty, and dynamics of HIV transmission in rural Haiti. In Han ten Brummelheis and Gilbert Herdt (eds.), *Culture and sexual risk: Anthropological perspectives on AIDS* (pp. 3–28). Amsterdam: Gordon & Breach.

Fettner, A.G., and W.A. Check (1984). *The truth about AIDS: Evolution of an epidemic*. New York: Holt, Rinehart & Winston.

Fishbein, Martin, Carolyn Guenther-Grey, Wayne Johnson, Richard Wolitski, Alfred McAlister, Cornelis A. Rietmeijer, Kevin O'Reilly, and The AIDS Community Demonstration Projects (1997). Intention to reduce AIDS risk behaviors: The CDC's AIDS Community

Demonstration Projects. In Marvin Goldberg, Martin Fishbein, and Susan E. Middlestadt (eds.), *Social Marketing* (pp. 123–46). Mahwah, NJ: Lawrence Erlbaum Associates.

Fisher, J.D., and W.A. Fisher (1992). Changing AIDS-risk behavior. *Psychological Bulletin*, 111, pp. 455–74.

Fisher, Walter (1987). *Human communication as narration.* Columbia, SC: University of South Carolina Press.

Fleshman, Michael (2001). AIDS prevention in the ranks. *Africa Recovery*, 15(1–2), pp. 16–17.

Folkers, Gregory K., and Anthony S. Fauci (2001). The AIDS research model: Implications for other infectious diseases of global health importance. *Journal of the American Medical Association*, 286(4), pp. 458–61 (25 July).

Foreman, M. (ed.) (1999). *AIDS and men: Taking risks or taking responsibility?* London: Panos/Zed Books.

Freeman, J. (2001). Concern about local setting is important. UN Special Session on HIV/AIDS, *Conference News Daily*, 25 June, p. 13.

Freire, Paulo (1970). *Pedagogy of the oppressed.* New York: Continuum.

Fumento, M. (1990). *The myth of heterosexual AIDS.* New York: Basic Books.

Gaitonde, Ishwas R. (2001). *A thief in the night: Understanding AIDS.* Chennai: East West Books.

Galavotti, Christine, Katina A. Pappas-Deluca, and Amy Lansky (2001). Modeling and reinforcement to combat HIV: The MARCH approach to behavior change. *American Journal of Public Health*, 91(10), pp. 1602–7.

Garrett, Laurie (1992). The next epidemic. In Jonathan Mann, D. Tarantola, and T. Netter (eds), *AIDS in the world* (pp. 106–23). Cambridge, MA: Harvard University Press.

——— (2000). *Betrayal of trust.* New York: Hyperion.

——— (2001). Opinion. UN Special Session on HIV/AIDS, *Conference News Daily*, 25 June, p. 20.

Gellert, G.A., P.C. Weismuller, K.V. Higgins, and R.M. Maxwell (1992). Disclosure of AIDS in celebrities. *New England Journal of Medicine*, 327(19), p. 1389.

Gilson, Lucy, Rashid Mkanje, Heiner Grosskurth, Frank Mosha, John Picard, Awena Gavyole, James Todd, Phillippe Mayaud, Roland Swai, Lieve Fransen, David Mabey, Anne Mills, and Richard Hayes (1997). Cost-effectiveness of improved treatment services for sexually transmitted diseases in preventing HIV-1 infection in Mwanza Region, Tanzania. *Lancet*, 350, pp. 1805–9 (20–27 December).

Glick, Deborah, Glen Nowak, Thomas Valente, Karen Sapsis, and Chad Martin (2002). Youth performing arts entertainment-education for HIV/AIDS prevention and health promotion: Practice and research. *Journal of Health Communication*, 7, pp. 39–57.

Goffman, Erving (1963). *Stigma: Notes on the management of spoiled identity*. New York: Penguin.

Goldstein, Sue, Shereen Usdin, Esca Scheepers, Aadielah Marker, and Garth Japhet (in press). Multimedia campaign for children's health in South Africa: The treatment of AIDS in *Soul Buddyz*. In Arvind Singhal and William Stephen Howard (eds.), *HIV/AIDS and African children: Health challenges and educational possibilities*. Athens, OH: Ohio University Press.

Gopinath, C.Y. (2000). *Question your relationships*. Nairobi: PATH.

Gottlieb, Michael S. (1998). Discovering AIDS. *Epidemiology*, 9(4), pp. 365–67.

———— (2001). AIDS: Past and future. *New England Journal of Medicine*, 344(23), pp. 1788–91.

Green, M.C., and T.C. Brock (2000). The role of transportation in the persuasiveness of public narratives. *Journal of Personality and Social Psychology*, 79(5), pp. 701–21.

Grosskurth, Heiner, Frank Mosta, James Todd, Ezra Mwijarubi, Arnold Klokke, Kesheni Senkoro, Phillippe Mayaud, John Changalucha, Angus Nicoll, Gina ka-Gina, James Newell, Kokugonza Mugeye, David Mabey, and Richard Hayes (1995). Impact of improved treatment of sexually transmitted diseases on HIV infection in rural Tanzania: Randomized controlled trial. *Lancet*, 346, pp. 530–36.

Guay, Laura A., Phillippe Musoke, Thomas Fleming, Danstan Bagenda, Melissa Allen, Clemensia Nakabiito, Joseph Sherman, Paul Bakaki, Constance Ducar, Martina Deseyve, Lynda Emel, Mark Mirochnick, Mary Glenn Fowler, Lynne Mofenson, Paolo Miotti, Kevin Dransfield, Dorothy Bray, Francis Mmito, and J. Brooks Jackson (1999). Intrapartum and neonatal single-dose Nevirapine compared with Zidovudine for prevention of mother-to-child transmission of HIV-1 in Kampala, Uganda: HIVNET 012 randomized trial. *Lancet*, 354, pp. 795–802 (4 September).

Gumucio Dagron, A. (2001). *Making waves: Stories of participatory communication for social change*. New York: Rockefeller Foundation.

Gupte, Pranay (2001). My top priority: Mobilizing world leaders. UN Special Session on HIV/AIDS. *Conference News Daily*, 26 June, p. 12.

Harris, D. (1991). AIDS and theory. *Linguafranca*, 1(5), pp. 16–19.

Harvey, Philip D. (1999). *Let every child be wanted: How social marketing is revolutionizing contraceptive use around the world*. Westport, CT: Auburn House.

Hawkins, P.S. (1993). Naming names: The art of memory and the NAMES Project AIDS Quilt. *Critical Inquiry*, 19, pp. 752–79.

Herek, Gregory M., and John P. Capitanio (1999). AIDS stigma and sexual prejudice. *American Behavioral Scientist*, 42(7), pp. 1130–47.

Herek, Gregory M., and Eric K. Glunt (1988). An epidemic of stigma: Public relations of AIDS. *American Psychologist*, 43(11), pp. 886–91.

Holland, J. (2001). Original AIDS quilt to hang in Manhattan. *The New York Times*, 1 December, p. A12.

Horton, D., and R.R. Wohl (1956). Mass communication and para-social interaction: Observation on intimacy at a distance. *Psychiatry*, 19(3), pp. 215–29.

Inciardi, J. (1992). *The War on Drugs II: The continuing epic of heroin, cocaine, crack, crimes, AIDS, and public policy*. Mountain View, CA: Mayfield.

Jacobson, Thomas L. (1993). A pragmatist account of participatory communication research for national development. *Communication Theory*, 3(3), pp. 214–30.

Japhet, Garth, and Sue Goldstein (1997a). *The Soul City experience in South Africa*. Audiotape recording of presentation made to the Second International Conference on Entertainment-Education and Social Change, Athens, Ohio. Columbus, OH: RoSu Productions.

——— (1997b). Soul City experience. *Integration*, 53, pp. 10–11.

Jha, Prabhat, Nico J.D. Nagelkerke, Elizabeth N. Ngugi, J.V.R. Prasada Rao, Bridget Willbond, Stephen Moses, and Francis A. Plummer (2001). Reducing HIV transmission in developing countries. *Science*, 292, pp. 224–25 (13 April).

Jibaja, M.J., P. Kingeny, N.E. Noff, Q. Smith, J. Bowman, and J.R. Holcomb (2000). Tailored interactive soap operas for breast cancer education of high-risk Hispanic women. *Journal of Cancer Education*, 15(4), pp. 237–43.

Johns Hopkins University Center for Communication Programs (JHU/CCP) (1999). *Men's participation in reproductive health in Africa: The Africa CUP Initiative*. Baltimore, MD: Johns Hopkins University Center for Communication Programs.

Jordan, M. (1996). India enlists barbers in the war on AIDS. *The Wall Street Journal*, 12 March, p. A14.

"Kaew" (2001). *The critical second: Life or death*. Bangkok: Dokya 2000.

Kalichman, Seth C. (1998). *Preventing AIDS: A sourcebook for behavioral interventions*. Mahwah, NJ: Lawrence Erlbaum Associates.

Kapila, Mukesh, and Maryan J. Pye (1992). The European response to AIDS. In Jaime Sepulveda, Harvey Fineberg, and Jonathan Mann (eds.), *AIDS prevention through education: A world view* (pp. 199–236). New York: Oxford University Press.

Kaul, Rupert, Francis A. Plummer, Joshua Kimani, Tao Dong, Peter Kimani, Timothy Reston, Ephantus Njagi, Kelly S. MacDonald, Job J. Bwayo, Andrew J. McMichael, and Sarah L. Rowland-Jones (2000). HIV-1-specific mucosal CD8+ lymphocyte responses in the cervix of

HIV-1-resistant prostitutes in Nairobi. *Journal of Immunology*, 164, pp. 1602-11.

Kelly, Jeffrey A., Janet S. St. Lawrence, S. Smith, H.V. Hood, and D.J. Cook (1987). Stigmatization of AIDS patients by physicians. *American Journal of Public Health*, 77, pp. 789-91.

Kelly, Jeffrey A., Janet S. St. Lawrence, Y.E. Diaz, L.Y. Stevenson, A.C. Houth, T.L. Bransfield, S.C. Kalichman, J.E. Smith, and M.E. Andrews (1991). HIV risk behavior reduction following intervention with key opinion leaders of population: An experimental analysis. *American Journal of Public Health*, 81, pp. 168-71.

Kelly, Jeffrey A., D.A. Murphy, K.J. Sikkema, T.L. McAuliffe, R.A. Roffman, L.J. Solomon, R.A. Winett, and S.C. Kalichman (1997). Randomized, controlled, community-level HIV-prevention intervention for sexual risk behaviour among homosexual men in U.S. cities. *Lancet*, 350, pp. 1500-1505.

Kinsella, J. (1989). *Covering the plague: AIDS and the American media.* New Brunswich, NJ: Rutgers University Press.

Klovdahl, Alden S. (1985). Social networks and the spread of infectious diseases: The AIDS example. *Social Sciences and Medicine*, 21(1), pp. 1203-16.

Knaus, Christopher Stephen, and Erica W. Austin (1998). The AIDS Memorial Quilt as preventative education: A development analysis of the Quilt as a preventative tool. Paper presented to the International Communication Association, Jerusalem, May 1998.

Korber, Bette, M. Muldoon, J. Theiler, F. Gao, R. Gupta, A. Lapedes, B.H. Hahn, S. Wolinsky, and T. Bhattacharya (2000). Timing the ancestor of the HIV-1 pandemic strains. *Science*, 288, pp. 1789-96 (9 June).

Kramer, Larry (1990). *Reports from the holocaust.* London: Penguin.

Lacey, Marc (2001). Where roads are paved with nothing but hope. *The New York Times*, 10 December, p. A4.

Lague, David (2002). Chinese researchers rediscover malaria remedy once seen as lost. *The Wall Street Journal* (Europe), 8-10 March, p. A7.

Lamont, James (2001). Long-distance drivers transport HIV worries to "truck girls." *The Financial Times*, 6 February, p. 3.

Lamptey, Peter R. (2002). Reducing heterosexual transmission of HIV in poor countries. *British Medical Journal*, 324, pp. 207-11 (26 January).

Lifson, Jeffrey D., and Malcolm A. Martin (2002). AIDS vaccines: One step forward, one step back. *Nature*, 415, pp. 272-73 (17 January).

Lincoln, C.E., and L.H. Mamiya (1991). *The black church in the African-American experience.* Durham, NC: Duke University Press.

Lippmann, Walter (1922). *Public opinion.* New York: Macmillan.

Lom, Mamadou Mika (2001). Senegal's recipe for success. *Africa Recovery*, 15(1-2), pp. 24-25.

Machlica, F. (1997). HIV/AIDS prevention strategies affecting special population groups. In D.C. Umeh (ed.), *Confronting the AIDS epidemic: Cross-cultural perspectives on HIV/AIDS education* (pp. 250–65). Trenton, NJ: Africa World Press.

Macintyre, Kate, Lisanne Brown, and Stephen Sosler (2001). "It's not what you know, but who you knew": Examining the relationship between behavior change and AIDS mortality in Africa. *AIDS Education and Prevention*, 13(2), pp. 160–74.

Maclure, Malcolm (1998). Inventing the AIDS virus hypothesis: An example of scientific versus unscientific induction. *Epidemiology*, 9, pp. 467–73.

Madraa, E., and M. Ruranga-Rubaramira (1998). Experience from Uganda. In A. Malcolm and G. Dowsett (eds.), *Partners in prevention: International case studies of effective health promotion practice in HIV/AIDS* (pp. 49–57). Geneva: UNAIDS.

Makgoba, Malegapura William, Nandipha Solomon, and Timothy Johan Paul Tucker (2002). The search for an HIV vaccine. *British Medical Journal*, 324, pp. 211–13 (26 January).

Malcolm, A., Peter Aggleton, M. Bronfman, Purnima Mane, and J. Verrall (1998). HIV-related stigmatization and discrimination: Its forms and contexts. *Critical Public Health*, 8(4), pp. 347–70.

Maldonado, M. (1990). Latinas and HIV/AIDS. *SIECUS Report*, 19(2), pp. 33–37.

Mane, Purnima, and Shubhada A. Maitra (1992). *AIDS prevention: The socio-cultural context in India*. Mumbai: Tata Institute of Social Sciences.

Mann, Jonathan M., and D.J.M. Tarantola (1998). HIV 1998: The global picture. *Scientific American*, pp. 82–83 (July).

Mann, Jonathan, D.J. Tarantola, and T.W. Netter (1996). *AIDS in the world*. New York: Oxford University Press.

Marseille, Elliott, James G. Kahn, Francis Mmiro, Laura Guay, Phillippa Musoke, Mary Glenn Fowler, and J. Brooks Jackson (1999). Cost-effectiveness of single-dose Nevirapine regimen for mothers and babies to decrease vertical HIV-1 transmission in Sub-Sahara Africa. *Lancet*, 354, pp. 803–9 (4 September).

McKee, Neill (1994). A community-based learning approach: Beyond social marketing. In Shirley A. White, K. Sadanand. Nair, and Joseph Ascroft (eds.), *Participatory communication: Working for change and development* (pp. 194–228). New Delhi: Sage Publications.

McKee, Neill, Mira Aghi, Rachel Carnegie, and Nuzhat Shahzadi (in press). Sara: A role model for African girls as they face HIV/AIDS. In Arvind Singhal and William Stephen Howard (eds.), *HIV/AIDS and African children: Health challenges and educational possibilities*. Athens, OH: Ohio University Press.

McKinlay, J.B., and L.D. Marceau (1999). A tale of three tails. *American Journal of Public Health*, 89, pp. 295–98.

——— (2000). Public health matters: To boldly go. *American Journal of Public Health*, 90(1), pp. 25–33.

McKusick, Leon, Thomas J. Coates, Stephen F. Morin, Lance Pollack, and Colleen Hope (1990). Longitudinal predictions of reductions in unprotected anal intercourse among gay men in San Francisco: The AIDS Behavioral Research Project. *American Journal of Public Health*, 80(8), pp. 978–83.

McMichael, A.J. (1995). The health of persons, populations, and planets: Epidemiology comes full circle. *Epidemiology*, 6, pp. 636–63.

McNeil, Donald G. (2001a). Indian company offers to supply AIDS drugs at low cost in Africa. *The New York Times*, 7 February, p. A1.

——— (2001b). Witnesses to an epidemic shrug off shame to fight a dangerous fear. *The New York Times*, 26 November, p. A12.

——— (2002). On stages and screens, AIDS educators reach South Africa's youths. *The New York Times*, 3 February, p. 6.

Melkote, Srinivas R., Sundeep R. Muppidi, and D. Goswami (2000). Social and economic factors in an integrated behavioral and societal approach to communications in HIV/AIDS. *Journal of Health Communication*, 5, pp. 17–28.

Metts, Sandra, and Mary Anne Fitzpatrick (1992). Thinking about safer sex: The risky business of "know your partner" advice. In Timothy Edgar, Mary Anne Fitzpatrick, and Vicki S. Freimuth (eds.), *AIDS: A communication perspective* (pp. 1–19). Mahwah, NJ: Lawrence Erlbaum Associates.

Ministerio da Saude (2000). *The Brazilian response to HIV/AIDS*. Brasília: Ministry of Health.

Mishra, Subhash (2000). Damned to death. *India Today*, pp. 40–41.

Morris, Martina (1997). Sexual networks and HIV. *AIDS*, 11(Supplement A), pp. S209–S216.

Moses, Stephen, Janet E. Bradley, Nico J.D. Nagelkerke, Allan R. Ronald, J.O. Ndinya-Achola, and Francis A. Plummer (1990). Geographical patterns of male circumcision practices in Africa: Association with HIV seroprevalence. *International Journal of Epidemiology*, 19(3), pp. 693–97.

Moses, Stephen, Francis A. Plummer, Elizabeth N. Ngugi, Nico J.D. Nagelkerke, Aggrey O. Anzala, and Jackonlah O. Ndinya-Achola (1991). Controlling HIV in Africa: Effectiveness and cost of an intervention in a high-frequency STD transmitter core group. *AIDS*, 5, pp. 407–11.

Mutume, Gumisai (2001). African leaders declare war on AIDS. *Africa Recovery*, 14(4), pp. 1, 20–23.

Nariman, H.N. (1993). *Soap operas for social change: Toward a methodology for entertainment-education television*. Westport, CT: Praeger.

Ncube, Japhet (2000). Sex: The shocking truth. *Drum*, 13 July, pp. 14–15, 24.

Nduati, Ruth, Grace John, Dorothy Mbori-Ngacha, Barbara Richardson, Julie Overbaugh, Anthony Mwatha, Jeckoniah Ndinya-Achola, Job Bwayo, Francis E. Onyango, James Hughes, and Joan Kreiss (2000). Effect of breastfeeding and formula feeding on transmission of HIV-1: A randomized clinical trial. *JAMA*, 283(9), pp. 1167–74 (1 March).

Neary, Dyan (2001). Holbrooke pushes business for involvement. UN Special Session on HIV/AIDS, *Conference News Daily*, 25 June, p. 4.

Nemapare, Prisca (2002). Health and nutritional risk factors among orphans in rural Zimbabwe. Paper presented to the international conference on HIV/AIDS and African Children, Athens, Ohio, April 2002.

Netter, Thomas W. (1992). The media and AIDS: A global perspective. In Jaime Sepulveda, Harvey Fineberg, and Jonathan Mann (eds.), *AIDS prevention through education: A world view* (pp. 241–53). New York: Oxford University Press.

Newton-Small, J. (2001). Beautiful islands in the Caribbean suffer the second highest level of AIDS in the world. UN Special Session on HIV/AIDS, *Conference News Daily*, 25 June, p. 8.

Ng, S.K.C. (1991). Does epidemiology need a new philosophy? A case study of logical inquiry in the acquired immunodeficiency syndrome epidemic. *American Journal of Epidemiology*, 133, pp. 1073–77.

Ngugi, Elizabeth N., Francis A. Plummer, J.N. Simonsen, D.W. Cameron, M. Brosire, P. Waiyaki, A.R. Arnold, and J.O. Ndinya-Achola (1988). Prevention of transmission of Human Immunodeficiency Virus in Africa: Effectiveness of condom promotion and health education among prostitutes. *Lancet*, 2, pp. 887–90 (15 October).

Niehoff, Arthur (1964). Theravada Buddhism: A vehicle for technical change. *Human Organization*, 23, pp. 108–12.

O'Hea, Erin L., Sara E. Sytsma, Amy Copeland, and Phillip J. Brantley (2001). The Attitudes toward Women with HIV/AIDS Scale (ATWAS): Development and validation. *AIDS Education and Prevention*, 13(2), pp. 120–30.

Olson, Elizabeth (2000). Red Cross says three diseases kill many more than disasters. *The New York Times*, 29 June, p. A17.

Okri, B. (1991). *The famished road*. New York: Oxford University Press.

Paiva, Vera (1995). Sexuality, AIDS, and gender norms among Brazilian teenagers. In Han ten Brummelheis and Gilbert Herdt (eds.), *Culture and sexual risk: Anthropological perspectives on AIDS* (pp. 79–96). Amsterdam: Gordon & Breach.

Paiva, Vera (2000). *Fazendo arte com a camisinha: Sexualidades jovens em tempos de AIDS.* São Paulo: Summus Editorial.

Pang, Augustine (1998). A is for AIDS, B is for baby, C is for courage. *The New Paper*, pp. 29–32.

———— (1999). Free from AIDS: New hope after five years. *The New Paper*, pp. 4–5.

Panos Institute (2000). *Beyond our means: The cost of treating HIV/AIDS in the developing world.* London: Panos Institute.

Papa, M.J., Arvind Singhal, Sweety Law, Suruchi Sood, Everett M. Rogers, and Corinne L. Shefner-Rogers (2000). Entertainment-education and social change: An analysis of parasocial interaction, social learning, collective efficacy, and paradoxical communication. *Journal of Communication,* 50(4), pp. 31–55.

Parker, Richard (1991). *Bodies, pleasures, and passions: Sexual culture in contemporary Brazil.* Boston: Beacon Press.

———— (1995). The social and cultural construction of sexual risk, or how to have (sex) research in an epidemic. In Han ten Brummelheis and Gilbert Herdt (eds.), *Culture and sexual risk: Anthropological perspectives on AIDS* (pp. 257–70). Amsterdam: Gordon & Breach.

Parker, Richard, and Veriano Terto (2001). *Solidariedade: A ABIA, Na virada do milenio.* Rio de Janeiro: ABIA.

Pasek, Beata (2001). Front line action in Poland. *Choices,* 10(4), pp. 18–19.

Pasick, R.J. (1995). Socioeconomic and cultural factors in the development and use of theory. In Karen Glanz, F.M. Lewis, and Barbara K. Rimer (eds.), *Health and health education: Theory, research, and practice* (pp. 425–40). San Francisco: Jossey-Bass.

Perloff, Richard M. (2001). *Persuading people to have safer sex: Applications of social science to the AIDS crisis.* Mahwah, NJ: Lawrence Erlbaum Associates.

Phillips, Michael M. (2001). To help fight AIDS, Tanzanian villages ban risky traditions. *Wall Street Journal,* 12 January, pp. A1, A12.

Phoolcharoen, W. (1998). Experience from Thailand. In A. Malcolm and G. Dowsett (eds.), *Partners in prevention: International case studies of effective health promotion practice in HIV/AIDS* (pp. 36–48). Geneva: UNAIDS.

Phusahat, Araya (2000). Development of and lessons learned from positive people groups and network. Best Practice Documentation on HIV/AIDS for Community Mobilization, Case Study 4. Bangkok: UNAIDS.

Piot, Peter (2001). The fight against HIV/AIDS: The UN at work. *Choices,* 10(4), p. 23.

Piotrow, Phyllis T., Rita C. Meyer, and B.A. Zulu (1992). AIDS and mass persuasion. In Jonathan Mann, D.J.M. Tarantola, and T.W. Netter (eds.), *AIDS in the world* (pp. 733–59). Cambridge, MA: Harvard University Press.

Piotrow, Phyllis T., D. Lawrence Kincaid, Jose Rimon II, and Ward Rinehart (1997). *Health communication: Lessons from family planning and reproductive health*. Westport, CT: Praeger.

Pisani, Elisabeth (1999). *Acting early to prevent AIDS: The case of Senegal*. Geneva: UNAIDS.

Population Reports (1989). *AIDS education: A beginning*. Baltimore, MD: Johns Hopkins University Center for Communication Programs, Population Information Program.

Punnyakamo, Sommai (2001). Coming to terms with truth. *Choices*, 10(4), p. 24.

Ramasundaram, S. (2002). Can India avoid being devastated by HIV? *British Medical Journal*, 324, pp. 182–85.

Ramasundaram, S., K. Allaudin, Bimal Charles, K. Gopal, P. Krishnamurthy, R. Poornalingam, and Dora Warren (2001). HIV/ AIDS control in India: Lessons from Tamil Nadu. Paper WG-5: 25, WHO Commission on Macroeconomics and Health, Geneva.

Ratzan, Scott C. (ed.) (1993). *AIDS: Effective health communication for the 90s*. London: Taylor & Francis.

Reeves, Patricia (2000). Coping in cyberspace: The impact of Internet use on the ability of HIV-positive individuals to deal with their illness. *Journal of Health Communication*, 5(Supplement), pp. 47–59.

Relv, M.V. (1997). Illuminating meaning and transforming issues of spirituality in HIV disease and AIDS: An application of Parse's theory of human becoming. *Holistic Nursing Practice*, 12(1), pp. 1–8.

Riviere, Pichon (1988). *O processo grupal*. São Paulo: Martins Fontes.

Rogers, Everett M. (1995). *Diffusion of innovations* (4th edition). New York: Free Press.

Rogers, Everett M., and Thomas M. Steinfatt (1999). *Intercultural communication*. Prospect Heights, IL: Waveland Press.

Rogers, Everett M., and J. Douglas Storey (1987). Communication campaigns. In Charles R. Berger and Steven H. Chaffee (eds.), *Handbook of communication science* (pp. 817–46). Thousand Oaks, CA: Sage Publications.

Rogers, Everett M., James W. Dearing, and Soonbum Chang (1991). AIDS in the '80s: The agenda-setting process for a public issue. Journalism Monographs, 126.

Rogers, Everett M., James W. Dearing, Nagesh Rao, Michelle L. Campo, Gary Meyer, Gary J.F. Betts, and Mary K. Casey (1995). Communication and community in a city under siege: The AIDS epidemic in San Francisco. *Communication Research*, 22(6), pp. 664–78.

Rogers, Everett M., Peter W. Vaughan, Ramadhan M.A. Swalehe, Nagesh Rao, Peer Svenkerud, and Suruchi Sood (1999). Effects of an entertainment-education radio soap opera on family planning behavior in Tanzania. *Studies in Family Planning*, 30(3), pp. 193–211.

Ronaldo (2001). HIV/AIDS does not recognize borders. *Choices*, 10(4), p. 26.

Root-Bernstein, Robert S. (1993). *Rethinking AIDS: The tragic cost of premature consensus*. New York: Free Press.

Rosenberg, Tina (2001). Patent laws are malleable, patients are educable, drug companies are vincible, the world's AIDS crisis is solvable: Look at Brazil. *The New York Times*, 28 January, pp. 26–31, 52, 58, 62–63.

Rosenfield, Alan, and Landon Meyer (2001). Let's not write off countries that face despairing futures. UN Special Session on HIV/AIDS, *Conference News Daily*, 27 June, p. 18.

Ruiz, M. (1995). Social merchandising: Using Brazilian television miniseries for drug-abuse and AIDS prevention. In H. Kirsch (ed.), *Drug lessons and education programs in developing countries*. New Brunswick, NJ: Transaction.

Salmon, Charles T., and Fred Kroger (1992). A systems approach to AIDS communication: The example of the National AIDS Information and Education Program. In Timothy Edgar, Mary Anne Fitzpatrick, and Vicki S. Freimuth (eds.), *AIDS: A communication perspective* (pp. 131–46). Mahwah, NJ: Lawrence Erlbaum Associates.

Salunke, Subhash R., Mohamed Slunke, Subhash K. Hira, and Madhukar R. Jagtap (1998). HIV/AIDS in India: A country responds to a challenge. *AIDS*, 12(Supplement B), pp. S27–S31.

Schoofs, Mark (1999). AIDS, the agony of Africa: Ending the epidemic. http://www/villagevoice.com/issues/9950/schoofs.php

—— (2002). A monkey's death complicates effort to find HIV vaccine. *Wall Street Journal*, 17 January, pp. A1, A6.

Sepkowitz, Kent A. (2001). AIDS: The first 20 years. *New England Journal of Medicine*, 344(23), pp. 1764–72.

Servaes, J.(1999). *Communication for development: One world, multiple cultures*. Cresskill, NJ: Hampton Press.

Shilts, Randy (1987). *And the band played on: Politics, people, and the AIDS epidemic*. New York: St. Martin's Press.

Singhal, Arvind (2001a). *HIV/AIDS and communication for behavior and social change: Program experiences, examples, and the way forward*. Geneva: UNAIDS.

—— (2001b). *Facilitating community participation through communication*. New York: UNICEF.

Singhal, Arvind, and William S. Howard (eds.) (in press). *HIV/AIDS and African children: Health challenges and educational possibilities*. Athens, OH: Ohio University Press.

Singhal, Arvind, and Everett M. Rogers (1989). *India's information revolution.* New Delhi: Sage Publications.

——— (1999). *Entertainment-education: A communication strategy for social change.* Mahwah, NJ: Lawrence Erlbaum Associates.

——— (2001a). *India's communication revolution: From bullock carts to cyber marts.* New Delhi: Sage Publications.

——— (2001b). The entertainment-education strategy in campaigns. In Ronald E. Rice and Charles Atkins (eds.), *Public communication campaigns* (pp. 343–56) (3rd edition). Thousand Oaks, CA: Sage Publications.

——— (2002). A theoretical agenda for entertainment-education. *Communication Theory*, 14(2), pp. 117–35.

Singhal, Arvind, and Peer J. Svenkerud (1994). Pro-socially shareable entertainment television programs: A programming alternative in developing countries. *Journal of Development Communication*, 5(2), pp. 17–30.

Singhal, Arvind, and Kant Udornpim (1997). Cultural shareability, archetypes, and television soaps: "Oshindrome" in Thailand. *Gazette*, 59, pp. 171–88.

Singhal, Arvind, Rafael Obregon, and Everett M. Rogers (1994). Reconstructing the story of *Simplemente María*, the most popular telenovela in Latin America of all time. *Gazette*, 54, pp. 1–15.

Singhal, Arvind, Li Ren, and Jianying Zhang (1999). *Audience interpretations of "Baixing," an entertainment-education television serial in China.* New York: Population Communications International.

Sood, Suruchi, and Everett M. Rogers (2000). Dimensions of parasocial interaction by letter-writers to a popular entertainment-education soap opera in India. *Journal of Broadcasting and Electronic Media*, 44(3), pp. 389–414.

Soul City (2000). The evaluation of Soul City 4: Methodology and top-line results. Paper presented to the Third International Entertainment-Education Conference for Social Change, Arnhem, the Netherlands, September 2000.

——— (2001). *Series 4: Impact Evaluation – AIDS.* Parkstown, South Africa: Soul City Institute for Health and Development Communication.

Specter, Michael (2001). India's plague. *The New Yorker*, 17 December, pp. 74–85.

Steinfatt, Thomas M. (2002). *Working at the bar: Sex work and health communication in Thailand.* Westport, CT: Ablex.

Steinfatt, Thomas M., and Jim Mielke (1999). Communicating danger: The politics of AIDS in the Mekong region. In William N. Elwood (ed.), *Power in the blood: A handbook on AIDS, politics, and communication* (pp. 385–402). Mahwah, NJ: Lawrence Erlbaum Associates.

Sthapitanonda-Sarabol, Parichart, and Arvind Singhal (1998). Glocalizing media products: Investigating the cultural shareability of the "Karate Kids" entertainment-education film in Thailand. *Media Asia*, 25(3), pp. 170–75.

———— (1999). Cultural shareability, role modeling, and para-social interaction in an entertainment-education film: The effects of Karate Kids on Thai street children. In Sue Ralph, J.L. Brown, and T. Lees (eds.), *Youth and global media* (pp. 205–17). Luton: University of Luton Press.

Stolberg, S.G. (1998). Eyes shut, black America is being ravaged by AIDS. *The New York Times*, 29 June, p. A1.

Stucky, Christina (2001). A house of hope in Botswana. *Choices*, 10(4), pp. 10–11.

Sussman, Edward (2002). Many HIV patients carry mutated drug resistant strains. *Lancet*, 359, p. 490 (5 January).

Svenkerud, Peer J., Rita Rahoi, and Arvind Singhal (1995). Incorporating ambiguity and archetypes in entertainment-education programming: Lessons learned from Oshin. *Gazette*, 55, pp. 147–68.

Svenkerud, Peer J., Arvind Singhal, and Michael J. Papa (1998). Diffusion of innovations theory and effective targeting of HIV/AIDS programs in Thailand. *Asian Journal of Communication*, 8(1), pp. 1–30.

Swain, Kristie Alley (2000). Religiosity-related barriers to AIDS dialogue among African-Americans: Implications for church-based interventions. Paper presented to the International Communication Association, Acapulco, June 2000.

Swarms, Rachel L. (2001). South Africa's AIDS vortex engulfs a rural community. *The New York Times*, 25 November, pp. A15–A16.

Sweat, Michael, Steven Gregorich, Gloria Sangiwa, Colin Furlonge, Donald Balmer, Claudes Kamenga, Olga Grinstead, and Thomas Coates (2000). Cost-effectiveness of voluntary HIV-1 counselling and testing in reducing sexual transmission of HIV-1 in Kenya and Tanzania. *Lancet*, 356, pp. 113–21 (8 July).

UNAIDS (1998a). *A measure of success in Uganda*. Geneva: UNAIDS.

———— (1998b). *AIDS education through Imams: A spiritually motivated community effort in Uganda*. Geneva: UNAIDS.

———— (1998c). *Social marketing: An effective tool in the global response to HIV/AIDS*. Geneva: UNAIDS.

———— (1999a). *Comfort and hope: Six case studies on mobilizing family and community care for and by people with HIV/AIDS*. Geneva: UNAIDS.

———— (1999b). *Acting early to prevent AIDS: The case of Senegal*. Geneva: UNAIDS.

———— (2000a). AIDS epidemic update: December, 2000. http://www.unaids.org/wac/2000/wad00/files/WAD_epidemic_report.htm

UNAIDS (2000b). *HIV and AIDS-related stigmatization, discrimination, and denial: Forms, contexts, and determinants.* Geneva: UNAIDS.

UNAIDS/Penn State (1999). *Communications framework for HIV/ AIDS: A new direction.* Edited by Collins O. Airhihenbuwa, Bunmi Makinwa, M. Frith, and Rafael O. Obregon. Geneva: UNAIDS.

Valente, Thomas W. (1997). On evaluating mass media's impact. *Studies in Family Planning,* 28(2), pp. 170–71.

Valente, Thomas W., and Uttara Bharath (1999). An evaluation of the use of drama to communicate HIV/AIDS information. *AIDS Education and Prevention,* 11(3), pp. 203–11.

Valente, Thomas W., Robert K. Foreman, Benjamin Junge, and David Valhor (1998). Satellite exchange in the Baltimore Needle Exchange Program. *Public Health Reports,* 113(S1), pp. 91–96.

Vaughan, Peter W., and Everett M. Rogers (2000). A staged model of communication effects: Evidence from an entertainment-education radio soap opera in Tanzania. *Journal of Health Communication,* 5(2), pp. 203–27.

Vaughan, Peter W., Alleyene Regis, and E. St. Catherine (2000). Effects of an entertainment-education radio soap opera on family planning and HIV prevention in St. Lucia. *International Family Planning Perspectives,* 26(4), pp. 148–57.

Vaughan, Peter W., Everett M. Rogers, Arvind Singhal, and Ramadhan M.A. Swalehe (2000). Entertainment-education and HIV/AIDS prevention: A field experiment in Tanzania. *Journal of Health Communication,* 5(Supplement), pp. 81–100.

Verghese, Abraham (1995). *My own country: A doctor's story.* New York: Vintage Books.

von Schoen Angerer, Tido, David Wilson, Nathan Ford, and Toby Kasper (2001). Access and activism: The ethics of providing antiretroviral therapy in developing countries. *AIDS,* 15(Supplement 5), pp. S81–S90.

Wallack, Lawrence (1990). Mass media and health promotion: Promise, problem, and challenge. In Charles A. Atkin and Lawrence Wallack (eds.), *Mass communication and public health* (pp. 41–50). Thousand Oaks, CA: Sage Publications.

Watts, J. (1998). Popular drama prompts interest in HIV in Japan. *Lancet,* 352, p. 1840.

Weiss, Helen A., Maria A. Quigley, and Richard J. Hayes (2000). Male circumcision and risk of HIV infection in Sub-Saharan Africa: A systematic review and meta-analysis. *AIDS,* 14, pp. 2361–70.

Whiteside, Alan, and Clem Sunter (2000). *AIDS: The challenge for South Africa.* Cape Town: Human & Rousseau and Tafelberg.

Wiener, B. (1993). AIDS from an attributional perspective. In J.B. Bryor and G.D. Reeder (eds.), *The social psychology of HIV infection* (pp. 287–302). Mahwah, NJ: Lawrence Erlbaum Associates.

Williams, David, Paul Cawthorne, Nathan Ford, and Saree Aongsonwang (1999). Global trade and access to medicines: AIDS treatments in Thailand. *Lancet,* 354, pp. 1893–95.

Wohlfeiler, Dan (1998). Community organizing and community building among gay and bisexual men: The STOP AIDS Project. In Meredith Minkler (ed.), *Community organizing and community building for health* (pp. 230–43). New Brunswick, NJ: Rutgers University Press.

Wolf, R. Cameron, Linda A. Tawfik, and Katherine C. Bond (2000). Peer promotion programs and social networks in Ghana: Methods for monitoring and evaluating AIDS prevention and reproductive health programs among adolescents and young adults. *Journal of Health Communication,* 5, pp. 61–80.

World Health Organization (WHO) (2001). *Controlling STI and HIV in Cambodia: The success of condom promotion.* Manila: WHO Regional Office.

Yep, Gus A. (1994). HIV/AIDS education and prevention for Asian and Pacific islander communities. *AIDS Education and Prevention,* 6, pp. 184–86.

———— (1997). Overcoming barriers in HIV/AIDS education for Asian-Americans: Toward more effective cultural communication. In D.C. Umeh (ed.), *Confronting the AIDS epidemic: Cross-cultural perspectives on HIV/AIDS education* (pp. 220–30). Trenton, NJ: Africa World Press.

Zambia Central Statistical Office & MEASURE Evaluation (1999). *Zambia Sexual Behaviour Survey 1998.* Chapel Hill, NC: University of North Carolina at Chapel Hill, MEASURE Evaluation Project.

Zhu, Twofu, Bette T. Korber, Andre J. Nahmias, Edward Hooper, Paul M. Sharp, and David D. Ho (1998). An African HIV-1 sequence from 1959 and implications for the origin of the epidemic. *Nature,* 391, pp. 594–97 (5 February).

Zillman, Dolf, and P. Vorderer (eds.) (2000). *Media entertainment: The psychology of its appeal.* Mahwah, NJ: Lawrence Erlbaum Associates.

Author Index

Subject Index

∎

About the Authors

■

Dr. Arvind Singhal is Presidential Research Scholar and Professor in the School of Interpersonal Communication, College of Communication, Ohio University, where he teaches and conducts research in the areas of diffusion of innovations, mobilizing for change, design and implementation of strategic communication campaigns, and the entertainment-education communication strategy.

He is co-author (with Professor Everett M. Rogers) of three previous books: *India's Communication Revolution: From Bullock Carts to Cyber Marts* (2001); *Entertainment-Education: A Communication Strategy for Social Change* (1999); and *India's Information Revolution* (1989). Their book *Entertainment-Education* received the National Communication Association's Applied Communication Division's Distinguished Book Award for 2000. In addition, he is the author of some 60 scholarly articles in such journals as the *Journal of Communication*, *Journal of Broadcasting and Electronic Media*, *Communication Monographs*, *Communicatoin Theory*, *Gazette*, *Journal of Health Communication*, among others. Dr. Singhal has won the Top Paper Award from the International Communication Association six times, the Baker Award for Research twice at the Ohio University, and numerous other teaching and research recognitions.

Dr. Singhal's research in the US and developing countries has been supported by the Ford Foundation, Rockefeller Foundation,

David and Lucile Packard Foundation, and the CDC, to name just a few. He has served as a consultant to international development agencies such as the World Bank, UNICEF, UNDP, UNAIDS, FAO, U.S. AID, FHI, and PATH.

Everett M. Rogers is Regents' Professor, Department of Communication and Journalism, University of New Mexico. He has been teaching in universities and conducting scholarly research for the past 45 years. He has served on the faculty of Ohio State University, Michigan State University, Stanford University, University of Southern California, and the University of New Mexico. Professor Rogers is particularly known for his book *Diffusion of Innovations*, published in its fifth edition. He has conducted research projects on various aspects of the diffusion of innovations in Colombia, India, Korea, Indonesia, Thailand, Brazil, Nigeria and Tanzania, and in Ohio, Iowa and Kentucky. He has taught in Germany, France, Ecuador, Singapore and Colombia.

Professor Rogers has recently authored or co-authored books on the history of communication study, technology transfer and the rise of technopolises, organizational aspects of health communication campaigns, media agenda-setting, intercultural communication, and on the entertainment-education strategy. He is also involved in research on the effects of programs to prevent drunk driving in New Mexico, with emphasis on cultural factors in such behavior change.

In 1996, Professor Rogers received an honorary doctorate from the Ludwig-Maximilians University of Munich, and in 1998 he was named the Wee Kim Wee Professor of Communication Studies at the Nanyang Technological University in Singapore.